Principles of Pharmacoeconomics

Second Edition

Principles of Pharmacoeconomics

Second Edition

J. Lyle Bootman, Ph.D.
Raymond J. Townsend, Pharm.D.
William F. McGhan, Pharm.D., Ph.D.

W HARVEY WHITNEY BOOKS COMPANY

Principles of pharmacoeconomics / [edited by] J. Lyle Bootman, Raymond
J. Townsend, William F. McGhan.
   p.   cm.
   Includes bibliographical references and index.
   ISBN 0–929375–17–3 (alk. paper)
   1. Chemotherapy—Economic aspects.   2. Pharmaceutical industry.
3. Pharmaceutical policy.   I. Bootman, J. Lyle.   II. Townsend.
Raymond J.   III. McGhan, William F.
RM263.P73   1996
338.4'361558—dc20   96–3346
                                                              CIP

HARVEY WHITNEY BOOKS COMPANY
4906 Cooper Rd., PO Box 42696, Cincinnati, OH 45242 USA

Table of Contents

Preface

During the next decade, the development of new drugs will be stimulated by an increased understanding of disease processes and the application of biotechnology discoveries. The use of these new clinical agents in practice will be increasingly determined not only by their effectiveness, but also by the cost of the technology. In essence, the rising costs of health care will force decisions to be made regarding both the effectiveness of the technology and the overall cost implications. Therefore, the purpose of this book is to present various techniques, tools, and strategies to evaluate the economic contribution of specific drug therapies at a policy level and for individual patient needs. This information is relevant for researchers, practitioners, and students of the science. However, the major audience for this book is the introductory student. It should not be considered a text for the advanced level student of pharmacoeconomics.

Additionally, it is our hope that this book will further stimulate pharmacists, physicians, and others to generate more pharmacoeconomic research in order to adequately apply the results to the prevention and treatment of disease. We believe that pharmacoeconomics as a discipline will not become a part of the mainstream of pharmacy education and practice until application of the research data takes place at the patient care level. The application of pharmacoeconomics to clinical practice and pharmaceutical care will be crucial to pharmacy's success in our future healthcare delivery system.

This book could not have been completed without the administrative assistance of the University of Arizona College of Pharmacy staff, especially Kathy Fitzgerald and Jeffrey Johnson. We also thank our families, colleagues, and friends for their support, love, and especially their understanding as we completed this task.

J. Lyle Bootman
Raymond J. Townsend
William F. McGhan

Contributing Authors

Judith T. Barr, Sc.D.
Associate Professor
Northeastern University
Bouve College of Pharmacy and
  Health Sciences
Boston, MA
Chapter 8

J. Lyle Bootman, Ph.D.
Dean and Professor
University of Arizona
College of Pharmacy
Tucson, AZ
Chapters 1 and 2

J. Gregory Boyer, Ph.D.
Department Head
International Director
Pharmacoeconomic Research
Glaxo Wellcome
London, UK
Chapter 7

Kathleen M. Bungay, Pharm.D.
Clinical Pharmacy Specialist
Department of Pharmacy
New England Medical Center
Boston, MA
Chapter 7

Elizabeth A. Chrischilles, Ph.D.
Assistant Professor
The University of Iowa
Preventative Medicine and Environmental
  Health
Iowa City, IA
Chapter 5

Stephen Joel Coons, Ph.D.
Associate Professor
Department of Pharmacy Practice and
  Director, Center for Pharmaceutical
  Economics
College of Pharmacy, The University
  of Arizona
Tucson, AZ
Chapter 6

Michael Dickson, Ph.D.
Professor and Chairman
University of South Carolina
College of Pharmacy
Department of Pharmacy Practice
Columbia, SC
Chapter 2

JoLaine R. Draugalis, Ph.D.
Associate Professor and Associate Director
Center for Pharmaceutical Economics
College of Pharmacy
The University of Arizona
Tucson, AZ
Chapter 15

Jean Paul Gagnon, Ph.D.
Director, Global Health
Economics Policy
Hoechst Marion Roussel
Kansas City, MO
Chapter 12

Jacqueline Gardner, Ph.D.
Associate Professor
School of Pharmacy
University of Washington
Seattle, WA
Chapter 9

Jan D. Hirsch, Ph.D.
Principal of Hirsch and Reid Consulting
Orange, CA; and
Assistant Clinical Professor
Division of Clinical Pharmacy
School of Pharmacy
University of California at San Francisco
San Francisco, CA
Chapter 11

Nelda Johnson, Pharm.D.
Project Director
Health Policy and Clinical Outcomes
Thomas Jefferson University Hospital
Philadelphia, PA
Chapter 11

Robert M. Kaplan, Ph.D.
Chief, Division of Health Care Sciences,
Professor, Department of Family and
  Preventive Medicine
School of Medicine, University of
  California–San Diego
La Jolla, CA
Chapter 6

Deborah S. Kitz, Ph.D.
Executive Director
Abington Surgical Center
Willow Grove, PA
Chapter 4

Lon N. Larson, Ph.D.
Associate Professor
College of Pharmacy and Health Sciences
Drake University
Des Moines, IA
Chapter 3

William F. McGhan, Pharm.D., Ph.D.
Professor and Senior Researcher
Institute for Pharmaceutical Economics
Philadelphia College of Pharmacy
 and Science
Philadelphia, PA
Chapters 1 and 4

David Nash, M.D., M.B.A.
Director, Health Policy & Clinical
 Outcomes
Thomas Jefferson University Hospital
Philadelphia, PA
Chapter 11

Jane T. Osterhaus, Ph.D.
Director of Pharmacoeconomic Research
Glaxo Wellcome
Research Triangle Park, NC
Chapter 10

Peter Penna, Pharm.D.
Director of Pharmacy Administration
Group Health
Renton, WA
Chapter 13

Eugene C. Reeder, Ph.D.
Professor
College of Pharmacy
University of South Carolina
Columbia, SC
Chapter 12

Lisa A. Sanchez, Pharm.D.
Vice President
Health Economics
Emron
Boston, MA
Appendix

Kevin A. Schulman, M.D.
Medical Director
Clinical Economics Research Unit
Assistant Professor of Medicine
Georgetown University Medical Center
Washington, DC
Chapter 14

Gerald E. Schumacher, Pharm.D., Ph.D.
Professor
Northeastern University
Bouve College of Pharmacy and
 Health Sciences
Boston, MA
Chapter 8

Paul E. Stang, Ph.D., PA-C1
Director of Epidemiology
SmithKline Beecham Pharmaceuticals
Philadelphia, PA
Chapter 9

Bruce Steinwald, M.B.A., Vice President
Director of the Outcomes Study Group
Health Technology Associates Inc.
Washington, DC
Chapter 7

Andy Stergachis, Ph.D.
Professor and Chairman
School of Pharmacy
University of Washington
Seattle, WA
Chapter 13

Sean D. Sullivan, Ph.D.
Assistant Professor
School of Pharmacy
University of Washington
Seattle, WA
Chapter 13

Raymond J. Townsend, Pharm.D., FCCP, FAPRS
Worldwide Director and Vice President
Pharmacoeconomic Research
Glaxo Wellcome Inc.
Research Triangle Park, NC
Chapters 1 and 10

John E. Ware, Jr., Ph.D.
Senior Scientist
The Health Institute
New England Medical Center
Boston, MA
Chapter 7

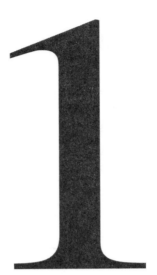

Introduction to Pharmacoeconomics

J. Lyle Bootman
Raymond J. Townsend
William F. McGhan

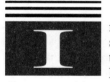n 1993, the US spent $935 billion on health care, representing approximately 15% of the nation's gross domestic product (GDP).[1] In addition, the Congressional Budget Office projected that the nation's health expenditures would reach $1.7 trillion, or 18%, of the GDP by the year 2000.[1] Drug expenditures accounted for approximately $75 billion in 1993, or approximately 8% of the national healthcare expenditures.[2] Although the proportion of GDP spent on total health care has climbed steadily, the percentage spent on outpatient prescriptions has remained at less than 10% over the past 30 years.[2] US consumers pay directly out of their own pockets for much of their medication costs. Even though private health insurance and government programs cover a growing portion of drug expenditures, approximately 36% of drug costs are still paid directly by consumers.[2] The cost of pharmaceuticals and pharmacy services have, therefore, become an important issue to patients, third-party payers, and governments alike. Today, and in the future, it is necessary to scientifically value the costs and consequences of drug therapy.

The basic value of drug therapy to prescribers and patients in the US is evidenced by the increased therapeutic use of prescriptions. Community pharmacists dispense approximately 1.7 billion prescriptions annually.[3] From the 1950s to 1990, the number of prescriptions dispensed per person per year in the US increased from 2.4 to 6.8. The nation's hospitals provide approximately $10 billion worth of drug and drug products to hospitalized patients.[4] Drugs available over-the-counter without prescription also serve an important role in the country's health care. The sales of nonprescription drugs has increased from $700 million in the 1950s to an expected $40+ billion by the end of the century.[5] These figures may be indicative of the value and perceived benefit that society attributes to medications. Most economists would acknowledge that a crude, lower-bound estimate of the value and benefits of drugs to consumers is the amount they spend on these products.

Pharmaceuticals and other therapeutic interventions have contributed to the important progress being made in the health status of the US population. Corresponding to the introduction of new drug entities during the past two decades, the mortality rates for several diseases have declined substantially.[6] Drugs account for only about 5% of the expenditures in hospital budgets, but drug therapy plays a crucial role in the efficient treatment of hospitalized patients. Many life-saving drugs are used by the average institutionalized patient. An average hospitalized patient receives six to eight different drugs on a typical day. Effective drug therapy helps to partially explain why the mean length of stay in hospitals was 7.2 days in 1992.[4]

Despite the general evidence supporting the use of pharmaceuticals, few data exist regarding the actual costs and benefits attributed to specific drug therapies. A primary reason is the lack of defined methodologies to evaluate medical interventions. Perhaps the current focus on reducing expenditures of pharmaceuticals and pharmacy services to save costs to the total healthcare system is inappropriate. A purpose of this book is to present economic and humanistic measurement methodologies that may be used not only to evaluate the outcomes of drug therapy, but also put them in perspective with other related healthcare expenditures.

Outcomes

The term "outcomes" is increasingly being used to describe the results and value of healthcare intervention. However, depending on perspective, the outcomes of health care are multidimensional. The clinician has traditionally been most concerned with clinical outcomes of treatments. More recently, healthcare payers and administrators have focused on the resource use or economic outcome of healthcare decisions. Patients, on the other hand, are becoming increasingly knowledgeable and involved in decisions regarding their own health care and are seeking more information regarding the humanistic outcomes of therapy. Patients want to know how their quality of life will be affected or just how satisfied other patients with their condition have been with various treatments.

As the healthcare marketplace is rapidly changing, there is a danger that the change will be driven primarily by the desire to contain cost. Clearly, cost-containment is an important objective. However, successful healthcare management as measured by the objectives of patients, physicians, and other healthcare providers, as well as by societal expectations, requires that the quality of care also be maintained. Outcomes measurement must take into account economic considerations while recognizing that acceptable clinical and humanistic outcomes are also important objectives. The true value of healthcare interventions, programs, and policy can be assessed only if all three dimensions of outcomes are measured and considered.

Definition of Pharmacoeconomics Research

Economics is about trade-offs and choices between wants, needs, and the scarcity of resources to fulfill these wants. When thinking of economics, most people think of the trade-offs between goods and services and money; however, the trade-off might also be expressed in humanistic terms. We are, therefore, careful to include both resource use and humanistic evaluations of drug therapy within pharmacoeconomic assessment.

Pharmacoeconomics has been defined as "the description and analysis of the costs of drug therapy to health care systems and society."[7] Pharmacoeconomic research identifies, measures, and compares the costs (i.e., resources consumed) and consequences (clinical, economic, and humanistic) of pharmaceutical products and services. Within this framework are included the research methods related to cost-minimization, cost-effectiveness, cost-benefit, cost-of-illness, cost-utility, and decision analysis, as well as quality-of-life and other humanistic assessments. In essence, pharmacoeconomic analysis uses tools for examining the impact (desirable and undesirable) of alternative drug therapies and other medical interventions.

Questions that pharmacoeconomics may help to address are as follows: What drugs should be included on the hospital formulary? What is the best drug for a particular patient? What is the best drug for a pharmaceutical manufacturer to develop? Which drug delivery system is the best for the hospital? How do two clinical pharmacy services compare? Which drugs should be included in a Medicaid formulary? What is the cost per quality year of life extended by a drug? Will patient quality of life be improved by a particular drug therapy decision? What is the best drug for this particular disease? What are the patient outcomes of various treatment modalities?

In essence, pharmacoeconomic analysis uses important tools for examining the outcomes or impact of drug therapy and related healthcare interventions.

Historical Perspective

The emerging discipline of pharmacoeconomics has become adopted as a health science discipline by the pharmaceutical industry, academic pharmaceutical scientists, and pharmacy practitioners worldwide. As stated previously, it is generally defined as the description and analysis of the costs and consequences of pharmaceuticals and pharmaceutical services and their impact on individuals, healthcare systems, and society. The research methods used by scientists in this discipline (e.g., cost-effectiveness, cost-utility, quality-of-life evaluations) are drawn from many areas—economics, epidemiology, medicine, pharmacy, the social sciences. In essence, pharmacoeconomic analysis uses such tools to examine the impact of alternative drug therapies and services on patient care outcomes. We believe that this discipline will have a significant impact on the delivery and financing of health care throughout the world. Furthermore, we believe that pharmacoeconomics may influence health care and the practice of pharmacy at a magnitude equivalent to the impact of clinical pharmacy and pharmacokinetics.

During the early 1960s, pharmacy began evolving as a clinical discipline within the healthcare system. It was during this time that the pharmaceutical science disciplines such as pharmaceutics, clinical pharmacy, drug information, and pharmacokinetics became a critical and integral part of pharmacy education and science. In the 1970s pharmacoeconomics developed its roots. In 1978 McGhan, Rowland, and Bootman, from the University of Minnesota, introduced the concepts of cost-benefit and cost-effectiveness analyses in the *American Journal of Hospital Pharmacy*.[8] Bootman et al.[9] also published an early pharmacy research article in 1979 in which cost-benefit analysis was used to evaluate the outcomes of individualizing aminoglycoside dosages in severely burned patients with gram-negative septicemia using sophisticated pharmacokinetic protocols. The actual term "pharmacoeconomics" did not appear in the literature until 1986 when the first of a two-part presentation by Townsend entitled "Post Marketing Drug Research and Development" was published describing the need to develop research activities in this evolving discipline.[10] To date, many of the efforts in this discipline have been directed toward the refinement of the research methods and their application to evaluating pharmaceutical services and specific drug therapies.

Pharmacoeconomics continues to evolve similarly to another relatively new pharmaceutical science—pharmacokinetics. Pharmacokinetics surfaced in the 1950s in US colleges of pharmacy, and in the 1970s it became an integral part of the pharmacy curriculum. Many of the theoretical models for pharmacokinetics are based on the physicochemical principles developed by physicists, chemists, and engineers. As a parallel, pharmacoeconomics has borrowed from the basic economic and social sciences for most of its theoretical models. McGhan, Rowland, and Bootman introduced course material related to pharmacoeconomics into the undergraduate and graduate pharmacy curricula as early as 1976 at the University of Minnesota. However, the educational content was emphasized at the graduate level, not at the undergraduate professional program levels. In the 1990s, we are beginning to see much of this material incorporated at the PharmD profession education level alongside the discipline of pharmacotherapy.

Furthermore, upon examining the evolutionary path of pharmacokinetics, it is clear that its application in the clinical setting was a driving force that assured its place in the professional pharmacy curriculum. We believe that pharmacoeconomics will obtain the same level of recognition when its application in the clinical setting is more complete. In other words, when pharmacy practitioners begin to apply the results of pharmacoeconomic research to therapeutic decision-making, thus positively influencing patient outcomes, the discipline will become an increasingly critical component of the pharmacy curriculum. Likewise, the successful implementation of "pharmaceutical care" will come about only with sufficient pharmacoeconomic research that adequately documents the degree to which the benefits of such care outweigh the costs associated with those services. In fact, the profession of pharmacy is unlikely to succeed in its role of providing pharmaceutical care without this critical body of knowledge. Pharmacists must become the key player in assuring that drug therapy and related pharmacy services are not only safe and effective but also provide real value in both economic and humanistic terms.

 ## Overview of Pharmacoeconomic Methodologies

The purpose of this section is to acquaint the reader with the basic methodologic approaches regarding the economic evaluation of drug therapy. By definition, pharmacoeconomic evaluations include any study designed to assess the costs (i.e., resources consumed) and consequences (clinical and humanistic) of alternative therapies. This includes such methodologies as cost-benefit, cost-utility, and cost-effectiveness (Table 1). Each of these methodologies will be discussed in more depth in later chapters. Review articles that discuss the application of these techniques

Table 1. Pharmacoeconomic Methodologies

METHODOLOGY	COST MEASUREMENT UNIT	OUTCOME UNIT
Cost-benefit	dollars	dollars
Cost-effectiveness	dollars	natural units (life-years gained, mmol/L blood glucose, mm Hg blood pressure)
Cost-minimization	dollars	assume to be equivalent in comparative groups
Cost-utility	dollars	quality-adjusted life-year or other utilities

to healthcare evaluations also may assist the interested reader in becoming more aware of the role of these tools.[8-30] The evaluation mechanisms delineated were oftentimes helpful in demonstrating the cost-impact of innovative treatments, therefore granting them greater acceptance by healthcare providers, administrators, and the public.

COST-MINIMIZATION ANALYSIS

When two or more interventions are examined and demonstrated or assumed to be equivalent in terms of a given outcome or consequence, costs associated with each intervention may be examined and compared. This typical cost-analysis is referred to as cost-minimization analysis. An example of this type of analysis with regard to drug therapy may be the evaluation of two generically equivalent drugs in which the outcome has been proven to be equal although the acquisition and administration costs of the two drugs may be significantly different.

COST-BENEFIT ANALYSIS

Cost-benefit analysis is a basic tool that can be used to improve the decision-making process in the allocation of funds to healthcare programs. Although the general concept of cost-benefit analysis is not overly complicated, many technical considerations require a degree of explanation and interpretation in order to understand how it can be or has been applied.

Cost-benefit analysis consists of identifying all of the benefits that accrue from the program or intervention and converting them into dollars in the year in which they will occur. This stream of benefit dollars is then discounted to its equivalent present value at the selected interest rate. On the other side of the equation, all program costs are identified and allocated through a specific year and, again, the costs are discounted to their present value. Then, if all relevant factors remain constant, the program with the largest present value of benefits less costs is the best in terms of its economic value.

Ideally, all benefits and costs resulting from the program should be included. This presents considerable difficulty, especially on the benefits side of the equation, as many benefits are either difficult to measure, difficult to convert to dollars, or both. For example, the benefits of improved patient quality of life, improved patient satisfaction with the healthcare system, and improved working conditions for the physician are not only difficult to measure but are extremely difficult to assign a dollar value to. This problem has been addressed by many researchers in health economics and has not yet been completely resolved. Generally, the analyst or researcher will convert as many benefits as possible into monetary units. The remaining variables are labeled as "intangible benefits" and left to decision-makers to include in their final deliberations. Cost-benefit analysis often has been used when comparing the value of dissimilar programs where the outcomes are in different units (e.g., cost-benefit of having a neonatal care program vs a cardiac rehabilitation program).

COST-EFFECTIVENESS ANALYSIS

Cost-effectiveness analysis is a technique designed to assist a decision-maker in identifying a preferred choice among possible alternatives. Generally, cost-effectiveness is defined as a series of analytical and mathematical procedures that aid in the selection of a course of action from various alternative approaches. Cost-effectiveness analysis has been applied to health matters where the program's inputs can be readily measured in dollars, but the program's outputs are more appropriately stated in terms of health improvement created (e.g., life-years extended, clinical cures).

An important point to be considered in both cost-benefit and cost-effectiveness analysis is that a program/treatment providing a high benefit (effectiveness) to cost ratio in terms of value to society as a whole may not be valued in the same way by all members of society. For example, drug therapy that reduced the number of patient-days in an acute care institution may be positive from a third-party payer's point of view but not necessarily from the view of the institution's administrator who operated under a fixed level of revenue and who depended on a fixed number of patient-days to meet expenses. What is viewed as cost-beneficial for society as a whole may be viewed differently by plan sponsors, administrators, health providers, governmental agencies, or even individual patients. One must consider whose interests are to be taken into account when using these analyses.

COST-UTILITY ANALYSIS

In examining Table 1, one can better appreciate the subtle differences between the techniques discussed to this point. Cost-utility analysis is an economic tool in which the intervention consequence is measured in terms of quantity and quality of life. It is much the same as cost-effectiveness analysis with the added dimension of a particular point of view, most often that of the patient. Quite often the results of a cost-utility analysis are expressed in the intervention cost per quality-adjusted life-year gained, or changes in quality-of-life measurement for a given intervention cost. Although cost-utility analysis has been used somewhat successfully to aid in decisions regarding healthcare programs (e.g., surgery vs chemotherapy), instruments that are reliable and sensitive enough to detect changes with drug treatments (e.g., one antihypertensive agent vs another) are still needed.

===== COST-OF-ILLNESS EVALUATION

Cost-of-illness studies are important to pharmacoeconomic evaluations of new therapies. By evaluating the humanistic impact of disease and the resources used in treating a condition prior to discovery of a new intervention, the pharmacoeconomist can effectively establish a baseline for comparison. Although the value and methodologies of cost-of-illness studies have been debated, they remain prevalent in the pharmacoeconomic literature.[28,29] As with all pharmacoeconomic evaluation, when conducting or evaluating cost-of-illness, it is important to carefully consider the design and intent of the study. There is value in having baseline information, but absolute conclusions regarding the value of an intervention versus an alternative can be made only after direct comparison.

===== Pharmacoeconomics and Drug Development

In 1985 the pharmaceutical industry spent over $4.1 billion for the development of new drugs; for 1994, that figure was estimated to be $13.8 billion. This figure represents approximately 18.8% of pharmaceutical sales.[2] This percentage is certainly higher than that found in other industries. It has been estimated that it takes $359 million and 12 years to bring a new drug to the market.[2] The process by which a drug is evaluated and developed for the marketplace is illustrated in Figure 1.

Because pharmacoeconomic data are becoming increasingly important to practitioners making drug formulary decisions, it is important to have these data as soon as possible after Food and Drug Administration approval. To do this, discussion and planning for pharmacoeconomic evaluation should begin during the early stages of drug development. A major question arises as to the ideal time to conduct pharmacoeconomic studies and the best process by which to do so. Pharmacoeconomic studies may be planned and conducted at the clinical development stage and at the Phase IV stage of postmarketing research. Basic research and development activities may be partially guided by preliminary pharmacoeconomic analyses. Therefore, studies may need to be conducted at several stages of pharmaceutical research. The following is a summary of the research activity for each phase.

===== PHASE I TRIALS

The objective of the initial clinical trials, or Phase I, is to determine the toxicity profile of the drug in humans. The first Phase I trials usually consist of administration of single, conservative doses to a small number of healthy volunteers. The effects of increasing the size and number of daily

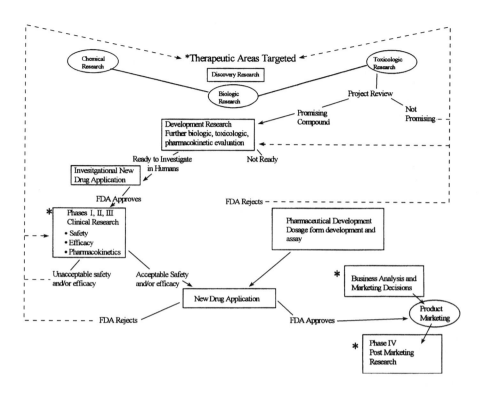

Figure 1. Research and development stages of a new drug. FDA = Food and Drug Administration. * = Pharmacoeconomic evaluations may be designed or conducted at these levels.

doses are evaluated until toxic effects surface or the likely therapeutic dosage is substantially exceeded. It is during this stage that cost-of-illness studies should be accomplished to aid in the decision of whether to further develop the drug and to gather background data for future pharmacoeconomic evaluations.

PHASE II TRIALS

In Phase II trials, the drug is administered to a limited number of patients with the target disease. Patients without complicating, coexisting medical conditions are preferred for these trials. This reduces the number of variables that could confound analysis of the drug's activity and permits the potential therapeutic benefit of the new drug to be more clearly demonstrated.

Even in carefully selected patients, however, demonstrating the efficacy of a new drug is not easy or certain. To provide unequivocal evidence of the drug's therapeutic benefit, it is necessary to compare its effectiveness with that of standard medically accepted treatments or, where ethically appropriate, with a placebo. These comparisons also are used to establish the optimal dosage range for therapeutic activity of the new drug. During this phase, cost-of-illness studies can begin or continue, as can preliminary development of quality-of-life and resource utilization instruments.

PHASE III TRIALS

In Phase III trials, larger numbers of patients are given the new drug in the established dosage range and in the final dosage form. This larger sample size refines the knowledge gained during Phase II and helps identify patients who might have rare reactions to the drug. Patient selection is still closely supervised in Phase III, although some patients with coexisting medical problems are intentionally included to allow assessment of complication in the drug's use.

Discussion, planning, and implementation of pharmacoeconomic studies during this level of research are important. The prospective clinical study that has incorporated a pharmacoeconomic evaluation during the final stages of efficacy evaluation is close to the ideal situation. Critics of these studies claim that pharmacoeconomic evaluations will hinder the new drug application process. Advocates of pharmacoeconomic evaluation correctly note that, unless a new drug treatment has no alternatives and is truly a break-through, the value of using it must be scientifically studied.

PHASE IV TRIALS

During the postmarketing phase, or Phase IV, retrospective and prospective pharmacoeconomic studies can be designed and conducted to gather data in support of the use of the drug. Postmarketing pharmacoeconomic studies are extremely important in that they allow study of the costs and consequences of drug therapy without the altered interventions that occur in strictly controlled clinical trials. During tightly controlled clinical trials, pharmacoeconomics can only put value on efficacy, and this only approximates the "real world." Once a product is on the market cost-effectiveness can be determined. (Note: efficacy studies answer Can it work?; effectiveness studies evaluate Does it work?)

As previously indicated, clinical trials are used to evaluate the efficacy and safety of therapies. The relationships between pharmacoeconomic evaluations and clinical trials are threefold:

1. The pharmacoeconomic evaluation may be a secondary objective of a trial designed primarily to study safety and efficacy.
2. The pharmacoeconomic evaluation may be the principal purpose of a clinical trial, or

3. A pharmacoeconomic evaluation may be done retrospectively using clinical data obtained in previous trials.

Once a drug is marketed, either retrospective or additional prospective pharmacoeconomic studies may be designed and conducted.

Epidemiologic studies are frequently used to study the efficacy and safety of drugs. Epidemiologic data with regard to the disease and treatment under investigation can yield highly important information for the economic evaluation of a specific drug therapy. Understanding the natural progression of the disease comorbidities and treatment enables estimation of the variables that may have pharmacoeconomic implications with regard to cost of illness and quality of life.

Epidemiology's role in pharmacoeconomic evaluations and considerations for conducting pharmacoeconomic research within clinical trials are the subject of two subsequent chapters in this book.

 ## Pharmacoeconomic Guidelines

Over the past few years, researchers and evaluators have called for pharmacoeconomic guidelines. The uses and subject of the proposed guidelines are as follows:

Methodological guidelines would guide researchers to appropriately design, conduct, analyze, and report economic and humanistic evaluations.

Reimbursement and pricing guidelines would outline the content, presentation, and evaluation of pharmacoeconomic data to determine or justify the price or reimbursement of a pharmaceutical product.

Approval guidelines would set out the standards acceptable to a particular government in order to obtain approval to market a new product.

Promotional guidelines would set the criteria for the use of pharmacoeconomic data in support of pharmaceutical promotion to prescribers and consumers.

Although the intent of the call for guidelines is understandable, at present, the science of pharmacoeconomic research is still developing. It would not be desirable to implement guidelines that would limit the development of knowledge in this area. Suffice it to say that the substance of any guidelines involving research must be well grounded in appropriate methodology and sound scientific principles.

 ## Challenges of Pharmacoeconomic Research

In the future we will be routinely challenged to do pharmacoeconomic research, although merely performing the research will not solve all of the problems all of the time. To be useful, appropriate pharmacoeconomic evaluations must be tailored to the specific problem and decision at hand. Our challenge, therefore, begins with looking beyond the obvious and easy solutions.

Cost-minimization analysis is useful when comparing interventions with identical clinical and humanistic outcomes, but this can be the exception rather than the rule for many clinical applications outside of true generic substitution. Cost-benefit analysis would, at first glance, be the answer to more complex problems, in that it would allow for evaluation of various interventions with multiple and dissimilar outcomes. Here, too, one must be careful to note the pitfalls and challenges associated with converting all of the benefits to monetary terms (how do you place a monetary value on reduced blood pressure, insulin control, or improvement in quality of life?). Allowing consequences to remain in natural and measurable terms means that cost-effectiveness analysis can be appropriate for many problems and help with many decisions when the outcomes of the interventions are measured in the same terms. But what about the patient and how the various treatments effect daily living and quality of life? Should decisions be made strictly on getting the best clinical outcome for the dollars spent? Perhaps then cost-utility analysis, which takes into account patient preference and quality of life, should be the gold standard of pharmacoeconomic research. Alas, here too are the problems of measuring quality of life and preference in a changing world.

Present and future controversies surrounding pharmacoeconomic research also include arguments for methodologies of valuations and discounting. What is the most appropriate perspective to take when valuing costs and consequences: the patient, the physician, or perhaps the third-party payer? What of ethics? Will we be able to justify our decisions solely on the numbers obtained through scientific research?

One of the biggest challenges ahead for pharmacoeconomic research lies in the education of those who are going to be evaluating the data derived from this research. Although the end users of pharmacoeconomic research data would like to have simple, clear-cut answers to their questions regarding the allocation of resources and the healthcare benefits derived from them, in actuality the answers are quite complex. Pharmacoeconomics remains an art as well as a science. Even though the science may be perfectly clear, applying that science must be done artfully using professional judgment. Just as it is impossible to set out an algorithm for the treatment of a disease that is appropriate for all patients, it would be impossible to set out an algorithm for making pharmacoeconomic decisions. In the end, the user of pharmacoeconomic research data must be able to evaluate the scientific appropriateness and robustness of the research and make a decision regarding its usefulness in a particular situation. To do this, evaluators will need to understand the basic principles of pharmacoeconomic research.

The challenges of pharmacoeconomic research are inexhaustible; many of them are addressed within the chapters of this book. The real challenge, however, is not in identifying the tools of pharmacoeconomic research, but rather in discovering how and when to use them.

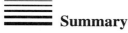

Summary

The overall costs of medical and pharmaceutical care continue to rise. The added value to society, individual healthcare institutions, and patients as weighed against cost has not been well established. The problem has become increasingly difficult to address because of the lack of understanding of methodologies for the evaluation of new and existing drug therapy. The remaining chapters of this text provide in-depth information on specific methodologies oftentimes used in pharmacoeconomic investigations.

References

1. US Congress, Congressional Budget Office. Economic implications of rising health care costs. Washington, DC: Government Printing Office, 1992.

2. The case for America's pharmaceutical research companies. Washington, DC: Pharmaceutical Research and Manufacturers of America, 1994.

3. La Piana Simonsen L. What are pharmacists dispensing most often? Top 200 drugs of 1992. Pharmacy Times, April 1993:29-44.

4. Scott L. Healthcare update. Mod Health 1994;24 (June 20):18.

5. Cowley CT, Hager M. Some counter intelligence. Newsweek 1990;115 (Mar 12):82-4.

6. Manasse HR. Medication use in an imperfect world: drug misadventuring as an issue of public policy. Am J Hosp Pharm 1988;46:929-44.

7. Townsend RJ. Postmarketing drug research and development. Drug Intell Clin Pharm 1987;21:134-6.

8. McGhan W, Rowland C, Bootman JL. Cost-benefit and cost-effectiveness: methodologies for evaluating innovative pharmaceutical services. Am J Hosp Pharm 1978;35:133-40.

9. Bootman JL, Wertheimer A, Zaske D, Rowland C. Individualizing gentamicin dosage regimens on burn patients with gram-negative septicemia: a cost-benefit analysis. J Pharm Sci 1979;68:267-72.

10. Townsend RJ. Post marketing drug research and development: an industry clinical pharmacist's perspective. Am J Pharm Educ 1986;50:480-2.

11. Bootman JL, Rowland C, Wetheimer A. Cost-benefit-analysis: a research tool for evaluating innovative health programs. Eval Health Prof 1979;2:129-54.

12. Bootman JL, Zaske D, Wetheimer AL, Rowland C. Individualization of aminoglycoside dosage regimens: a cost analysis. Am J Hosp Pharm 1979;36:368-70.

13. Stason WB, Weinstein M. Allocation of resources to manage hypertension. N Engl J Med 1977;296:732-9.

14. Weisbrod BA, Huston JH. Benefits and costs of human vaccines in developed countries: an evaluative survey. Washington, DC: Pharmaceutical Manufacturers Association, 1983.

15. Haaga JG. Cost-effectiveness and cost-benefit analysis of immunization programs in developing countries: a review of the literature. Washington, DC: Pharmaceutical Manufacturers Association, 1983.

16. Wagner JL. Economic evaluations of medicines: a review of the literature. Washington, DC: Pharmaceutical Manufacturers Association, 1983.

17. Dao TD. Cost-benefit and cost-effectiveness analysis of pharmaceutical intervention. Washington, DC: Pharmaceutical Manufacturers Association, 1983.

18. Vinokur A, Cannell CF, Eraker SA, Juster TF, Lepkowski JM, Mathiowetz N. The role of survey research in the assessment of health and quality-of-life outcomes of pharmaceutical interventions. Washington, DC: Pharmaceutical Manufacturers Association, 1983.

19. Little AD. Beta-blocker reduction of mortality and reinfarction rate in survivors of myocardial infarctions: a cost-benefit study. Washington, DC: Pharmaceutical Manufacturers Association, 1983.

20. Little AD. Use of beta blocker in the treatment of glaucoma: a cost-benefit study. Washington, DC: Pharmaceutical Manufacturers Association, 1983.

21. Little AD. Use of beta blockers in the treatment of angina: a cost-benefit study. Washington, DC: Pharmaceutical Manufacturers Association, 1983.

22. Dao TD. Cost-benefit and cost-effectiveness analyses of drug therapy. Am J Hosp Pharm 1985;42:791-802.

23. Drummond MF, Stoddart GL, Torrance GW. Methods for the economic evaluation of health care programmes. New York: Oxford University Press, 1987.

24. Klarman H. Application of cost/benefit analysis to health services and the special case of technological innovation. Int J Health Serv Res 1974;4:325-52.

25. Klarman H. Present status of cost-benefit analysis in the health field. Am J Public Health 1967;57:1948-58.

26. Rice DP. Measurement and application of illness costs. Public Health Rep 1969;84: 95-101.

27. Crystal R, Brewster A. Cost-benefit and cost-effectiveness analysis in the health field: an introduction. Inquiry 1966;3:3-13.

28. Drummond M. Cost-of-illness studies. PharmacoEconomics 1992;2(1):1-4.

29. Davey PJ, Leeder SR. The cost of migraine. More than just a headache? PharmacoEconomics 1992;2(1):5-7.

30. MacKeigan LD, Bootman JL. A review of cost-benefit and cost-effectiveness analyses of clinical pharmacy services. J Pharm Marketing Management 1988;2(3):63-84.

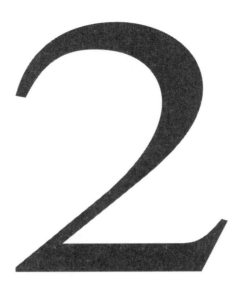

Pharmacoeconomics: An International Perspective

Michael Dickson
J. Lyle Bootman

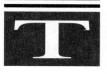he application of economic analysis to pharmaceuticals is part of a larger global trend to maximize the value received for money spent on healthcare services. Figure 1 shows a 30-year upward trend in healthcare expenditure as a percentage of gross domestic product in selected countries. Figure 2, which traces pharmaceutical expenditure as a percentage of gross domestic product, shows a slightly less consistent trend than that shown in Figure 1, but nevertheless, there is a clear upward trend. Governments are attempting to moderate these trends to keep expenditures within socially acceptable limits. The efforts of several national governments have given mixed results (Poullier JP. From cash registers to sophisticated purchasing: the changed health role of governments. Presented at the Adam Smith Institute Conference on International Health Care Reforms: Its Impact on the Pharmaceutical and Health Care Industries, Brussels, November 22, 1993).

Figure 3 is useful for understanding why some observers believe the attention focused on pharmaceuticals is misplaced. It shows that pharmaceutical expenditure, as a percentage of total healthcare expenditure, is relatively steady or declining. This association, and the belief that pharmaceutical products are a "cost-effective" therapy, has created the argument that more, not less, should be spent on pharmaceuticals. Two economic questions arise: (1) How much should be spent on pharmaceuticals? and (2) Which pharmaceutical products give the greatest value for money spent? The first question must be addressed by politicians; the second is the subject of this chapter. A variety of attempts to apply the concept of economic evaluation to pharmaceuticals in several countries are reviewed.

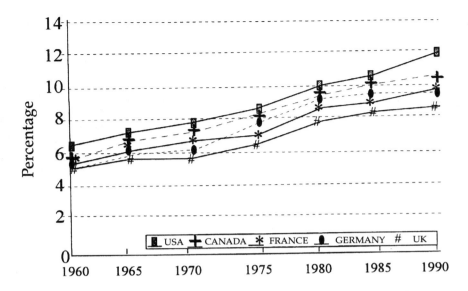

Figure 1. Total healthcare expenditure as a percentage of gross domestic product. OECD Health Data File, 1993; OECD:Paris.

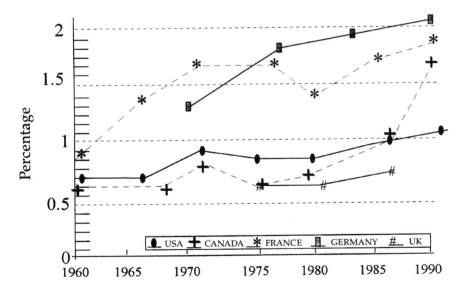

Figure 2. Pharmaceutical expenditure as a percentage of gross domestic product. OECD Health Data File, 1993; OECD; Paris.

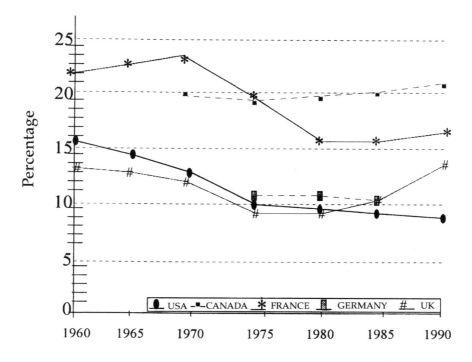

Figure 3. Expenditure on pharmaceuticals as a percentage of total healthcare expenditure. OECD Health Data File, 1993; OECD: Paris.

In most industrialized countries, with the notable exception of the US, the government is the primary payer for the vast majority of healthcare services, usually including pharmaceuticals. Many of these governments have a long history of price control (or restraint) for health care, but the trends shown earlier have persisted. Therefore, the search for mechanisms to constrain rising healthcare costs (including pharmaceuticals) continues. Pharmaceuticals are a small and generally decreasing part of total healthcare expenditures, but they still attract the attention of government regulators for at least four reasons: (1) absolute expenditure continues to grow, (2) pharmaceuticals are viewed as products rather than services, (3) some products are perceived to have little value, and (4) there is a concern that new biotechnology products will push pharmaceutical expenditure to an unprecedented level. All of these are issues that contribute to the current environment for an emphasis by regulators and payers on value for money. All countries are faced with the same problem: an increasing demand for care to be paid for with stable or diminishing resources.

The diversity of healthcare systems coping with this same problem offers a chance to review the variety of approaches that have been developed, and the extent of their adoption. Pharmaceuticals present an unusual, if not unique, opportunity to make international comparisons because molecules don't change when they cross borders. To this extent the object of comparison is equivalent, but it is important to remember the difficulties posed by differences in cultures, medical tradition, regulatory environments, and pharmaceutical presentations (e.g., dosage forms, package sizes, strengths). With an appreciation of these issues, this chapter has three objectives:

- To examine the extent to which pharmacoeconomics is used globally by governments to exercise control over prescription pharmaceuticals.
- To illustrate the application of pharmacoeconomics in pharmaceutical marketing, and
- To speculate on how global trends may develop in the near future.

Events in this arena are moving rapidly and it is not possible to write the ending to this story. This chapter can only provide a picture of the situation as it currently exists in selected countries.

Potential Intervention Points

Pharmaceutical regulations of any kind are typically applied at any of three places. Pharmacoeconomic regulation, if it occurs, is likely to be instituted in a similar manner. It also should be clear that pharmacoeconomic regulations will *not* replace existing controls. They will be added to the regulatory machinery rather than replacing older mechanisms. The unambiguous goal is to constrain pharmaceutical expenditure using the rationale that economic analysis will permit regulators to obtain value for money. Methods and specific implementations may differ across countries, but the likely points of regulation will be marketing approval, pricing decisions, and determination of reimbursement status.

MARKETING APPROVAL

Currently, most governments (e.g., the US, Canada, and countries of the European Union) prohibit the application of a need clause, often called a fourth hurdle. In the past, a need clause was sometimes used to deny marketing approval for some new products on the premise that they were not needed. Need clauses existed in Nordic countries, but these have been removed to be consistent with European Union guidelines.

If pharmacoeconomic guidelines were applied to the marketing approval process, the rationale would be that new products should pass a threshold test for value. Such thresholds are difficult to express, and more difficult to justify. There also is the problem of what to do with products previously approved for marketing. In summary, it seems unlikely that pharmacoeconomic analysis will become a significant part of the marketing approval process, which has traditionally, and universally, been grounded in the principles of safety, efficacy, and quality.

▬▬▬ PRICING DECISIONS

For those countries that set product prices, it would be possible to incorporate pharmacoeconomic data into this decision. Principles of economic analysis could be implemented by requiring producers to submit appropriate data with their product pricing dossier. This approach avoids associating the fourth hurdle (need) with marketing approval and allows product differentiation based on relative value (e.g., higher value could yield a higher price).

The seemingly scientific nature of this process weakens when attempting to establish a link between value and price. Value can be quantified to demonstrate the relative superiority of one product over another or to support the position that a threshold has been reached. The leap from this position to a particular price remains an exercise in persuasion. Regulators tend to believe that pharmaceutical producers choose methods and comparisons that favor their own view. Conversely, producers argue that regulators will use pharmacoeconomic analysis to justify lower prices rather than recognizing the value created by their producers. Use of pharmacoeconomic data for pricing decisions potentially creates another point of contention between regulators (payers) and producers.

▬▬▬ REIMBURSEMENT STATUS

It is common for governments to create reimbursement (consumer cost-sharing) schedules for pharmaceuticals based on any of several scales—price, therapeutic category, recipient income, and the like. Pharmacoeconomic regulation could be used to refine these scales or create another method for scaling consumer cost-sharing. Some would argue that a pharmacoeconomic approach would speed up the price-setting process by removing obstacles associated with differences of opinion. However, the difficult decisions are only transferred to the reimbursement step. Incorporating pharmacoeconomic data into reimbursement decisions has the advantage of rationalizing the consumer cost-sharing decision, and perhaps dealing with the commonly occurring dilemma of how much consumer economic burden is too much.

For example, pharmacoeconomic data could be used in the French reimbursement system in which there are three levels of reimbursement based on a product's classification: 100%, 65%, and 35%. Pharmacoeconomic analysis could be used to classify products or set levels of reimbursement with, or without, reference to the pricing system. Such an approach would create a relative value-based formulary.

A confirmation of the strategies outlined above is seen in recent proposals for revision to the Dutch healthcare system. One proposal would use value for money criteria, among others, to assess the value of existing medicines and determine the extent to which they should be reimbursed.[1]

Global Status of Pharmacoeconomic Regulation

Currently, only the governments of Australia, Canada, and Ontario have incorporated specific economic evaluation criteria into their pharmaceutical regulations. As discussed later, there have been nongovernmental guidelines published in some countries, and a few European countries have vague statements regarding the economic dimensions of prescribed medicines. The most specific guidelines are from the three governments mentioned above. Australia was the first country to take this step, which makes it a model for others to examine, if not to emulate.

Australia

BRIEF HISTORY OF THE *GUIDELINES*

The current Australian *Guidelines* were preceded by a background paper by Evans et al. in which the purpose, methods, and implications of economic analysis on pharmaceuticals for Australia were described. (Unpublished data. Evans D, Freund D, Dittus R, Robertson J, Henry D. The use of economic analysis as a basis for inclusion of pharmaceutical products on the pharmaceutical benefits scheme. December 1989). In their conclusions, the authors acknowledged the complexity and difficulty of using economic analysis to make decisions about pharmaceuticals. They advised: "Staff training will be a priority; flexibility will be necessary during the development and introduction of formal requirements, and the pace of development must be controlled carefully."

Over a year later Drummond observed that "the implementation of the guidelines will place considerable demands both on the industry and the Commonwealth itself."[2] He expressed the belief that "implemented sensibly they could form the basis for better decisions about the rational diffusion and use of medicines . . . if implemented inappropriately, the guidelines will be nothing more than an expensive way of slowing down the entry of new medicines."[2]

The final *Guidelines* were published in 1992, became effective in 1993, and were scheduled for revision in 1994 (as of yet, the revisions have not been published).[3] They are best understood in the overall context of the Australian healthcare system, including the prescription drug benefit.

AUSTRALIAN HEALTHCARE SYSTEM

Australian health care is funded from three sources: the commonwealth, states and local governments, and private spending (health insurance and out-of-pocket expenditure). In 1984, the Medicare Act created a universal system of health insurance that provides basic medical and hospital coverage for all Australians and includes a pharmaceutical benefit for out-of-hospital drugs. Private insurance may cover those products not provided by Medicare.

The Pharmaceutical Benefits Scheme (PBS), a commonwealth agency, pays for most prescription pharmaceuticals. Prescriptions in Australia are regulated by the PBS for over 90% of all products dispensed. Only those products listed by the PBS are eligible for full or partial payment. To be listed by the PBS, a product must first receive marketing approval. The product is then reviewed by the Pharmaceutical Benefits Advisory Committee (PBAC) which, among other duties, advises the Minister of Health, Housing, and Community Services on whether, and how, the product should be listed. Recently, a Pharmaceutical Benefits Pricing Authority was established to advise the Minister on prices at which products should be listed. Since the latter is not a statutory body, it is the PBAC that continues to have final responsibility for price recommendations to the PBS.

GUIDELINES

The new economic analysis guidelines are implemented through the PBAC as part of its existing analysis for the purpose of recommending a price to the PBS. Pharmaceutical manufacturers are advised that submissions are necessary for branded products (generically equivalent products are specifically exempted from the economic analysis provision) for three purposes:

- to obtain a PBS listing for a new product,
- to receive an amended listing for an existing product, and
- to support a request for a substantial price increase.

The economic analysis is conceived as a desktop analysis based on available data, rather than relying on obtaining new data from field studies, although the latter are not completely ruled out. Applicants are reminded that the PBAC is primarily concerned with *comparative* benefits and costs. Thus, the choice of a comparator product, or other therapy, is a critical step in the analysis that will be presented to the PBAC.

The global nature of the pharmaceutical industry is acknowledged because the *Guidelines* address the question of using data from overseas trials. Data from overseas trials may be used if they are "of sufficient quality and are a reasonable basis for economic analyses relevant to the Australian health care system. However, an economic analysis performed overseas will often not be suitable because of major differences in costs, health care practices and the way in which health care is funded."[3] Applicants are reminded that economic analysis should be limited to the disease under study and not subsequent conditions. Finally, applicants are discouraged from including indirect costs such as those associated with employment and productivity. The reasoning for this position is elaborated in the background paper by Evans et al. that argues for a societal viewpoint in the analysis (unpublished data).

The *Guidelines* describe all aspects of a submission to the PBAC, but the three discussed here are specific to the economic analysis. It is, of course, impossible to totally separate economic aspects of the PBAC submission from other components.

Outcomes of Therapy. Applicants are asked to place the new product in one of four categories which will then determine how the analysis is conducted. In making the decision, applicants are asked to distinguish between efficacy and effectiveness. The possibilities are:

A) A breakthrough drug for an indication for which there currently is no drug therapy,
B) A drug that has significant advantages over existing drugs, either in greater effectiveness or less toxicity,
C) A drug with greater effectiveness and greater toxicity than existing products, and
D) A drug that is equivalent to existing therapies in effectiveness and toxicity.

Analyzing products in category A may be problematic if there is no suitable existing drug therapy to be used as a comparator. In these cases, traditional management becomes the comparator. The analysis for drugs in groups B and C is more conceptually clear, but problems may arise in the analysis of adverse reactions. For category D drugs, the analysis must clearly demonstrate equivalency with (or at least be no worse than) the comparator. Thus, choice of a comparator is critical to conduct of the analysis and its results.

The *Guidelines* recognize a variety of possible outcome variables, but express a preference for measures of the final outcome of therapy. Clearly, this is not always possible and intermediate outcome indicators are permitted as measures of final outcome (e.g., blood pressure as an intermediate measure for an antihypertensive agent). Quality of life and quality-adjusted life-years are recognized as legitimate outcome measures, but both require special attention to provide the PBAC sufficient data for assessing the validity and reliability of reported results. Indirect medical benefits also can be used to support the application, but as noted earlier, data on employment and productivity are *not* encouraged.

Assessment of Outcomes. The *Guidelines* require detailed information as to the reason for choosing the clinical trial data included in the submission, as well as convincing arguments for the inclusion of data from overseas clinical trials. The applicant also must compare subjects from the clinical trials to typical Australian patients with conditions relevant to use of the new product (effectiveness vs efficacy). The expectation is that data included in the analysis will be relevant in all important respects, and age and gender distribution are specifically mentioned. Finally, the choice of comparator therapy must be justified. The *Guidelines* state: "The comparator should be the therapy which most prescribers would replace in practice."[3] The formulation, dosage, and duration of therapy for the comparator must conform to the product information regarding optimal use for the particular indication (regardless of how it is most commonly used).

Economic Basis of the Submission. The *Guidelines* specify which form of economic analysis to use for particular types of outcomes.[a] The submission must specify whether the population of the study is real or hypothetical, and report the relevant demographic characteristics. The time horizon for disease treatment will depend on the particular situation. The period chosen must be appropriate (e.g., analyses for hypertensive agents and those for agents to treat acute infections will have different time horizons). The outcomes specified earlier must be quantified over the appropriate time period for each therapy studied. This is often difficult to do with clinical trial data, and applicants probably will be given considerable latitude if it is adequately justified.

Net direct medical and nonmedical costs are to be estimated over the relevant time periods for the therapies studied. The present value of net costs and outcomes are to be reported using an annual discount rate of 5%. Finally, the submission should report the net direct cost of treating patients in the study groups. A sensitivity analysis is required and marginal cost analysis also may be needed depending on the situation.

SUMMARY

In summary, The Australian *Guidelines* are consistent with much of the current thinking regarding pharmacoeconomic analysis. The major area of contention is the exclusion of indirect costs from the analysis. Pharmaceutical manufacturers would be likely to argue for inclusion of this component; thus far, however, that position has not prevailed.

---

[a]The four traditional methods are explicitly mentioned: cost-minimization, cost-effectiveness, cost-utility, and cost-benefit. The salient features of each approach are mentioned with respect to its applicability. Although cost-benefit analysis is included, it is *not* encouraged.

Canada

BRIEF HISTORY OF THE GUIDELINES

The development of pharmacoeconomic guidelines in Canada apparently began in 1991 with the publication of draft guidelines by the Ontario Ministry of Health. The draft guidelines were revised by the Ministry of Health, and in 1992 became the basis for further development by an interprovincial working group.[4] After further revisions the working group guidelines formed the foundation for The Collaborative Workshop on Pharmacoeconomics in June 1993.[5] The Ontario Ministry of Health, drawing on the Collaborative Workshop experience, revised and published its final draft guidelines in November 1993.[6]

The Interprovincial Working Group proposed establishing a federal agency known as the Canadian Agency for Pharmaceutical Information Assessment (CAPIA). CAPIA would have been responsible for developing national standards for comparative economic analysis of pharmaceuticals. It also would have served as a clearing house for pharmacoeconomic information, but provinces would maintain responsibility for selecting products to be provided in their individual benefit programs. At a workshop in Montreal immediately following the Collaborative Workshop, it was suggested that CAPIA functions could be made the responsibility of an existing agency.[7] Later, the CAPIA proposal was turned over for review to the Canadian Coordinating Office for Health Technology Assessment (CCOHTA), but it was not immediately adopted. By 1994 both Ontario and CCOHTA had published pharmacoeconomic guidelines. Before presenting these guidelines it will be helpful to understand basic aspects of the Canadian and the Ontario healthcare systems.

CANADIAN AND ONTARIO HEALTHCARE SYSTEMS

In the Canadian system, provinces are responsible for providing healthcare services. Comprehensive health care is universally available and transferable among provinces. Provinces are responsible for providing care, which is financed by a provincial–federal cost-sharing formula. Unlike hospital and physician services, the federal government does *not* set guidelines for prescription drug benefits, but all 10 provinces offer some type of pharmaceutical benefit. In the absence of federal guidelines it is not surprising to find considerable variability among provincial drug benefit packages.

In Ontario, a prescription drug benefit is provided for the elderly ($\geq$65 years), those receiving custodial or nursing home care, and those receiving certain types of public assistance payments.[8] Only products listed in the *Ontario Drug Benefit Formulary/Comparative Drug Index* will be paid for by the Ministry of Health. Consumer cost-sharing is not required for prescriptions covered under the plan.

Price restraint on pharmaceuticals is exercised to some degree at the federal level by the Patented Medicine Prices Review Board. This board limits the launch price of new products and price increases on existing products. The board has authority over all patented products (both over-the-counter and prescription drugs), but not for unpatented products. It is not involved in the drug approval process. Pharmaceutical prices for any particular product can differ across provinces because of provincial initiatives to negotiate better prices in an effort to control pharmaceutical expenditures.

Producers are faced with two pricing hurdles in Canada. First, they must adhere to federal Patented Medicine Prices Review Board guidelines and, second, respond to provincial government requests for price quotes. A product could meet the federal requirements, but fail to be listed on a provincial formulary if the company bid is considered too high relative to competitors' prices in that province. Pharmacoeconomic guidelines will add additional information requirements on pharmaceutical firms.

===== ONTARIO *GUIDELINES* FOR ECONOMIC ANALYSIS OF
===== PHARMACEUTICAL PRODUCTS

The Drug Quality and Therapeutics Committee (DQTC) advises the Ontario Minister of Health on products to be listed in the *Formulary*. The DQTC has traditionally considered information on effectiveness, safety, and cost which has been modified by the Ontario *Guidelines* to include pharmacoeconomic data (referred to in the *Guidelines* as cost-effectiveness data).[9] Thus, the *Guidelines* do not represent new authority, but a modification of existing rules.

Components of an Economic Analysis. The *Guidelines* specify seven components of an economic analysis that can be used to satisfy the cost information requirement of the DQTC. A full cost-effectiveness analysis includes[9]:

1. All relevant costs and clinical outcomes.
2. An incremental analysis. Differences between the new product and the comparator (another product or alternative therapy) are to be obtained.
3. Costs and clinical outcomes to be discounted over time at the rate of 5%.
4. Clear identification of the perspective of the decision-maker. The societal perspective is to be adopted, but the data are to be presented in a disaggregated fashion so that direct medical costs to the provincially funded healthcare system are separate from the costs of the societal perspective. The societal perspective includes all direct and indirect costs (e.g., lost wages).

5. Identification of all sources of data.
6. A sensitivity analysis.
7. The incremental cost-effectiveness ratios from item 2 compared with ratios for other interventions to measure relative economic attractiveness.

Although the organization is different, the Ontario *Guidelines* are quite similar to those of Australia. An important difference is the treatment of nonmedical indirect costs (see item 4) that are included in Ontario (e.g., items such as lost wages). The Australian *Guidelines* discourage the inclusion of this component.

Requirement for Cost-Effectiveness Analysis and Suggested Format of a Report. All submissions to the DQTC must include an economic analysis or a justification of why it is absent. The *Guidelines* include a detailed 18-point checklist by which the submission will be evaluated. Applicants are expected to provide clear and succinct answers to each of the questions, but the best way to answer the questions is left to the applicant. As with the Australian version, the Ontario *Guidelines* emphasize, and give details on, the importance of quality of the evidence, choice of comparator, time horizon, measuring outcomes, and generalizability of the sample to patients served by the Ontario *Formulary*.

The Ontario *Guidelines,* unlike the Australian *Guidelines*, suggest an approach for interpreting the cost-effectiveness ratios. No thresholds for action are given, but different results are ordinally arranged (e.g., dominant, economically attractive, economically unattractive ratios). There is a suggestion that future research may provide a method for using the ratios to make allocation decisions. The applicant's report also must provide an economic impact analysis similar to that required in Australia. Final decisions will be based on incremental cost-effectiveness ratios and a measure of the overall impact on Ontario healthcare resources.

Finally, the Ontario *Guidelines* recognize possible sources of bias in studies conducted or funded by the pharmaceutical firm making the submission. They argue that it would be best if a contract exists between the company and the investigators, but recognize this is not always possible. The minimum expectation is that supporting documents will disclose the authors of the analysis and their source of funding. Item 17 on the worksheet reads as follows: "Who performed the analysis? Did the authors of the report sign a letter indicating their agreement with the entire document presented? Does the report indicate that the authors had independent control over the methods and right to publish the analysis regardless of its results?"[9]

In summary, the Ontario and Australian *Guidelines* are quite similar, but there are differences in perspective of the analysis that affects the treatment of nonmedical indirect costs. Both guidelines attempt to provide another tool for evaluating pharmaceuticals that will be paid for by government programs. The mechanisms of decision-making may be different in the two jurisdictions, but the economic analysis data appear to be quite similar. Given the infancy of both programs, it is far too early to assess whether they will achieve the desired effects.[10]

CANADIAN *GUIDELINES* FOR ECONOMIC EVALUATION OF PHARMACEUTICALS

Unlike the Ontario *Guidelines*, the Canadian *Guidelines* are not related to a specific government agency for which a submission is being prepared. Recall that prescription benefit programs are managed by provinces in Canada. Therefore, the CCHOTA-stated purpose of the Canadian *Guidelines* is somewhat different: "One of the purposes of these guidelines is to facilitate the building of knowledge about individual drug products and their alternatives. To the extent that the *Guidelines* produce more comparable studies, the process of aggregating those studies in meta analyses and building the requisite knowledge base should be enhanced and facilitated."[11]

All of the major topics covered in the Australian and Ontario *Guidelines* are included in the Canadian *Guidelines*. Also included in these *Guidelines* is explicit language about the decision-maker, which is somewhat separate from the concept of perspective. On this issue, the text indicates: "The primary audience (decision maker) for the study should be identified. Secondary target audiences can also be listed."[11] Later, under the heading of "perspective," the view is expressed that: "All studies should report from a comprehensive societal perspective. That perspective should be transparently broken down into those of other relevant viewpoints, including that of the primary decision maker."[11]

This level of detail regarding transparency and disaggregation of the data is found throughout the Canadian *Guidelines*. In summary, the Canadian *Guidelines* are similar to those for Ontario and Australia, but are more detailed. A comparison on specific points for these guidelines, as well as others, is found in Table 1.

Europe

The situation in Europe is quite diverse because of the diversity of healthcare systems and approaches to the pricing and reimbursement for prescription drugs. To date, no European country has adopted guidelines as explicit as those of Australia, Canada, or Ontario.[12] There are several countries that have official mandates to encourage consideration of economic criteria in healthcare decision-making, but none has explicit pharmacoeconomic guidelines. German law, for example, requires that reference

Table 1. Comparison of Pharmacoeconomic Guidelines, January 1995

CRITERIA	AUSTRALIA	CANADA	ONTARIO	UK	PhRMA
Perspective	government	society	society	society	choice[a]
Discount rate	5%	5%	5%	6%[b]	choice[a]
Time horizon	disease dependent	long range	choice	choice	choice
Comparator	replaced product	existing practice	least expensive[c]	choice[a]	choice
Sensitivity	yes	yes	yes	yes	yes
Incremental analysis	yes	yes	yes	yes	yes

PhRMA = Pharmaceutical Research and Manufacturers of America.
[a]Choice must be stated and justified.
[b]Use the rate recommended by the Treasury, currently 6%.
[c]Least expensive currently available strategy and most commonly used alternative.

prices exploit savings in the marketplace and the French Commission de la Transparence is expected to consider how a product will contribute to "improved medical care" when setting prices.

The only consistent policy among European Union Member States is the separation of marketing approval decisions from pricing and reimbursement decisions. Marketing approval is always kept separate and based only on safety, efficacy, and quality.

The economic pressures on European healthcare budgets suggests a considerable potential for the use of economic analysis to evaluate prescription pharmaceuticals. For example, the UK Minister of Health has observed: "'Value for money' is probably the main issue to be addressed in discussions between the pharmaceutical industry and government, and the UK government will be looking closely at economic evaluation of medicines."[13]

A joint working party of the Joint Strategy Group of the Government and the Association of the British Pharmaceutical Industry took up the task of establishing a framework for economic evaluation of pharmaceuticals and published their report in early 1994. The preface to their statement of guidelines makes it clear that economic analysis should not be required: "There should be no formal requirement to conduct economic evaluation of pharmaceuticals. The DoH [Department of Health] would like to see cost-effectiveness studies made available for new products but sees this as a matter for purchasers, prescribers and the companies concerned."[14] This approach contrasts sharply with that in Australia and Ontario, which both require some form of economic evaluation for pharmaceuticals. In this respect, the UK guidelines are more like those published by the CCHOTA.

The UK *Guidelines* also are similar to the Canadian *Guidelines* with respect to perspective. As in Canada, the societal viewpoint is preferred in the UK, and the data are to be presented in disaggregated form to allow for use by different decision-makers. Other aspects of the UK *Guidelines* are shown in a comparative fashion in Table 1.

It appears that harmonization of European economic evaluation guidelines for pharmaceutical products is not likely in the near future, even though enormous progress has been made on the harmonization of the drug approval process in the European Union. This situation is potentially problematic for pharmaceutical firms operating in several European markets. If each country adopts different guidelines, the pathway to market will become cluttered with new obstacles just as the European Union is attempting to harmonize marketing approval for prescription pharmaceuticals.

The Drummond et al. survey documented that even in the absence of economic evaluation criteria there have been numerous economic studies of pharmaceuticals in Europe.[12] Most of the studies were funded by pharmaceutical firms and, according to the authors, were not full economic evaluations. These results were used by companies for purposes other than satisfying government regulatory demands. Often they were used to meet the demands of formulary committees or other nongovernmental bodies with the authority to limit access to pharmaceuticals.[15]

United States

There is, at this time, no US government requirement to provide pharmacoeconomic data. The Food and Drug Administration (FDA) has become involved in the issue because it has jurisdiction over promotional claims for pharmaceutical products. Recently there has been a greater interest in claims regarding cost-effectiveness and outcomes associated with products. The FDA has reviewed these claims prior to product launch and made decisions on a case-by-case basis.[16] To understand this situation, and its future direction, requires an appreciation of the US healthcare system.

US HEALTHCARE SYSTEM

As in some other countries, the marketing approval process in the US is based on safety and efficacy with no consideration given to economic criteria. But, the US regulatory environment is different from that of other industrialized countries because there is no government-funded universal health insurance coverage. There are federal- and state-funded healthcare benefits (e.g., Medicare, Medicaid) for segments of the population, but the US healthcare market in general is characterized by a large private sector dominated by insurers and managed-care providers. Healthcare providers are beginning to consider methods for using economic data in the preparation of formularies and reimbursement strategies. However, none have adopted guidelines as detailed and sophisticated as those discussed above. The absence of national requirements provides maximum choice for everyone concerned, but also the potential for unnecessary duplication of effort by pharmaceutical firms. In the US, as in Europe, there are numerous economic evaluations conducted by pharmaceutical companies for a variety of purposes.

A potential template for pharmacoeconomic regulations in the US can be found in the most recent version of the Health Security Act (HR 3600/1757), which was *not* passed by Congress. This proposal would have established an Advisory Council on Breakthrough Drugs (Title I, Subtitle F) for the purpose of judging the reasonableness of prices for new drugs. Among the six factors to be considered by the Advisory Council were the following directly related to conducting economic evaluation of pharmaceutical products.[17]

- Cost-effectiveness relative to the cost of alternative course of treatment options, including nonpharmacologic medical interventions.

- Improvements in quality of life, including ability to return to work, ability to perform activities of daily living, freedom from attached medical devices, and other appropriate measures of quality-of-life improvements.

While not explicitly identified as such in the text, these criteria are equivalent to specification of comparators and perspectives as identified in guidelines for other countries. Although the legislation did not become law, these kinds of initiatives often find their way into subsequent proposals. As such, they offer a view of what might be expected in the future if pressure for demonstrating value for money continues to grow. The proposal for a committee to examine launch prices of new drugs signals a serious attempt to cope with new drug prices and reflects the trends presented in Figures 1 and 2. In this context, the inclusion of cost-effectiveness and quality-of-life measures recognizes that pharmaceuticals should be valued by more than price.

More recently, the Pharmaceutical Research and Manufacturers of America (PhRMA) released a draft of its own guidelines that are intended to provide guidance for companies conducting pharmacoeconomic studies. PhRMA clearly regards their role as setting standards for voluntary compliance. They state: "The following principles should be used to provide guidance for the conduct and evaluation of pharmacoeconomic studies intended for use in the promotion of pharmaceuticals."[18]

Not surprisingly, the PhRMA document covers many of the same topics found in other guidelines. But, they are related more to the quality of the studies performed and avoid making policy statements (e.g., specifying a perspective or discount rate). With respect to perspective, the PhRMA *Principles* state only that it must be specified and explained. A preference for one perspective is not stated. Other parameters of economic evaluation, such as, the discount rate, time horizon, analytical methods to be used, and the use of foreign data, are left to those doing the study with the expectation that they will be clearly specified (transparent) and appropriate to the research intent. The PhRMA *Principles* are consistent with the pluralistic character of the US healthcare market and their constituency. Other aspects of the *Principles* are summarized in Table 1.

Marketing Implications

Regulations can compel economic evaluations by companies when governments control markets, but there are some instances in which markets provide incentives beyond the regulatory structure. Two examples will illustrate this point.

It was noted earlier that the UK does not require economic analysis of pharmaceuticals reimbursed by the National Health Service. However, recent changes in the payment methods for general practitioners (GPs) have created an interest in pharmacoeconomic data. Fund Holding GPs are general practitioners who have agreed to accept certain practice constraints in exchange for greater flexibility in the use of National Health Service–allocated funds. The purpose is to provide incentives for GPs to be responsive to patient needs. Fund Holding GPs have a budgeted amount for prescribing for patients, certain hospital expenses, and office staffing. Money may be shifted among line items at the discretion of the Fundholding GP to meet patient needs. GPs quickly realized that generic prescribing can be used to preserve funds in the prescribing budget for use elsewhere. Brand name pharmaceutical firms with higher-priced brand name products have been affected by these incentives.[19] They see the need to provide economic data demonstrating that their products are more cost-effective than other treatments and will save money in the long run (e.g., through lower hospitalization rates and lower total cost of therapy).

It could be argued that economic analysis guidelines are necessary, even in this situation, to ensure that studies are conducted properly and consistently. An alternative view is that markets will determine what products are appropriate and useful. Regardless, it is clear that economic evaluation data are finding a place in prescribing decisions in the absence of government regulation on specific product prices.

The US market offers an example in the form of large managed-care organizations that are developing extraordinary buying power for pharmaceuticals. There is a trend in the private sector toward more sophisticated economic thinking about pharmaceuticals as one treatment modality in a strategy for total disease management. The interest is in controlling total cost of care, not just the pharmaceutical budget. Since pharmaceuticals are often the most cost-effective form of therapy, there is a built-in incentive to increase pharmaceutical use. However, these buyers also have the power to demand lower prices based on their purchase volume and other incentives. The market environment is further complicated because some payers have "carved out" the pharmaceutical benefit from the general health benefit causing the buyer's attention to focus only on pharmaceutical unit price. It is an understatement to say that the US healthcare marketing environment is confusing.

Pharmaceutical manufacturers are attempting to respond by developing economic data to demonstrate two points. First, to illustrate to a buyer the cost associated with selected diseases (e.g., breathing disorders, hypertension, diabetes) for which drug therapy is an important component of treatment. Second, to demonstrate the superiority of a particular product and to justify a price that may be higher than that of generic competitors or substitute therapies. Buyers are growing more capable of assessing the information provided to them and are beginning to develop the expertise necessary to make sound judgments. However, this concept is not universally accepted.

The use of pharmacoeconomic data for marketing purposes has raised the issue of potential bias because most of the studies are conducted or funded by pharmaceutical firms. The perception of bias is always a possibility when pharmaceutical firms support pharmacoeconomic research on their own products. The Australian, Canadian, and Ontario *Guidelines* have specified methods for disclosing responsibility for the research and independence of the investigators. In the US, a set of ethical principles has been published by an independent academic group, not affiliated with the pharmaceutical industry, to address the potential for bias.[20] They argue that competitive markets create pressure for bias which, therefore, requires adoption of standards to insure integrity of scientific information. They stated that, "Identifying studies that have followed protocols designed to reduce bias would allow readers to recognize the likelihood of bias in studies not so designated. As a result, competitive pressures would be channeled toward less biased, more useful research. Adherence to these standards would generate a seal of approval that could in itself be valuable in selling pharmaceuticals in an increasingly skeptical and competitive marketplace."[20]

The six standards of practice presented by the authors are similar to those found in the Australian, Canadian, and Ontario *Guidelines*. They include:[20]

- establishing written agreements between companies and institutions (not individuals),
- proper selection of comparators, based on the situation,
- transparency of the company–investigator relationship,
- provisions on the control of data in step-wise funded projects,
- a preference for conservative assumptions, and
- a commitment to publish valid results regardless of their promotional value.

Concern over the potential for bias caused the editors of the *New England Journal of Medicine* to enunciate a policy on publication of cost-effectiveness analysis.[21] Their concerns fall into three areas: (1) the relationship between industry funding and the investigators, (2) written assurance of the authors' independence regarding conduct of the research and publication of its results, and (3) complete disclosure of all the data used in the analysis, all assumptions, and any model used in the analysis. Letters to the editor in a subsequent issue of the *Journal* suggest much disagreement with this policy.[22] Correspondents generally fault the policy for focusing on the source of funding rather than the quality of the work. These and other actions by the private sector in the US have created an environment for economic evaluation that is similar to that of other countries where study criteria are mandated by the government.

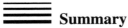

Summary

Currently only two governments (Australia and Ontario) have pharmacoeconomic guidelines that must be used for conducting government-mandated studies. The Canadian federal government has published guidelines, but it does not require submission of data. There has been a joint statement of principles by the UK Department of Health and the Association of the British Pharmaceutical Industry, but the UK does not require pharmacoeconomic studies. In the US, PhRMA has published guidelines for conducting studies and reporting results. The FDA does not require pharmacoeconomic data for marketing approval of a product, but cost-effectiveness claims must be supported by data submitted to the FDA.

Regardless of the regulatory conditions, product-related pharmacoeconomic study results are used by a limited number of decision-makers. Pharmaceutical firms use the results for promotional purposes and to satisfy the information requirements of decision-makers. Generally, there are three types of decisions to which these data are applied. When making decisions on pricing and reimbursement, pharmacoeconomic data are used to help establish the relative value of products. The data also are used to make decisions regarding access to pharmaceutical products. For example, a pharmacy and therapeutics committee may use the data to make formulary decisions or to further restrict access to a product. The additional restrictions might take the form of restrictions on prescribers (e.g., requiring a specialist consult) or step-care requirements.

Future developments in the use of pharmacoeconomic data depend on changes in the existing marketing environment. Important determinants would include the following:

- FDA action. If the FDA decides to adopt guidelines for pharmacoeconomic studies different from those for clinical trials, it will remove the current confusion created by the absence of a standard. Conversely, new standards could impose constraints in the marketplace as well as increasing the administrative burden of marketing new products.
- US healthcare reform. If healthcare reform is pursued, it is likely that some reform of the pharmaceutical market will occur. One possibility is resurrection of the health technology assessment agenda described earlier. Because the US market represents a substantial portion of global pharmaceutical sales, this new regulatory action would have profound global implications.

- Global healthcare reform. The data presented early in this chapter suggest that health expenditure is a continuing concern of many governments. Global competitiveness depends in part on a sound domestic economy, which could be disturbed by excessive healthcare expenditure. Therefore, the prospect exists for pharmacoeconomic guidelines to be adopted by other countries as well as being tightened where they now exist.
- Cost of technology. The cost of bringing a new pharmaceutical product to market continues to rise. Payers are demanding that rising costs be balanced by rising benefits. The pharmacoeconomic movement addresses the question of balance between the upward spiral in research and development costs and the value they provide. If costs continue to rise, the demands of payers for demonstrating value will get louder.

The role of product-related pharmacoeconomics is becoming more clear as the discipline develops. Even as the techniques are being refined, they are being advocated as having a wider role in health care at the system level. Thus, we see the emphasis on outcomes management. The direction and driving force behind these changes continues to be the recognition that consumers, at all levels, want value for money.

References

1. Radical changes ahead in Holland. Scrip Worldwide Pharmaceutical News. No. 1861. London: PJB Publications, 1993; October 5:20.

2. Drummond M. Australian guidelines for cost-effectiveness studies of pharmaceuticals: the thin end of the boomerang? PharmacoEconomics 1991; (suppl 1); 61-9.

3. Guidelines for the pharmaceutical industry on preparation of submissions to the pharmaceutical benefits advisory committee (including submissions involving economic analysis). Canberra, Australia: Commonwealth Department of Health, Housing and Community Services, August 1992.

4. Detsky A. Guidelines for economic analysis of pharmaceutical products: a draft document for Ontario and Canada. PharmacoEconomics 1993;3:354-61.

5. Schubert F, ed. Proceedings of the Canadian collaborative workshop on pharmacoeconomics. Amsterdam: Excerpta Medica, November 1993.

6. Ontario guidelines for economic analysis of pharmaceutical products. Toronto: Ontario Ministry of Health, November 22, 1993.

7. Brogan T. Pharmacoeconomics: the Canadian experience. Scrip Magazine. No. 19. November 1993:18.

8. Ontario drug benefit formulary comparative drug index No. 33. Toronto: Ontario Ministry of Health, 1993:viii.

9. Ontario guidelines for economics analysis of pharmaceutical products. Toronto: Ontario Ministry of Health, 1994.

10. Mitchell A. The Australian perspective on the development of pharmacoeconomic guidelines. In: Schubert F, ed. Proceedings of the Canadian Collaborative Workshop on Pharmacoeconomics. Quebec, Canada, June 21, 1993. Amsterdam: Excerpta Medica, November 1993.

11. Guidelines for economic evaluation of pharmaceuticals: Canada. 1st ed. Ottawa: November 1994:1.

12. Drummond M, Ruttin F, Bienna A, Pinto CG, Horisberger B, Jönsson B, et al. Economic evaluation of pharmaceuticals. PharmacoEconomics 1993;4:173-86.

13. Value for money warning in UK. Scrip Worldwide Pharmaceutical News. No. 1879. 1993; December 7:7.

14. Strategy Group of the Government and the Association of the British Pharmaceutical Industry. Guidance on good practice in the conduct of economic evaluations of medicines. London: Association of the British Pharmaceutical Industry, May 1994.

15. Johnson JA, Bootman JL. Pharmacoeconomic analysis in formulary decisions: an international perspective. Am J Hosp Pharm 1994;51:2593-8.

16. Bonastia CJ. What is the FDA's position on pharmacoeconomic data in promotion? Outcomes Measurement Management 1994;5(6):1-2.

17. New pricing criteria in Clinton text. Scrip World Pharmaceutical News. No. 1880. London: PJB Publications, 1993; December 10:13.

18. Principles for pharmacoeconomic research. Washington, DC: Pharmaceutical Research and Manufacturers of America, February 16, 1995.

19. Reluctant 'yes' on PPRS. Scrip Worldwide Pharmaceutical News. No. 1851. London, PJB Publications, 1993;August 31:2.

20. Hillman AL, Eisenberg JM, Pauly MV, Bloom B, Glick H, Kinosian B, et al. Avoiding bias in the conduct and reporting of cost-effectiveness research sponsored by pharmaceutical companies. N Engl J Med 1991;324:1362-5.

21. Kassirer JP, Angell M. The *Journal's* policy on cost-effectiveness analyses (editorial). N Engl J Med 1994;331:669-70.

22. Correspondence. N Engl J Med 1995;332:123-5.

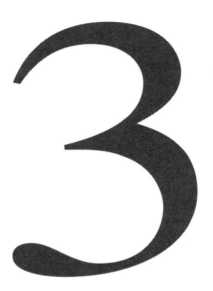

3

Cost Determination
and Analysis

Lon N. Larson

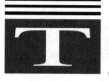he price of a drug product is not the same as the cost of drug therapy. One objective of this chapter is to clarify this difference by defining and describing the concept of cost. A second is to describe how the cost of a therapy or service is determined. Unlike price, which is usually quite easily obtained, cost is more difficult to measure. The ultimate purpose of this chapter is to enable the reader to quantify the cost of a given program or service; in other words, to identify the resources used in a therapy and to assign monetary values to those resources.

The chapter begins with a brief description of production in the healthcare system and the definitions of cost-related terminology. This is followed by a description of the elements in the cost of illness and cost of therapy. The third section of the chapter provides a five-step approach to determining the cost of a therapy or service. The fourth section discusses issues in valuing resources in pharmacoeconomic analyses. Finally, in Appendix I, review and thought-provoking questions that can be used to assess the methods of cost determination are presented.

The concept of cost deals with the resources that are used or consumed in the production of a good or service. Production in the healthcare system is a two-step process. The ultimate products of the healthcare system are therapies that cure, prevent, or alleviate disease and, thereby, affect health status. In producing these therapies, several services may be used—prescription drugs, laboratory tests, hospital stays, physician visits, surgical procedures. Stated differently, these services are the inputs in a production process that produces therapies as its outputs. These services, in turn, require basic resources such as personnel, equipment, facilities, and supplies. In other words, healthcare services can be viewed as intermediate goods—they consume basic resources and, in turn, they are consumed in the production of therapies. In some pharmacoeconomic analyses, determining the basic inputs is important. For instance, to determine the cost of once-a-day dosing, the basic inputs of labor and equipment should be specified. In contrast, to calculate the cost of treating an illness with drug therapy, determining the services used (i.e., the intermediate rather than the basic inputs) is appropriate.

Several cost-related terms need to be understood. These include cost, direct and indirect cost, fixed and variable cost, average and marginal cost, and opportunity cost. *Cost* is defined as the magnitude of resources consumed.[1] The cost of a product or service is the monetary value of resources consumed in its production or delivery. Resources include labor, plant and equipment, and supplies.

A *direct cost* involves a transfer of money. If money is exchanged for the use of a resource, this is a direct cost. An *indirect cost,* in contrast, is an unpaid resource commitment.[1] No money is exchanged. An example of an indirect cost is unpaid assistance from a family member. Also, lost time from work is an indirect cost because output is lost due to the absence. Note that the economist and the accountant have different definitions of the term "indirect cost." The economic view is presented here. In accounting, indirect cost refers to overhead or shared expenses that are used in the production of several products. The allocation of shared costs, or the accountant's indirect cost, is discussed later.

Resource use may or may not be affected by the volume of output. A *fixed cost* does not change with an increase or decrease in output. In contrast, a *variable cost* does vary or change with a change in the volume of output.[2] To illustrate, an employee's salary is a fixed cost, but a sales commission is a variable cost. Similarly, depreciation of plant and equipment is fixed, whereas cost of goods sold (drug products in the case of a pharmacy) is variable.

Average cost is the resources consumed per unit of output. It is derived by dividing total cost by volume or quantity of output. *Marginal cost* is the change in total cost of producing one additional (or one less) unit of output.[2] Because fixed cost remains unchanged as output increases, marginal cost may be viewed as the average variable cost. Thus, if a program involves principally variable costs, its average and marginal costs are similar. If, however, a program has a large amount of fixed costs (relative to variable costs), its marginal cost is less than its average cost.

Opportunity cost is defined as the amount that a resource could earn in its highest valued alternative use; it is the value of the alternative that must be foregone when something is produced.[3] Opportunity cost is the best measure of the value of a resource.[4] In a competitive marketplace, the price of a good or service—set through the interaction of supply and demand—is its opportunity cost. However, some healthcare services are relatively immune from price competition and using price as a proxy for opportunity cost is hazardous. Inpatient hospital care, which is discussed in more detail later, is an example. Other resources have no market prices—volunteer help, unpaid family assistance at home—and their opportunity cost is estimated by calculating potential earnings from another endeavor.

What are some of the implications of these definitions? First, cost should not be confused with charge or price.[5] Cost is the magnitude of resources consumed in producing a good or service. Price is what the customer is asked to pay for the good or service. A good example is hospitals where the charge for a service may not reflect resources consumed because of cross-subsidization between departments (e.g., the very expensive aspirin). Second, cost is not the same as out-of-pocket payment. Often, the cost of a service is viewed as what the patient must pay out of pocket. This assumes that any third-party payment or charity care is without cost, and that is not the case. Third, cost should not be confused with flow of money. To illustrate, assume that a new program is started and is staffed with existing personnel. Even though the personnel budget is unchanged, there is still a labor cost, or resource commitment, to the program. The personnel resource is consumed. The assumption is made that the time spent on this program could have been spent in another productive venture (i.e., the opportunity cost of a foregone alternative).

Cost of Illness and Cost of Therapy

An illness consumes resources and, thus, it has a cost.[6] The cost of an illness is the sum of three components: (1) the medical resources used to treat the illness, (2) the nonmedical resources associated with it, and (3) lost productivity due to illness or disability (indirect costs). A fourth category, the intangible cost of pain and suffering, is often unquantifiable. Medical resources are the services used to treat the illness, and they include hospital care, professional services, drugs, and supplies. Nonmedical resources are out-of-pocket expenses for goods and services outside the medical care sector. Transportation to the site of treatment, lodging for family during treatment, and hiring a person to help with home care are examples of nonmedical services. These are direct costs because money is exchanged. Even though they are nonmedical in nature, they are considered part of the cost of the illness because their use is caused by the illness. The illness also may cause decreased productivity because of temporary or permanent disability. As mentioned above, this lost productivity is an indirect cost because no money is exchanged. (The productivity may be measured as lost wages, even if the person was paid through sick leave or another benefit program.)

A medical therapy is intended to cure, prevent, or reduce the severity of an illness. As it does, the cost of the illness is reduced and this reduction in the cost of the illness is the benefit of the therapy. However, a therapy uses or consumes resources. As with the cost of illness, the cost of a treatment also may be classified as medical, direct nonmedical, and indirect. To illustrate with a simple example, chronic renal dialysis may be performed at a clinic or at home. The medical resources used in clinic dialysis include equipment, facilities, and medical personnel. In addition, travel expense to the facility is a direct nonmedical expense. Finally, if the patient must miss work, the lost productivity is an indirect cost of the treatment. In comparison, home dialysis also includes equipment and supplies (medical costs), but facility fees and transportation costs are absent. However, home dialysis requires a trained helper. The helper's time (whether paid or not) is a cost of treatment. If the helper is paid, it is a direct cost; if unpaid, it is indirect. All of these items should be included in a comparison of the cost of the dialysis alternatives.

A therapy can cause other resources to be consumed. These also are considered as part of the total cost of the therapy. One of these is the resources used in treating adverse effects of the therapy. For example, chronic dialysis may cause anemia, the treatment of which will consume medical resources. In addition, dialysis prolongs life. During the additional years of life, the patient may be treated for other medical problems unrelated to dialysis. The costs of treating these diseases are included as a cost of dialysis because they would not have been incurred if the patient had died of endstage renal disease.

This is how cost is operationally defined in cost-benefit analysis. The cost of a therapy includes medical resources, nonmedical resources, and indirect costs that are used in producing the therapy itself, in treating its adverse effects, and treating any illness that occurs if life is extended. Similarly, the benefit in cost-benefit analysis is the reduction or savings in the three components (medical, nonmedical, indirect) of the cost of illness. The therapy may eliminate the need for other medical services and it may increase productivity by reducing morbidity and disability (indirect benefits).

Many pharmacoeconomic applications focus exclusively on medical costs and omit nonmedical and indirect costs. This may be appropriate if the scope of the analysis is limited to the healthcare system or if the alternatives do not differ with respect to these resources.

Cost in cost-effectiveness analysis (or cost-utility analysis) can take on a slightly different connotation. Weinstein and Stason operationally define cost as the net effect on medical resources.[7] They include four categories of medical resources in their definition: (1) the medical resources used by the therapy itself, (2) the medical resources used to treat adverse effects, (3) the medical resources used during additional years of life, and (4) the medical resources saved when the therapy negates the need for other services. The first three were discussed above. The fourth component actually is a savings or a reduction in the cost of the therapy. In essence, the cost of a therapy is its net effect on medical resource consumption.

Finally, a slightly different variation of cost was used by Thompson et al.[8] In their study of an arthritis therapy, the cost portion of the cost-effectiveness ratio included: (1) the cost of the therapy, (2) the additional medical cost arising from the therapy (e.g., services to monitor the patient), (3) medical cost averted, (4) cost of transportation, (5) paid and unpaid assistance in the home, and (6) changes in earned income. In contrast to Weinstein and Stason, Thompson et al. expanded cost to include nonmedical and indirect resources.

The inclusion of indirect cost (e.g., lost earnings) in the cost of a cost-effectiveness ratio is arguable.[9] If it is included as part of cost, the success of the therapy reduces the total cost by reducing lost earnings. The success also is reflected in the effectiveness portion of the ratio, measured as years of life saved or improved quality of life. The success of the therapy is now double-counted, affecting both the numerator (cost) and denominator (effectiveness) of the ratio. What is the correct approach? There is no set answer. If indirect cost and the measure of effectiveness are not highly correlated (i.e., relatively unrelated to each other), including indirect cost is easier to justify than if they are highly correlated.

A Framework for Determining Costs

The framework for determining the cost of a therapy or service encompasses five steps: (1) specifying the "ingredients," or inputs, (2) counting the units of each resource or input, (3) assigning dollar values to the ingredients so that values approximate opportunity cost, (4) adjusting for differences in timing, and (5) allowing for uncertainty.

SPECIFYING THE INGREDIENTS

The initial step in determining the cost of a therapy or program is to identify the resources consumed by the program; that is, the ingredients used to produce the therapy or service.[10] The goal is to develop a comprehensive list of the inputs that are used in producing it. In the case of a therapy, what medical services are used: hospital care? physician visits? prescription drugs? What nonmedical services or indirect costs are involved? For a service, what types of personnel are required? what equipment and supplies?

A key point is that to be meaningful, an economic evaluation must include all relevant resources and not just the ones that are obvious and/or easy to identify and measure. The ingredients approach of identifying the inputs separately from assigning a dollar value to them is a means to reduce the likelihood of overlooking relevant items. It may turn out that some resources are insignificant in the analysis and can be dropped. However, this should be a conscious decision, made only after the resource has been identified and assessed.

In determining the relevance of resources, the analyst must specify the scope or perspective of the analysis. Economic evaluations may assume the viewpoint of a single provider, insurer, the healthcare system, or society. An example will help clarify this point. Consider a Medicare patient as she moves through the various levels of care from hospital to extended-care facility to home. From the hospital's perspective, its relevant costs are those incurred during the hospital stay. For instance, the hospital welcomes a drug therapy that can reduce the length of stay and/or other services during the stay. An earlier discharge, however, may mean that more intensive and more costly nursing home care is required. This is relevant from the perspectives of the healthcare system and Medicare; it is irrelevant to the hospital. Finally, assume that the patient is discharged home and a family member assumes the role of caregiver. From society's perspective, the caregiver's time is a cost; however, the cost is outside the realm of the healthcare system and is not covered by Medicare. Thus, the cost of a healthcare program depends on one's perspective.

COUNTING UNITS

For each resource, a unit of use or unit of consumption should be specified. The magnitude of resource consumption is measured or counted in that unit. For instance, the use of a drug product may be measured in doses, physician services may be measured in procedures, and inpatient services may be measured in days. It is helpful to count and to report units separately from assigning monetary values because monetary values can vary. If units are counted and reported separately, the impact of a different monetary value can be easily estimated. For instance, a service may reportedly consume $100 worth of pharmacist time per patient; this is less revealing than if it is reported as 4 hours of pharmacist time valued at $25 per hour.

ASSIGNING DOLLAR VALUES

Once the resources used in a program have been identified and counted, they are assigned a monetary value. This is often quite complex. As a general rule, the time and effort spent in assigning a monetary value should be proportional to the importance of that resource. Major resources or cost items should receive more attention than minor items.

Several factors enter into this valuation process. In general, the best measure of a resource's value is its opportunity cost. One issue is the relationship between opportunity cost and market price. A second issue is the relationship between opportunity cost and average cost. A third issue is that some resources may be shared among several activities or programs and, therefore, must be allocated. These issues are in the next three sections.

Opportunity Cost and Market Price. Although opportunity cost is the true cost of consuming a resource, market prices are probably the best indicator of value and should be used if available.[4] Market prices are appropriate for prices that are established through price competition. For some health services, however, there is little competition and market prices may not be appropriate. Hospital charges, for instance, can be misleading because they may bear little (if any) relationship to resources consumed. If market price is not appropriate, a value must be derived from financial records or cost-accounting data. Similarly, for resources that have no price (e.g., volunteers, unpaid assistance from a family member, lost homemaker productivity), the opportunity cost must be estimated.

Opportunity Cost and Average Cost. As mentioned earlier, marginal cost is the change in total cost that results from producing one additional unit of output. In general, marginal cost is a better indicator of opportunity cost than is average cost. Marginal cost also is a better indicator of resource value than average cost because the fixed expenses—which are included in the average cost—are consumed, even in the absence of the additional unit. Likewise, when a unit of output is not produced (e.g., a shortened hospital stay), the resources saved are equal to the marginal cost of the avoided output rather than its average cost. The problem is that, unlike average cost, the marginal cost is almost never known; it is not reported in nor easily derived from accounting reports.

Allocating Shared Resources. If a resource is consumed exclusively in the production of a single product or service, it is referred to as a direct cost in accounting. However, a resource also may be shared among several programs or departments; that is, it is not exclusively associated with one product or service. Cost allocation systems are designed to distribute these shared expenses appropriately among product lines or revenue departments (i.e., the final outputs).[4,5]

Although the details of allocation systems are beyond the scope of this chapter, one fundamental issue is the basis by which an overhead expense is to be allocated. Costs can be allocated in numerous ways, including on the basis of square feet, time spent, and revenue generated. For example, in determining the cost of space for a program that does not have its own separate facility, "housing" expenses (e.g., rent, utilities) are tied to area and are logically allocated on the basis of square feet. If personnel are shared among multiple products, the cost associated with each of the products may be allocated on the basis of time spent on each one. In allocating administrative expenses (e.g., pharmacy director/manager) shared by many products, payroll expense or revenue generated may be used as a basis for allocation.

The key point is that if a resource is used by multiple programs or services, the cost of that resource should be allocated among the programs. The cost should not be attributed to only one program, nor should it be omitted from others. If a pharmacist begins a new service, the personnel cost is not zero simply because the pharmacist was already on the payroll.

ADJUSTING FOR DIFFERENCES IN THE TIMING OF COSTS

A time preference is associated with money. We prefer to receive dollars now rather than later because they can generate benefits or returns in the interim. For the same reason, we prefer to pay out dollars later rather than now. In other words, a dollar today is worth more than a dollar tomorrow. As a simple example, suppose a lottery winner had the choice of receiving $1 million today or $1 million spread over 20 years; in all likelihood, the total sum would be taken today, so as to allow more time to enjoy and/or invest the winnings.

Because current and future dollars are not valued the same, future costs must be discounted to reflect their current value when a program extends over multiple years.[11] The present value (PV) can be calculated by multiplying the future cost (FC) by the discount factor (DF). The discount factor is dependent on two variables: the number of years into the future that the expense is incurred (n) and the discount rate (r). Thus, discounting can be expressed by the formula: $PV = FC \times DF(n,r)$. (Mathematically, the discount factor is equal to $1/(1 + r)^n$, where r is the discount rate and n is the year incurred.)

The present value of a multiyear cost stream is the sum of the present value of the costs for each year. An example may help. Let's assume that a hypothetical treatment regimen has costs as follows: $3,000 in the first year, $2,000 in the second year, and $1,000 each year thereafter. Over three years, the unadjusted cost is $6,000. With a discount rate of 6%, the discount factors for costs incurred at the end of years 1-3 are as follows: year 1, $1 \div 1.06 = 0.943$; year 2, $1 \div (1.06)^2 = 0.890$; year 3, $1 \div (1.06)^3 = 0.840$. The value of the cost stream over three years is: ($3,000 \times 0.943$) + ($2,000 \times 0.890$) + ($1,000 \times 0.840$) = $5,449.

The impact of two assumptions should be noted. In this calculation, we assumed that the expenses were incurred at the end of each period; therefore, the first-year costs (12 months in the future) were discounted using the factor for $n = 1$; the costs for the second year (24 months out) were discounted by the factor for $n = 2$; and so on. An equally acceptable assumption is that the expenses are incurred at the beginning of each year. Thus, the first-year costs are current—not future—and do not need to be discounted. The second-year costs (12 months in the future) are discounted with the factor of n = 1; for the third year (24 months out), the factor of n = 2 is used. In this case, the cost stream would be: ($3,000 × 1.0) + (2,000 × 0.943) + (1,000 × 0.890) = $5,776.

The second assumption relates to the discount rate. Using a higher discount rate reduces the present value of future dollars. For instance, with a 10% discount rate, the discount factors for the end of years 1–3 are 0.909, 0.826, and 0.751, respectively. In our example, this discount rate would have resulted in a present value of (3,000 × 0.909) + (2,000 × 0.826) + (1,000 × 0.751) = $5,130.

A key issue is which discount rate to use. There is no set rule as to the best discount rate to use in economic evaluations. Theoretically, the discount rate may reflect the rate of return possible in private-sector investments, or it may reflect the social rate of time preference. The latter is society's collective time preference, as measured by the real interest rate (interest rate minus rate of inflation) on long-term government securities. In practice, sensitivity analysis is frequently used in which a range of rates are used in the calculations. Two recommendations in selecting the range of discount rates are government-recommended rates (5%, 7%, 10%) and the rates used in previous studies.[4]

The relationship between discounting and inflation should be clarified. They are different concepts. As mentioned above, discounting is based on the time preference for money. Discounting is appropriate whenever a program or therapy extends over multiple years—even if the inflation rate is zero. Inflation is the change in price. If data are collected over multiple years, the prices may need to be adjusted to a uniform price to account for inflation. This is not discounting. If the analysis is longitudinal, following the same subjects more than one year, the cost in future years is discounted for time preference. Consequently, a discount rate is used that is based on the real interest rate (the rate excluding inflation). Similarly, when projecting or estimating the cost in future years from current prices, no estimate is made for inflation. For example, if the current price of long-term drug therapy is $300 per year, that same price is used in estimating future cost and then discounted by the real interest rate.

===== **ALLOWING FOR UNCERTAINTY**

Oftentimes, cost or resource consumption is not known with certainty; assumptions are made and estimated figures are derived. A method to compensate for this uncertainty is sensitivity analysis. In a sensitivity analysis, the economic evaluation is reworked using different assumptions or estimates of the uncertain costs.

Sensitivity analysis can be viewed as a "what if" analysis: What if a price increase (decrease) for a drug product is assumed? What if a different hospital per diem is used? What if different manpower requirements are assumed? Again, sensitivity analysis is essential for any cost that is not known with certainty. To assume that assumptions and estimates are factual can lead to erroneous conclusions.

Pharmacoeconomic Applications

This part of the chapter is devoted to exploring methods of determining the costs of various services of importance in pharmaceutical-related evaluations: personnel time, drug product costs, physician services, and hospital costs.

PERSONNEL TIME

Some economic evaluations, notably those dealing with a service, require the time spent on specific activities. For instance, the time devoted to dosage preparation and administration may be needed in assessing drugs with different dosing schedules or in evaluating drug distribution systems. Similarly, an evaluation of a clinical service requires the amount of personnel time needed to perform the service.

Work measurement techniques can be used to acquire this information. Two techniques are of relevance in cost determination: work sampling and stopwatch time study.[12] In work sampling, momentary observations are made at preselected times. After sufficient observations, the percentage of time devoted to each activity (including idle time) can be determined (i.e., the number of observations for an activity divided by the total number of observations). Work sampling is especially useful with nonrepetitive tasks that are not entirely uniform from occurrence to occurrence.

Stopwatch time studies, on the other hand, are useful with repetitive tasks that are of short duration. This method directly measures the time required to complete a task or activity; for instance, the time to type a label or mix a solution. Again, several observations of several persons are required to derive an average time for an average worker. After the time has been determined using one of these two techniques, the appropriate wage rates can be applied to derive the final labor costs.

One cautionary note is in order pertaining to opportunity cost; specifically, the opportunity cost of labor may not be reflected in the payroll. For example, if a hospital implements a new service without adding any personnel, this does not mean that the labor cost of the service is zero. Rather, the labor devoted to the program has an opportunity cost because it could have been devoted to other activities. Thus, the market value of the labor devoted to the program is rightfully considered a cost of the program. Similarly, a program may free up personnel time, but not affect the payroll. A notable example is switching from a drug requiring three times a day dosing to one that requires once daily dosing; obviously, nursing time is reduced. In this case, the payroll may be unaffected, but the nursing time saved can be devoted to other activities.

DRUG PRODUCTS

Drug products may have multiple prices. Buying groups, contractual agreements, quantity discounts, and competitive bidding have resulted in several prices for the same drug. In economic evaluations, an appropriate price to use is the average wholesale price (AWP). Even though the AWP is oftentimes higher than the actual acquisition cost, it is a standard price that is available to all purchasers. Thus, findings based on AWP may be more applicable to other settings than findings based on a special contract price. Further, AWPs enable more realistic comparisons between products of different manufacturers. Again, the actual acquisition costs may be tempered by special contracts with one manufacturer, but not another.

Drug products are a good example of the advantage of separating units from prices in measuring and reporting the cost of a therapy. If the number of doses used is known, the appropriate price for that setting or institution can be applied. This cannot be done if only the monetary value of the drug product is reported.

PHYSICIAN SERVICES

For physician services—office visits and surgical procedures as well as outpatient laboratory and radiology services—two alternatives are frequently used in economic evaluations. One is to use the amount charged; in essence, this is the market price for the service. The second is to use the allowable charge (or usual and customary charge) of a third-party payer. It is important that the third-party fee schedule be reflective of cost and not be artificially low or discounted.

HOSPITAL SERVICES

Assigning value to hospital services is among the most difficult tasks in pharmacoeconomic evaluations; it also is often one of the most critical. An error in valuing hospital services given their magnitude relative to other medical services can easily overwhelm other costs and result in misleading conclusions. Again, a cardinal rule is: the more important (larger) a cost item, the more time and effort its valuation deserves. Thus, hospital services—the most expensive of all healthcare services—deserve special attention in pharmacoeconomic analyses.

The distinction between cost and charges was noted earlier. The amount charged is the price of a service, whereas the cost is the magnitude of the resources consumed in producing it. A couple of factors can cause the charge for a service to be potentially quite different from its cost. One is cost-shifting between departments. Some services in hospitals are priced much higher than their cost (e.g., drugs), while others may be priced lower than their cost (e.g., room and board). A second is the difference between average and marginal cost for hospital services.

Charges can be converted to costs using cost-to-charge ratios. These ratios vary from hospital to hospital. (These ratios typically use allocated costs rather than direct costs and, consequently, include overhead expenses.) A ratio is determined for each department or revenue center within the hospital. This ratio, multiplied by the charge figure from a given department, gives the underlying cost.

In a pharmacoeconomic analysis, the specific method of valuing hospital services will depend on the nature of the study and on the data available.[4] Again, the analyst seeks to determine which resources have been used (saved) and what is their opportunity cost? Three options will be considered here: an overall per diem encompassing all hospital services, utilization and cost of specific services, and payment rates by diagnosis-related group (DRG).

An overall per diem cost may be deceiving. The per diem figure is simply the average daily cost; that is, the sum of all costs (routine as well as ancillary services) divided by the number of patient days. There are two problems with using per diem costs. One, is that it is an average of all fixed and variable costs. It is not equivalent to the marginal cost. As a hospital experiences one additional (or one less) patient day, the resources consumed (saved) are equal to the marginal cost and not the average cost. Two, a per diem assumes that all days are equal in terms of resource consumption. In actuality, the initial days of a stay are almost always more intensive in the use of ancillary services than are the latter days. Let us assume that one treatment alternative is associated with an average length of stay that is one day less than an alternative treatment. To use the per diem cost of the hospital (or one of its units) as the value of that day saved will likely overstate the resources actually saved.

A second, more refined option is to separate routine services from ancillary (or medical) services. Routine services are those that are relatively standard across all patient days (e.g., room, dietary, laundry, administration). For these services, the average daily cost applies to each day. (It is not equal to marginal cost, and sensitivity analysis to account for this is appropriate.) Ancillary or medical services—such as pharmacy, laboratory, and radiology—vary by patient. Therefore, it is appropriate for the use of each of these services to be measured or estimated separately. In the example above, the savings of a one-day reduction in length of stay would consist of two components: the reduced need for routine services and the reduced use of each ancillary service.

A third valuation is the payment rate for DRGs. This can be useful if it is indicative of actual costs and not artificially low because of political or noneconomic factors. This global payment rate is useful in valuing admissions avoided or incurred. However, when comparing two treatment alternatives for a given DRG, the global payment rate is not very useful. For instance, if a treatment can be performed on an outpatient basis, the DRG payment rate may be a useful measure of the inpatient resources saved. When comparing two inpatient treatments for the same DRG, however, the payment rate is meaningless (although a cost system based on DRGs could be revealing).

In sum, one must be cautious in valuing the resources consumed (saved) in hospital services. Sensitivity analysis, using various assumptions, is certainly appropriate, if not essential.

Summary

This chapter has provided an overview of the major issues involved in determining and analyzing the cost of a service or therapy. Measuring and placing a monetary value on the resources consumed by a service or therapy are a central part of an economic evaluation. Determining and analyzing the cost of a service or therapy involves five steps: specifying the ingredients (identifying the resources consumed), counting units, assigning monetary values, adjusting for time, and sensitivity analysis. Whether performing a study or critiquing one, careful attention should be given to the following question. What is the cost—the magnitude of resources consumed—by the alternatives being compared? In other words, what resources are consumed and at what opportunity cost? See Appendix I for a listing and analysis of some published articles. The questions following each article are intended to guide the reader's assessment of the cost determination performed in each study being described.

APPENDIX I. ARTICLES, COMMENTS, AND QUESTIONS REGARDING ASSESSMENT OF COST DETERMINATION

Article: Thompson MS, Read JL, Hutchings C, Paterson M, Harris ED. The cost effectiveness of auranofin: results of a randomized clinical trial. J Rheumatol 1988;15:35-42.
Comment: Note especially the sections entitled Economic Data and Effects on Costs and Tables 2 and 3. This was a clinical trial that assessed the cost of treating arthritis with and without auranofin.
Questions: (1) What medical resources were included in the cost of the therapeutic alternatives? What nonmedical resources were included? (2) How was the quantity consumed of each resource determined? (3) How

was each resource priced or valued? (4) Was the price of auranofin adjusted for inflation or time preference?

Article: Schulman KA, Glick HA, Rubin H, Eisenberg JM. Cost-effectiveness of HA-1A monoclonal antibody for gram-negative sepsis. JAMA 1991;266:3466-71.
Comment: Note especially the sections entitled Methods and Costs. This study applied economic data to the results of a clinical trial.
Questions: (1) Whose perspective was used? (2) What medical resources were included? (3) How was hospital use measured? How was it assigned monetary value? (4) Were the costs of adverse effects addressed? The costs of adjunctive services? (5) The medical services required in the additional life-years saved were not included. Should they have been?

Article: Canafax DM, Gruber SA, Chan G, Miles CJ, Matas AJ, Najarian JS, et al. The pharmacoeconomics of renal transplantation: increased drug costs and decreased hospitalization costs. Pharmacotherapy 1990;10: 205-10.
Comment: Note especially the section entitled Cost Analysis and Tables 1-4. This study compared the costs of care for one year after transplantation for two groups of patients who had received transplants during two different time periods and who had received different therapies.
Questions: (1) What services or resources were included? Were any relevant ones omitted? (2) How were the resources counted and valued? (3) Charges were adjusted for inflation (based on the hospital's changes in prices). Should prices also have been adjusted for time preference?

Article: Calvo MV, Del Val MP, Alvarez MM, Dimingues-Gil A. Decision analysis to assess cost-effectiveness of low-osmolality medium for intravenous urography. Am J Hosp Pharm 1992;49:577-84.
Comment: Note especially the section entitled Cost Analysis and Table 2. This is a decision-analytic study.
Questions: (1) Acquisition cost and adverse effects were included, preparation costs were not. Is this justified? (2) What resources were included? (3) How were the resources counted and valued?

References

1. Jacobs P. Economic dimensions of the healthcare system. In: The economics of health and medical care. 3rd ed. Gaithersburg, MD: Aspen, 1991:47-8.
2. Jacobs P. Behavior of healthcare costs. In: The economics of health and medical care. 3rd ed. Gaithersburg, MD: Aspen, 1991:125-31.
3. Jacobs P. Economic measurement: cost-benefit and cost-effectiveness analysis. In: The economics of health and medical care. 3rd ed. Gaithersburg, MD: Aspen, 1991:353.

4. Drummond MF, Stoddart GL, Torrance GW. Cost analysis. In: Methods for the economic evaluation of health care programmes. New York: Oxford University Press, 1987:41-53.

5. Finkler SA. The distinction between cost and charges. Ann Intern Med 1982;96:102-9.

6. Drummond MF. Cost-of-illness studies: a major headache? PharmacoEconomics 1992;2:1-4.

7. Weinstein MC, Stason WB. Foundations of cost-effectiveness analysis for health and medical practices. N Engl J Med 1977;296:716-21.

8. Thompson MS, Read JL, Hutchings C, Paterson M, Harris ED. The cost effectiveness of auranofin: results of a randomized clinical trial. J Rheumatol 1988;15:35-42.

9. Drummond MF, Stoddart GL, Torrance GW. Cost-effectiveness analysis. In: Methods for the economic evaluation of health care programmes. New York: Oxford University Press, 1987:78–9.

10. Levin HM. Cost-effectiveness analysis in evaluation research. In: Guttentag M, Struening EL, eds. Handbook of evaluation research, Beverly Hills, CA: Sage Publications, 1975:89-122.

11. Spiro HT. Finance for the nonfinancial manager. New York: Wiley and Sons, 1977: 70-6.

12. Roberts MJ. Work measurement. In: Brown TR, Smith MC, eds. Handbook of institutional pharmacy practice. 2nd ed. Baltimore: Williams & Wilkins, 1986:90-110.

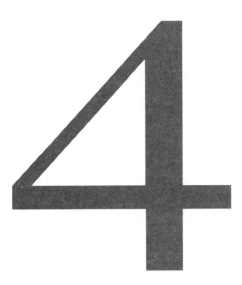

Cost-Benefit Analysis

William F. McGhan
Deborah S. Kitz

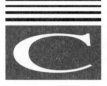ost-benefit analysis (CBA) is a method for comparing the value of all resources consumed (costs) in providing a program or intervention against the value of the outcome (benefits) from that program or intervention.[1,2] In essence, CBA may be thought of as the "yield" of an "investment." Will the benefits of a program exceed the cost of implementing it? Which program will produce the greatest net benefit?

CBA is a tool that can be used to guide the decision-making process in the allocation of funds for health and other programs.[3-7] Although the overall concept of CBA is simple, many of the methodologic considerations require a certain degree of technical understanding in order to apply CBA appropriately.

CBA requires that the costs and benefits both be valued in the same units, usually dollars. If a particular pharmaceutical regimen decreases the need for serum concentration monitoring, the dollar value of the eliminated tests is the benefit. Similarly, if the benefit is lives saved, a dollar value can be assigned to those lives.

Questions Cost-Benefit Analysis Can Answer

Single or multiple interventions may be assessed via CBA. For a single intervention, CBA may be used to determine whether a positive or predetermined minimum return will result from the intervention. For example, will a vaccine program result in savings of at least $75 per patient for a managed healthcare program?

Multiple programs with similar or unrelated outcomes may be examined with CBA. Patrick and Woolley,[8] for example, conducted a CBA of three approaches to a pneumococcal vaccine program provided by a health maintenance organization (HMO). They evaluated the strategies of vaccinating no one, vaccinating all enrollees, or vaccinating all enrollees determined to be at high risk. For each approach, they determined the probability of disease, probability of adverse effects from the vaccine, cost of treating each of these events, and other costs for the HMO and for the patients. The CBA indicated that a program of vaccinating only those patients considered to be at high risk was most appropriate, even when the HMO's costs for identifying high-risk patients were included.

CBA of programs with unrelated outcomes is useful when funds are limited and only one program may be implemented. Should a hospital develop a cephalosporin surveillance program or a cholesterol-lowering program for employees? Which will generate the greatest benefit relative to the cost of implementing each program? Should a city government invest in a prenatal nutrition program, an AIDS awareness program, or three new community health centers?

CBA evolved from the need to ascertain estimates of the costs and benefits of public investment projects, like bridges and dams. Expenditures for health care should produce net social benefits for the public. CBA techniques can be applied to make such resource allocation decisions in the healthcare field. Economists have reminded us that medical care is both an investment good and a consumption good. When considered as an investment good, medical care is an investment in human capital.[6,7,9] In economic terms, for example, the present value of a person's lifetime productivity (earnings) is often considered the appropriate measure of the potential benefit from any investment in human capital.

A major function in any planning process is the formulation of alternative ways to achieve desired objectives and then choosing among those alternatives. Many times, decisions are made on the basis of intuition and personal judgment. CBA—by requiring precise definitions and objectives, identifying criteria for judging results, quantification of the results of each alternative, and examination of the effects of assumptions and uncertainties—provides a foundation based on quantifiable data for decision-making.

Ideally, all benefits and costs generated by the program should be included in any CBA. This may present considerable challenges, particularly in assessing benefits. Benefits of many interventions or programs are difficult to measure, difficult to convert to dollars, or both. For example, benefits such as improved patient comfort, improved patient satisfaction with the healthcare system, improved working conditions for the physician, and so on, are not only difficult to measure but are extremely difficult to convert into dollars.[10-16] Even though a complete economic evaluation may not be possible, an important advantage of CBA is that it forces those responsible for the analysis to quantify as many aspects of the intervention as possible. Vague qualitative judgments or personal hunches should not play any role in CBA.

MEASURING BENEFITS

The economic benefits of a health program or intervention typically are classified as direct, indirect, and intangible.

Direct Benefits. Direct benefits are defined as that portion of averted costs currently borne that are associated with spending for health services; they represent potential savings in the avoided use of health resources. Savings may occur in care avoided prior to diagnosis and hospitalization, during hospitalization or treatment, during convalescent care, and during continued medical surveillance. In particular, as Rice suggested, direct benefits may accrue from saving "expenditures for prevention, detection, treatment, rehabilitation, research, training, and capital investments in medical facilities as well as professional services, drugs, medical supplies, and nonpersonal health services."[17,18] Most often, direct benefits may be assessed and assigned dollar values with relatively little difficulty.

Indirect Benefits. Indirect benefits represent potential increased earnings or productivity gains that would not have been possible without the particular healthcare program. Despite extensive explanation in the literature, indirect benefits can be difficult to measure. They are often calculated from the avoidance of earnings and productivity losses that would have been borne without the health program in question. Rice[17,18] provides a systematic method of measuring indirect benefits. Her estimates include wage and productivity losses resulting from illness, disability, and death based on age and gender for major causal categories of morbidity and mortality. The approach of valuing a patient's life by calculating gross discounted earnings is known as the "human capital" approach.

Drummond et al. discuss a number of methods for valuing indirect costs and consequences.[19] The various approaches to valuation are as follows:

1. Market valuations by using costs (prices or wages) as they
   - are paid to the individual patient,
   - exist in the marketplace, or
   - are imputed (e.g., imputing the value of housewife's time by referencing wages paid to domestic help).
2. Contingent valuation, which is usually the patient's willingness to pay or trade-offs of time or money for relief from various probabilities of illness or adverse effects.

3. Practitioners' or policy-makers' views or actions on what they believe are appropriate expenditures for various disorders.
4. Court awards (although these are sometimes based on lost earnings).
5. An individual's expenditures on life and health insurance.

Intangible Benefits. Intangible benefits of health or a particular intervention are difficult to measure. These include the psychological benefits of health, such as satisfaction with life or health.[20,21] Quantification of such intangible benefits poses an almost insuperable task. How many dollars should be assigned to the value of an increased satisfaction with life or freedom from pain? Several techniques for valuing intangible benefits are available, and Mishan[22] emphasizes that an attempt should be made to account for the extremely valuable "spillover" effects of medical care programs.

DISCOUNT RATES

Costs and benefits of a medical program may occur over a period of many years. For example, the benefits of a lead paint removal program occur over many years as cases of lead toxicity and learning problems are avoided. Dollar values must be assigned to these benefits in the year in which they will occur. This stream of benefit dollars is then discounted to its equivalent present value (value in today's dollars) at a selected interest rate. On the other side of the equation, all costs of the program are identified, assigned to a specific year and discounted to their present value at the same interest rate. Then, other things being equal, when selecting among several programs, the program with the largest present value of benefits minus costs is the "best" in terms of its present economic value.

A challenge in CBA is to determine the proper interest rate for discounting future benefits and costs. Prest and Turvey[16] recommend that the selection of a rate be based on similar projects, followed by sensitivity analysis (varying a key factor such as the discount rate to determine whether the conclusion changes) to determine the effect of a range of discount rates. The problem of selecting an appropriate discount rate and other methodologic considerations is discussed in further detail later in this and other chapters.

All benefits and costs that occur at different times must be adjusted to reflect comparable dollar values. This is accomplished by converting dollar amounts into present values through the use of an interest rate referred to as the discount rate. Although most economists agree that discounting should be emphasized, there is much discussion as to the appropriate rate for a given situation. The consequences of choosing a high or low discount rate are clear: a low discount rate favors projects with benefits accruing in the distant future, whereas a high rate favors projects with costs in the distant future.[22-24] One commonly used rate is the current yield on long-term government bonds. This seems practical as it represents a risk-free long-term alternative use of funds by a tax-free institution and, therefore, appears valid for evaluating long-term health proposals. Theoretical support can be found in the literature for practically any figure between the pure time-reference (risk-free) rate, which can be as low as 4%, and the corporate return on capital, approximately 20%.[25-29]

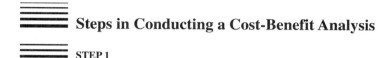

Steps in Conducting a Cost-Benefit Analysis

STEP 1

The first step in conducting a CBA is to identify clearly the intervention(s), program(s), or therapeutic regimen(s) to be evaluated. Patrick and Woolley[8] included identifying high-risk patients and treating adverse effects from the vaccine as part of the pneumococcal vaccine evaluation. The "program" went beyond administering vaccines and treating disease. For a cephalosporin surveillance program, it is not adequate simply to state that a program will be implemented. Will pharmacists become effectively incorporated into the hospital's infectious disease team? Will all requests for cephalosporin be screened? Will the program be for third-generation cephalosporins only? What are the specific components of the program?

STEP 2

The second step is to identify and value all of the resources consumed, or costs of providing each intervention, program, or regimen. Different types of resources should be recognized. In their CBA of an outpatient parenteral antibiotic program, Poretz et al.[30] included expenses for training patients to self-administer drugs, physician visits, and supplies.

A hospital pharmacy would include expenses for personnel time (salaries and employee benefits), office space, computer hardware and software, additional telephone lines, and general supplies in a CBA of a cephalosporin surveillance program. A comprehensive comparison of two pharmaceutical therapy regimens would include costs for purchasing each drug, supplies consumed in administering each agent, salary and employee benefit expenses for personnel time (pharmacists, nurses, physicians) consumed in preparing and delivering the drug, and hospital resources used to treat untoward effects of each regimen. Shapiro et al.[31] conducted this type of CBA of placebo versus cefazolin prophylaxis in women undergoing vaginal or abdominal hysterectomy and included expenses for hospital days, bacterial cultures, and antimicrobial agents. Complications of a particular therapy and expenses for treatment, increased length of hospital stay, and increased indirect costs should also be assessed in a CBA.[32]

STEP 3

Benefits are identified and valued in the third step. Benefits of the cephalosporin surveillance program might include decreased use of third-generation cephalosporins (i.e., attempting to lower the drug purchasing budget with equally efficacious drugs), a lower incidence of drug interactions, and an associated decreased use of resources needed to treat untoward events. For the hospital, the value of these benefits is their true cost savings. For the comparison of two pharmaceutical regimens, the benefits to the hospital of the regimen requiring a shorter duration of treatment would include cost savings from the decreased length of stay, assuming the hospital is reimbursed only on a fixed-price basis (e.g., diagnosis-related groups). If a fee-for-service payment system is used, a shorter length of stay benefits the third-party payer but may actually decrease revenue for the hospital.

Recall that if the benefit of an intervention is lives saved, a monetary value must be assigned to those lives. Similarly, the benefit may be fewer days of work missed. Actual or estimated patient salary information may be used to assign a dollar value to these days.[30-33]

STEP 4

The fourth step in CBA is to sum the value of all the costs and then sum all the benefits of each program, intervention, or regimen. Total costs then may be subtracted from total benefits to determine net benefits:

Net Benefits = Total Benefits − Total Costs

Some investigators prefer to compute a cost-to-benefit ratio, while others prefer to calculate a benefit-to-cost ratio. Although the analytic approach is commonly called CBA, calculating a benefit-to-cost ratio frequently is appropriate because the total benefits are usually expected to exceed total costs, producing a ratio of greater than 1:1.

Benefit-to-Cost Ratio = Total Benefits ÷ Total Costs

If initial estimates of the benefit (yield) of an investment in a program (cost) must exceed a minimum dollar value before it is approved for implementation, net benefits would be calculated. A hospital pharmacy may determine that the net benefit of a biotechnology surveillance program must be at least $50,000 annually. In this case, net benefits should be calculated. Alternatively, a benefit-to-cost ratio should be computed if the criterion for implementing a program is that the benefits must be at least twice as great as the cost (i.e., 2:1 benefit-to-cost ratio), regardless of the absolute value of the benefits and costs. By comparing benefit-to-cost ratios of multiple programs, the program that produces the greatest yield relative to the investment, can be identified. In some ways, hospital budget allocation decisions between expanding an outpatient pharmacy service versus a walk-in clinic versus a trauma program, for example, implicitly could compare the benefit-to-cost ratio for each program. The formula for the benefit-to-cost ratio is as follows:

$$\text{Benefit-to-Cost Ratio} = \frac{\sum_{t=1}^{n}[B_t/(1+r)^t]}{\sum_{t=1}^{n}[C_t/(1+r)^t]}$$

where B_t = total benefits for time period t, C_t = total costs for time period t, r = discount rate, and n = number of time periods. The decision criterion is as follows:

If B/C > 1, then benefits exceed costs and the program is socially valuable.

If B/C = 1, then benefits equal costs.

If B/C < 1, then benefits are less than costs; therefore, the program is not socially beneficial.

The major problem with selecting this method is in choosing r, the discount rate.

Another formula used in CBA relates to the concept of net present value (NPV), as represented in the formula below.[35]

$$\text{Benefits} - \text{Costs} = \text{NPV} = \sum_{t=1}^{n}[(B_t - C_t)/(1+r)^t]$$

Table 1 presents a simplified example of the type of data used in CBA. This exemplifies the importance of including cost items beyond just the acquisition expense for a drug. Administration costs and the cost of adverse drug reactions also should be assessed. On the benefits side, days back at work and extra months or years of life must be assessed and converted into dollar values.

Table 1. Simplified Cost–Benefit Analysis Applied to Drug Therapy

	COST ($)	
VARIABLE	DRUG A	DRUG B
Cost		
acquisition cost	300	400
administration	50	0
monitoring	50	0
adverse effects	100	0
Subtotal	500	400
Benefit		
Days at work	1000	1000
Extra months of life	2000	3000
Subtotal	3000	4000
Benefit-to-cost ratio	3000/500	4000/400
	= 6:1	= 10:1

Table 2. Sample Comparisons Using Different Cost–Benefit Approaches

PROGRAM	COSTS (t_0) ($)	BENEFITS (t_1) ($)	BENEFIT-TO-COST RATIO[a]	NET PRESENT VALUE[b] ($)	INTERNAL RATE OF RETURN[c] (%)
A	10,000	15,000	1.5:1	5,000	50
B	100,000	180,000	1.8:1	80,000	80

t_0 = time at the beginning of the intervention; t_1 = time at one time period later.
[a]Benefit-to-cost ratio = benefits ÷ costs.
[b]Net present value = benefits − costs.
[c]Internal rate of return = (benefits − costs) ÷ costs.

Table 2 illustrates that the cost–benefit mathematical formulas can be misleading, depending on the potential differences in the magnitude of dollars and time involved when comparing the costs and benefits of competing programs. Table 2 presents simplified versions of the different cost–benefit mathematical approaches to illustrate how the decision factors can vary. From these options, the formula that is most appropriate at a given institution must be selected. The results of all three formulas should be presented when comparing programs.

In the example provided in Table 2, program A might represent a proposal for a medium-size computer in the pharmacy and program B might represent a large computer system with multiple decentralized terminals. Although program B has a higher cost–benefit ratio and rate of return, it is an expensive system and the pharmacy may not want to commit such a substantial amount of funds. Numerous other examples could be considered here that change the results from the various formulas and make it more difficult to select between programs.

It should be emphasized that, for the limited investment streams presented in this example, the calculations have been greatly simplified. The calculations and comparisons become more complex as benefits are accrued at different increments of time and as costs and benefits are properly discounted with the more complete formulas presented earlier.

Perspective of the Analysis

An important consideration in conducting a CBA and other types of clinical economic evaluations is the perspective of the analysis. For whom are the costs and benefits being assessed? The patient? Department manager? Third-party payer? Practitioner? Society?[34-36]

Different resources are considered costs and benefits, and the dollar value of each may vary depending on the perspective from which the analysis is conducted. A pharmacy department may include expenses for a portable computer as part of their costs for an outpatient parenteral therapy program. However, these costs may be irrelevant to the patient. Similarly, a patient who is able to return to work considers this a benefit of the outpatient program. This factor does not have any financial impact on the hospital or pharmacy. Likewise, patients may incur out-of-pocket expenses for transportation to outpatient follow-up visits. These costs do not have any direct impact on the third-party payer, hospital, pharmacy department, or clinician.

Bootman and McGhan[36] point out that a factor considered to be a benefit from one perspective may be a cost from another perspective. For example, a hospital may view decreased inpatient days as a benefit (under fixed-price payment) of having an outpatient parental therapy program. However, a patient covered by health insurance that includes a higher co-payment for outpatient care and 100% coverage for inpatient care would view the decreased inpatient days as a cost. Although insurers would consider the change from inpatient surgical care to outpatient lithotripsy for renal stones a benefit, urologists may consider this a loss, particularly if the payment for lithotripter services is lower than that for surgical care. In the same way, outpatient drugs to dissolve gallstones may be a savings to society but a cost (loss) to hospitals.

Koplan and Preblud[37] included costs from different perspectives in their clinical economic evaluation of the mumps vaccine. For children with mumps, they included estimates of wages lost by parents staying home with the children, expenses for transportation to office visits, cost of the vaccine, and acute care costs. Although they did not place a dollar value on the ability to return to work, Rosenfeldt et al.[38] and Nevitt et al.[39] did include the ability to return to work as a "benefit" of coronary bypass surgery and total hip arthroplasty, respectively.

Under fixed-payment systems for hospital care, the importance of specifying the perspective from which the analysis is being conducted is magnified. These payment systems mean that high patient care expenses generated by the hospital no longer increase third-party payer payments. Extensive and unnecessary use of biotechnology, for example, may generate high patient care costs for the hospital, but do not affect third-party payments. On the other hand, pharmaceutical therapy that shortens the length of stay or eliminates the need for serum drug concentration monitoring may generate savings for the hospital. From the insurer's perspective, however, savings do not accrue; the payment is fixed. The insurer's costs may increase, however, if a patient receives inpatient care when ambulatory or home care is feasible and effective.

Fixed-price payment also imposes a relatively new requirement on CBA and other clinical economic analyses performed from the perspective of the hospital: true costs must be assessed. True costs are the value of the resources used in providing a service.[40] Charges, which usually bear no consistent relationship to costs and often are set to maximize revenue, are irrelevant in assessing hospital expenses or savings under fixed-price payment.

Determining the hospital cost for a service is usually a complex task. Assessing the cost of different modes of intravenous antibiotic therapy, for example, may involve time and motion studies of personnel activities (and assigning salaries and employee benefits) devoted to reconstituting and administering the drug, and hospital expenses for supplies used in each mode. In fact, Foran et al.[41] used an independent accounting firm to observe staff activities and supplies used and assign dollar values to these resources in an evaluation of drug dosing frequencies. Although determining hospital costs may be a time-consuming, detailed process, it is a critical element of any clinical economic analysis.

The perspectives from which the analyses will be conducted should be considered in the initial study design. More than one perspective may be included in the analysis. However, attention should be devoted to distinguishing the value of costs and value of benefits from each perspective.

Making Assumptions

Frequently, investigators find it necessary to use secondary data sources or make assumptions about the value of one or more variables in a clinical economic evaluation. This occurs most often when the clinical economic analysis is not being performed in conjunction with the clinical evaluation or when no acceptable historical data are available. In the example of the outpatient parenteral therapy program, a hospital may have to estimate annual mileage for a supply delivery van. Information about the hospital's catchment area and experience of other hospitals may guide the estimates.

Sensitivity analysis is a method of determining whether the conclusion of an economic evaluation changes when the value of one variable is varied as all other variables are held constant. Will the benefit-to-cost ratio fall below one if expenses for computer use are higher than estimated? If personnel expenses for the cephalosporin surveillance program are actually 25% higher than projected, will the net benefits of the program be negated? In other words, sensitivity analysis allows determination of whether the original conclusions are upheld through the range of variation in the value of the variables in question. Does the benefit-to-cost ratio remain above one through the range of variation? Do the net benefits remain positive? If the conclusions are upheld through the sensitivity analysis, there is a higher degree of acceptability in the conclusions. However, if the conclusions change, efforts should be made to determine the true value of the variable in question or to state explicitly that the conclusions are "sensitive" to the value of that single variable.

Koplan and Preblud,[37] for example, varied the incidence of disease, discount rate, and costs per vaccine dose. Under all reasonable ranges of each variable, they found that the benefit-to-cost ratio of the mumps vaccine remained above one. Thus, they were confident of the general findings regarding the economic aspects of the mumps vaccine.

Eisenberg and Kitz[33] included sensitivity analysis in their economic evaluation of outpatient antibiotic treatment for osteomyelitis. Initially, they used information from a previous report indicating that 50% of patients could return to their normal routines (e.g., work, school) during outpatient parenteral antibiotic therapy. To determine whether the general conclusions were sensitive to the value of this variable, they reanalyzed the data with 0% and 100% "return to routine" rates. The original conclusions were upheld under these values of this variable: benefits would accrue to patients from an outpatient program regardless of the return to routine rate.

Patrick and Woolley[8] included sensitivity analysis in their CBA of three approaches to pneumococcal pneumonia vaccine for a health maintenance organization population. Their overall conclusions about identifying and immunizing high-risk patients did not change when they varied the cost of the vaccine, duration of the program, likelihood of adverse effects, cost of illness, and several other factors.

One approach to sensitivity analysis is to increase and decrease the assumed value of the variable by a significant percent (e.g., 50% or 100%). Another approach is to select the mean (e.g., for salaries) for the initial analysis, and then repeat the analysis with the lowest and highest value of the variable.

Cost-Benefit or Cost-Effectiveness Analysis

Cost-benefit and cost-effectiveness analyses are both useful tools for assessing the clinical economic impact of medical care programs or interventions. There are, however, several important distinctions between the two approaches.

First, CBA may be applied to single or multiple programs, whereas cost-effectiveness analysis usually is used to compare two or more programs. Second, CBA may be used to compare programs with disparate outcomes. In contrast, cost-effectiveness analysis is a method for identifying the least costly approach to achieving a similar outcome. Third, CBA requires that all the outcomes or benefits be assigned a dollar value. The outcome or effect is not valued financially in cost-effectiveness analysis. Many investigators find it distasteful to place a monetary value on a benefit such as lives saved and, thus, prefer cost-effectiveness analysis.

Which approach should you use?[1,2,42] It depends. A general guideline is that cost-effectiveness analysis is most appropriate when a single effect or outcome can be defined. An effect might be providing antibiotic prophylaxis for patients undergoing surgery for nonperforated appendicitis or providing postsurgical analgesic therapy. CBA is usually most appropriate when a single program is to be evaluated or when funds are limited and budget allocation decisions must be made among programs with unrelated outcomes. McGhan et al.[1,2] pointed out that CBA is a particularly powerful technique for evaluating clinical pharmacy services. Are the costs of implementing a service offset by savings (benefits) from the service? These types of questions will be asked with increasing frequency as hospital administrators and healthcare managers respond to cost-containment pressures created by fixed-price payment programs.

Cost-Benefit Analysis in the Literature

As will be noted throughout this section, many of the CBAs in the pharmacy arena have focused on the use of antibiotics. Poretz et al.[30] conducted a CBA of an outpatient parenteral therapy program with ceftriaxone for patients with serious infections. They conducted a telephone survey to determine expenses for training sessions, supplies, physician visits, and transportation to follow-up visits. Income information and days of work missed by patients and companions were used to assess productivity losses. Data also were gathered regarding third-party payer coverage for components of care. The benefit-to-cost ratio of this outpatient therapy program was about 3.7:1, average total weighted benefits were approximately $6,600, and costs were about $1,800. The authors noted that insurance coverage was less comprehensive for outpatient care than for inpatient care, suggesting that analysis of these types of programs from the patient perspective should consider out-of-pocket expenditures for direct medical care routinely covered when provided on an inpatient basis.

A type of CBA of another outpatient parenteral therapy program was conducted by Kunkle and Iannini.[43] Their analysis was limited to an estimate of per diem hospital costs (excluding ancillary services), a conservative estimate of daily patient wages, and an estimate of nursing time consumed in delivering intravenous antibiotics.

Shapiro et al.[31] incorporated a CBA in a clinical trial of antibiotic prophylaxis for hysterectomy. This approach to conducting an economic evaluation is attractive because data regarding untoward effects, treatment failures, and other clinic parameters are collected concurrently with economic data. A danger of this approach, however, is that particular aspects of therapy, such as serum concentration monitoring, may occur simply because of the clinical trial. Such monitoring would not be part of standard clinical practice and may inadvertently be included in the economic assessment. It is necessary to exclude from the cost and benefit calculations the clinical trial-related expenses that would not occur in normal practice.

Identifying these factors may be difficult, particularly if little information is available about routine practice with a new pharmaceutical agent.

The CBA performed by Shapiro et al.[31] included expenses for operative site or urinary tract infections and febrile morbidity occurring during hospitalization or within six weeks after discharge following abdominal or vaginal hysterectomy. Although the authors used charge rather than cost data to assess expenses for hospital days, cultures, and antibiotic agents, the results indicated that the net benefit of prophylaxis versus placebo was about $100 per patient for abdominal hysterectomy and nearly $500 for vaginal hysterectomy.

Conafax et al.[44] examined the economic aspects of two immunosuppressive drug regimens following human lymphocyte antigen-identical renal transplants. Although charge rather than true cost data were used to value some medical services, the authors found that the cyclosporine regimen was less costly when rehospitalization and other expenses were considered for a one-year period following transplant. This occurred despite higher drug purchase expenses for cyclosporine.

Vaccination programs also have been evaluated through CBA. In addition to Patrick and Woolley's[8] evaluation of pneumococcal pneumonia vaccines, Koplan and Preblud[37] conducted a CBA of mumps vaccine for children in the US. They included data on disease incidence, vaccine efficacy, mumps, encephalitis, hearing loss, and death, and found a benefit-to-cost ratio of at least 7.4:1.

Summary

CBA is an approach to clinical economic assessment. It requires that both costs and benefits be measured in the same units, usually dollars. A single intervention may be evaluated or multiple interventions with different outcomes may be compared with CBA. Net benefits or benefit-to-cost ratio are computed to determine the yield of an "investment" in a diagnostic, therapeutic, or screening intervention.

References

1. McGhan WF, Lewis NJ. Guidelines for pharmacoeconomic studies. Clin Ther 1992; 3:486-94.

2. McGhan W, Rowland C, Bootman JL. Cost-benefit and cost-effectiveness: methodology for evaluating clinical pharmacy service. Am J Hosp Pharm 1978;35:133-40.

3. Crystal R, Brewster A. Cost-benefit and cost-effectiveness analysis in the health field: an introduction. Inquiry 1966;3:3-13.

4. Kissick WL. Cost-benefit studies in health planning in the U.S.A. Health Economics 1969:39-44.

5. Klarman H. Application of cost/benefit analysis to health services and the special case of technological innovation. Int J Health Ser Res 1974;4:325-52.

6. Klarman H. Present status of cost-benefit analysis in the health field. Am J Public Health 1967;57:1948-58.

7. Smith W. Cost/effectiveness and cost/benefit for public health programs. Public Health Rep 1968;83:899-906.

8. Patrick KM, Woolley FR. A cost-benefit analysis of immunization for pneumococcal pneumonia. JAMA 1981;245:473-7.

9. Pigou AC. Socialism versus capitalism. London: Macmillan Press, 1947.

10. Peters GH. Cost/benefit analysis and public expenditures. Paper 8. London: Institute of Economic Affairs, 1968.

11. Osteryoung J. Capital budgeting: long-term asset selection. Columbus, OH: Grid, 1974.

12. Silvers JB, Praholed CK. Financial management of health institutions. New York: Spectrum Publications, 1974.

13. Van Horne JC. Financial management and policy. Englewood Cliffs, NJ: Prentice-Hall, 1974.

14. Klarman H. Application of cost-benefit analysis to health services technology. J Occup Med 1974:172-86.

15. Schulbert HC, Sheldon CA, Baker F. Program evaluation in the health field. New York: Behavioral Publications, 1969.

16. Prest AR, Turvey R. Cost-benefits analysis: a survey. Econ J 1965;75:683-735.

17. Rice DP. Measurement and application of illness costs. Public Health Rep 1969; 84:91-101.

18. Rice DP. Estimating the cost of illness. Health Economics Series. No. 6. Washington, DC: US Government Printing Office, 1966.

19. Drummond MF, Stoddart GL, Torrance GW. Methods for the economic evaluation of health care programmes. New York: Oxford University Press, 1987.

20. Rinehard K, Felsman F, and Moody L. Time loss and indirect economic cost caused by disease among Indian and Alaskan natives. Public Health Rep 1970;85:402.

21. Ridker RG. Economic cost of air pollution. New York: Praeger, 1967.

22. Mishan EJ. Evaluation of life and limb: a theoretical approach. In: Harberger A, ed. Benefit/cost analysis. Chicago: Aldine-Atherton, 1971:103-23.

23. Packer AH. Applying cost-effectiveness concepts to the community health system. Operations Res 1968;16:227-53.

24. Klarman H. Economics of health. New York: Columbia University Press, 1965.

25. Marglin SA. The social rate of discount at the optimal rate of investment. J Econ 1963;77:95-111.

26. Baumol WJ. On the discount rate for public projects. In: Haveman R, Margolia J, eds. Public expenditures and policy analysis. Chicago, IL: Markham, 1970:273-90.

27. Amadio J, Mueller J, Grey R. Benefit/cost ratio. Public Health Report, Illinois Department of Public Health, Southern Illinois University. Carbondale and Jackson County Health Department, 1976.

28. Joehnk M, McGrail GR, Degal NJ. Application of a benefit/cost model to family practice. National Technical Information Service. No. HRP-0007312. Washington, DC: Department of Health, Education and Welfare, 1975.

29. Cohn E. Public expenditures analysis. Lexington, MA: DC Heath, 1972.

30. Poretz DM, Woolard D, Eron LJ, et al. Outpatient use of ceftriaxone: a cost-benefit analysis. Am J Med 1984;10:77-83.

31. Shapiro M, Schoenbaum SC, Tager IB, Munoz A, Polk BF. Benefit-cost analysis of antimicrobial prophylaxis in abdominal and vaginal hysterectomy. JAMA 1983;249:1290-4.

32. Crane VS. Pharmacoeconomics: therapeutic and economic considerations in treating critically ill patients. DICP Ann Pharmacother 1990;24 (suppl):S24-7.

33. Eisenberg JM, Kitz DS. Savings from outpatient antibiotic therapy for osteomyelitis: economic analysis of a therapeutic strategy. JAMA 1986;255:1584-8.

34. Mishan EJ. Cost-benefit analysis. New York: Hold, Rinehart and Winston, 1976.

35. McGowan JE. Cost and benefit: a critical issue for hospital infection control Am J Infect Control 1982;10:100-8.

36. Bootman JL, McGhan WF. A perspective on the cost-benefit of drug therapy. Clin Res Pract Drug Reg Aff 1985;3:53-69.

37. Koplan JP, Preblud SR. A benefit-cost analysis of mumps vaccine. Am J Dis Child 1982;136:362-4.

38. Rosenfeldt FL, Lambert R, Burrows K, Stirling GR. Hospital costs and return to work after coronary bypass surgery. Med J Aust 1983;1:260-3.

39. Nevitt MC, Epstein WV, Masem M, Murray WR. Work disability before and after total hip arthroplasty: assessment of effectiveness in reducing disability. Arthritis Rheum 1984;27:410:21.

40. Finkler SA. The distinction between costs and charges. Ann Intern Med 1982; 96:102-9.

41. Foran RM, Brett JL, Wulf PH. Evaluating the cost impact of intravenous antibiotic dosing frequencies. DICP Ann Pharmacother 1991;25:546-52.

42. Jolicoeur LM, Jones-Crizzle AJ, Boyer JG. Guidelines for performing a pharmacoeconomic analysis. Am J Hosp Pharm 1992;49:1741-7.

43. Kunkel MJ, Iannini PB. Cefonicid in a once-daily regimen for treatment of osteomyelitis in an ambulatory setting. Rev Infect Dis 1984;6:S865-9.

44. Conafax DM, Gruber SA, Chan GLC, et al. The pharmaeconomics of renal transplantation: increased drug costs with decreased hospitalization costs. Pharmacotherapy 1990; 10:205-10.

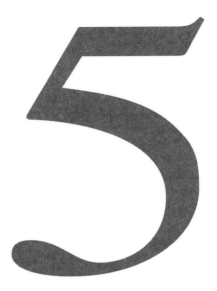

Cost-Effectiveness
Analysis

Elizabeth A. Chrischilles

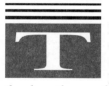he major objectives of this chapter are to: (1) define the concept and basic framework of cost-effectiveness analysis (CEA), (2) enumerate the steps involved in a proper CEA, and (3) illustrate these with examples from the drug therapy literature. Several concepts involved in CEA were developed in previous chapters (e.g., direct/indirect costs, sensitivity analysis, discounting), and will be discussed as they apply to CEA of drug therapy.

Cost-Effectiveness Analysis Defined

Like cost-benefit analysis (CBA), CEA is an approach used for identifying, measuring, and comparing the significant costs and consequences of alternative interventions. With respect to drug therapy, these alternative interventions may be two or more different drugs or classes of drugs. The goal may be to compare drug treatment with one or more types of nondrug treatment for a particular condition.

Unlike CBA, which values all effects of an intervention in monetary terms, CEA measures some effects in nonmonetary terms. For this reason, some believe that CEA is less comprehensive than CBA, since it excludes the valuation of life. However, although CBA includes the market value of life, it excludes the nonmarket value of life. CEA, on the other hand, includes both aspects implicitly but quantitatively in nonmonetary measures, such as life-years saved, disability-days avoided, quality-adjusted life-years gained, and episodes of nephrotoxicity avoided. It is because of this nonmonetary measurement of health outcome that it has often been said that

CEA cannot be used to compare interventions with different health outcomes. For example, if two drugs each have associated costs of $2,000, but one prevents 100 days of disability and the other saves one life, a traditional CEA can not be used to compare the two drugs because it does not provide a single metric along which to measure these very different outcomes.

THE BASIC FRAMEWORK AND VARIATIONS ON THE THEME

Beyond the general statements above, the definition of CEA becomes difficult because of its dynamic nature. Traditionally, CEA has quantified all costs of providing a service or treatment in monetary terms, while measuring consequences as nonmonetary health outcomes. The traditional CEA does not include the economic consequences of a particular service.[1-3] For example, a CEA might include reduced morbidity, such as avoided complications of therapy, but it would not include the economic consequence associated with those avoided complications (i.e., the avoided costs of diagnosing and treating complications). Methodologic developments during recent years have resulted in several variations of the basic CEA framework. Whereas the traditional design of CEA studies involved assessment of the costs of providing an intervention and some nonmonetary measure of health effects, modern examples of CEA taken from prominent medical journals have established a new standard for CEA.

In the modern CEA, aspects of CBA, cost-utility analysis, and CEA are combined to create a hybrid economic evaluation.[4-7] Such studies generally subtract cost savings induced by an intervention from the costs of the intervention itself (and add costs induced by the intervention) to arrive at a net cost. Nonmonetary consequences, such as mortality, disability, and effects on quality of life, are handled as they would be in traditional cost-effectiveness or cost-utility analyses. This allows the investigator to incorporate quality-of-life, nonmonetary health effects and economic consequences as well as costs of providing the intervention in a single economic evaluation. Such comprehensive evaluations have fallen under the rubric of CEA in most medical journals. The remainder of this chapter addresses this new, more comprehensive standard for CEA.

MISUSE OF THE TERM

Cost-consciousness in health care has resulted in widespread use of the term "cost-effective." Unfortunately, this has not been accompanied by a clear understanding of the term. Doubilet et al.[8] have summarized the misuse of the term in the medical literature. Studies that equate cost-effectiveness with cost savings and those that declare an intervention to be cost-effective based only on effectiveness data are equally erroneous. Either interpretation considers only half of the term.

RECOMMENDED USE OF THE TERM

Cost-effectiveness should be used to imply value for money. Table 1 illustrates very generally some possible combinations of net cost and net health benefits that might be discovered with a CEA of drug A versus drug B. If the net costs associated with drug A are lower than those with drug B and drug A also is associated with greater net health benefit (cell X_3), drug A is clearly more cost-effective than drug B. Cell X_2 also has an obvious interpretation: drug B is more cost-effective than drug A in this case. Cells X_1 and X_4 are more difficult to interpret. In cell X_1, drug A has greater net health benefit but is more costly than drug B; in cell X_4, drug A is associated with less net health benefit but is less costly than drug B. In either case, the question of whether the additional health benefit is worth the additional cost (or whether the decreased cost is worth the decreased health benefit) must be answered. For example, in a study of the cost-effectiveness of antimicrobial choices for nosocomial pneumonia, Weinstein et al.[9] estimated that ceftizoxime had a lower expected cost per patient but would result in the loss of an additional 0.44 years of life expectancy compared with the regimen of mezlocillin plus gentamicin. They estimated that the latter regimen would cost an additional $1,026 per year of life expectancy gained. In the era of high-cost, high-tech pharmaceuticals, enhanced effectiveness in the face of increased cost is a common occurrence. In the above case, the authors considered the increased effectiveness of the combined regimen to be worth the increased cost.

Principles of CEA

Warner and Luce[1] and Dao[2] have outlined the basic steps that apply to all CEA settings (Figure 1). Although they may seem obvious, failure to follow these steps has been detrimental to many analyses.[10]

Table 1. Costs and Effectiveness of Drug A Compared with Drug B

COSTS OF DRUG A	EFFECTIVENESS OF DRUG A	
	HIGHER THAN DRUG B	LOWER THAN DRUG B
Higher than drug B	X_1	X_2
Lower than drug B	X_3	X_4

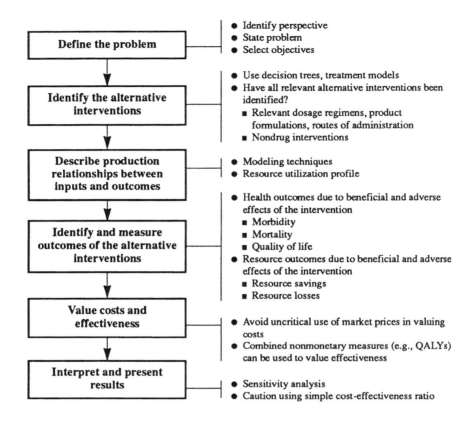

Figure 1. Basic steps of cost-effectiveness analysis. QALY = quality-adjusted life-year.

DEFINING THE PROBLEM

There are three steps to problem definition. A prerequisite for successful CEA is that the analyst understands the point of view or perspective from which the analysis is to be conducted. The next step is to state the basic problem being addressed. Third, specific objectives should be selected against which the alternative interventions are to be evaluated.

Perspective. Different decision-makers have legitimate differences in perspective that can affect what should be included in the analysis. A societal perspective (the aggregate of all society members, present and future) requires that all direct and indirect costs be addressed, as well as direct and indirect benefits and all intangible effects. Perspectives that are more narrow than that of society include those of the hospital, insurer, and patient.

Since these perspectives are narrower in scope, it is logical that they might not consider some costs and benefits important to society as a whole. Patients are concerned with costs only to the extent that they are responsible for payment. The insured individual pays only when there are deductibles, coinsurance, and limits on coverage. These are often only a small portion of the total costs. The patient, however, is extremely concerned with risks of productivity losses, morbidity, mortality, and quality of life. The hospital, on the other hand, is concerned only with costs prior to discharge and, as a result, effects on patient productivity and rehabilitation costs are typically not included for this perspective. From the perspective of the insurer, only those costs within the scope of coverage are relevant. As a result of including different cost and benefit components for each different viewpoint, conflicting decisions may arise from analyses conducted from differing perspectives.

Deciding which perspective to use is not always a straightforward task. The conventional view is to take the societal perspective, as the goals of CEA historically have been to determine what society should do with regard to resource allocation. However, this may not accurately reflect the primary concerns of a given patient, hospital, or insurer. A more narrow view is to accept that the proper perspective is that of the individual or organization for whom the analysis is being conducted. The latter approach is often too restrictive since, regardless of the point of view of the decision-maker for whom the analysis is being conducted, it is likely that they will need to know how others will assess the situation. Policy recommendations will have to be adopted, implemented, enforced, and perhaps withstand litigation by agencies, institutions, and individuals who have their own perspectives. One solution to the dilemma is to provide modules or subanalyses that reflect the perspectives of the various interested parties.[2] Luft[11] further expanded on this notion and suggested weighting the various subanalyses by the influence each group has in the decision-making process. This would allow the analyst to predict what would happen given the power distribution of interested parties. Regardless of the approach taken, the decision regarding the perspective (or perspectives) to be taken must be made prior to beginning the CEA.

Perception of the Problem. The real starting point of the analysis is in identifying the problem that needs to be solved. Traditional healthcare CEAs have started with a specific health problem (e.g., morbidity, disability, mortality) associated with a certain disease. Analysts are then motivated to identify and compare a wide variety of preventive and therapeutic modalities with respect to relative cost-effectiveness. More recently, a specific intervention strategy (e.g., a specific drug, surgical procedure, piece of equipment) has often served as the starting point. The problem to be solved is whether the intervention in question, say drug X, is cost-effective rather than to determine the most cost-effective alternative for reducing morbidity and/or mortality from a particular condition. CEAs of drug therapy have typically reflected this type of problem orientation.[6,12-15] Because the analyst begins with a given pharmaceutical intervention in mind, the drug(s) in question can be studied for single or multiple conditions.

Although both problem orientations are legitimate and can arrive at identical CEAs, the latter orientation carries a risk of "missing the forest for the trees."[1] For example, orientation toward comparative cost-effectiveness of cefaclor with amoxicillin for the treatment of acute otitis media might cause the analyst to overlook the fact that other drugs such as amoxicillin/clavulanate or trimethoprim/sulfamethoxazole are reasonable alternatives that should be investigated simultaneously. More generally, orientation toward comparative cost-effectiveness of drug X with other drugs in its class might cause the analyst to overlook the possibility that some other drug, no treatment, a nondrug treatment, or a preventive approach to the condition are reasonable alternatives that could be investigated simultaneously.

Thus, in conducting CEA of drug therapy, the analyst must always contemplate the implications of the problem orientation. If the problem is formulated in terms of a specific drug or drug class, consideration should be given to documentation in the medical literature of the acceptability of alternatives to the drug or drugs in question. It is quite proper to focus on drug–drug comparisons if the condition in question is known to require drug therapy. An example of the latter situation is illustrated by a CEA of alternative drug therapy approaches for long-term treatment of proximal venous thrombosis.[14]

Selection of Objectives. Specific objectives are next selected for comparing the effectiveness of alternative interventions. In other words, a decision must be made about how effectiveness will be evaluated. The previously established perspective of the analysis and problem statement will have laid the groundwork for this decision.

Selection of an appropriate, measurable objective (or objectives) is not always easy. Careful attention must be paid to the link between the health problem in question and the specific objective. Warner and Luce[1] have used the example of morbidity and mortality resulting from myocardial infarction (MI) to illustrate the importance of this phase of CEA. Clearly, both morbidity and mortality resulting from MI are important aspects of the health problem. Approaches to reducing the problem would vary depending on which of the two objectives the analyst selects: decreasing the mortality rate of those having an MI versus reducing the incidence of MIs. The first objective would suggest a variety of emergency treatment alternatives, whereas the latter suggests preventive approaches. The point is that selection of either objective does not allow consideration of intervention approaches suggested by the other. That is, preventive efforts would be expected to have little impact on mortality rates of those who did experience an MI and emergency treatment interventions would have little effect on the incidence of MIs.

In the above example, a dilemma exists. Whenever such a seeming incompatibility of possible objectives exists, the analyst has three choices: (1) to select one objective, thereby reducing the scope of the analysis; (2) to include both objectives, realizing the resulting analysis may be inconclusive because of the lack of a common unit of measure; or (3) to identify some other measurable objective that incorporates both concerns. In the case of MIs, a reasonable solution might be to select quality-adjusted life-years as an objective. Both preventive and treatment approaches are consistent with this measure.

An example of the difficulties involved in selecting objectives is fairly specific to drug formulary decisions. Gagnon and Osterhaus[16] have described in detail the aspects of CEA as they apply to formulary decision-making. In such situations, the pharmacy and therapeutics committee is typically considering addition, deletion, or restricted use of a particular drug. Thus, the problem orientation is intervention-based rather than health problem-based. Most drugs are used for more than one indication, and each indication may have different relevant health outcomes. Since a decision to add, delete, or restrict the use of a drug must consider all its potential uses, the pharmacy and therapeutics committee does not have the option of selecting a single measure from several seemingly incompatible measures. Either multiple objectives or some composite objective must be identified.

To ensure the appropriateness of the selected objectives, the analyst should be confident that the objective(s) chosen reflect the most important dimensions of the health problem(s) and are relevant to the alternative interventions that will be compared. Furthermore, a measure should be selected that is sensitive to the actual differences likely to be encountered between interventions. For example, if the percent of patients cured with alternative drug regimens is expected to be similar, but time to healing or symptom resolution or recurrence rates are expected to differ, an objective that reflects the latter measures should be selected.

IDENTIFYING THE ALTERNATIVES

The concept of cost-effectivenss is most meaningful when it is used in a relative manner. In other words, instead of addressing the cost-effectiveness of drug A alone, we examine the cost-effectiveness of drug A compared with that of drugs B and C. For example, if drug A is associated with costs of $10,000 for every life saved compared with no treatment, is it cost-effective? The answer will depend on the subjective value system of the decision-maker. On the other hand, if it can be said that drug A has lower net costs and equal or greater net health benefits than drug B, we can objectively say that drug A is the more cost-effective alternative. Of course, this comparison of alternative interventions does not ensure objectively interpretable results. For example, what if drug A is found both more costly and to have better net health benefit than its alternatives (e.g., cell X_1 in Table1)? In this case, the need for value judgment is apparent and the decision cannot be entirely objective. Note, however, that even in this latter case in which the decision is more subjective, the information about costs and effectiveness of the other alternatives will lead to a more informed decision than if only the costs and effectiveness of drug A had been considered.

A well-defined problem and concrete objectives provide boundaries on the variety of alternative means of attacking the problem. In general, the narrower the problem and objectives, the fewer relevant alternatives there will be. For example, if the problem is the consequences of ulcer disease, all alternatives must be directed at those consequences. If the objective is to increase healing rates of patients with active ulcers, preventive alternatives would be excluded.

In drug therapy CEAs, several types of interventions might be compared. In the simplest case, individual drugs may be compared with each other for a single condition. The drugs in question do not necessarily have to be from different drug classes, but they are usually different with respect to some relevant pharmacologic property. For example, Holloway et al.[13] compared the cost-effectiveness of gentamicin and tobramycin based on the premise that gentamicin has a greater nephrotoxic potential. Interventions being compared also may be from different classes of drugs (e.g., beta-blockers vs. thiazide diuretics for initial treatment of hypertension. When classes of drugs are compared, a single drug from each class is often selected as a representative for that class.

Interventions may be compared across multiple disease conditions, as is required for many formulary decisions.[16] For example, the histamine$_2$-blockers cimetidine, ranitidine, and famotidine might be compared for both treatment of existing ulcers and prophylaxis of recurrent ulcers. Depending on the scope of the problem and specific objectives being addressed, it may be necessary to include nondrug therapy (e.g., surgery) or even no therapy as alternative interventions. For example, in a CEA of isoniazid for the prevention of tuberculosis, the policy of avoiding drug therapy among other tuberculin reactors, who are at low risk for activation, was evaluated.[7]

Other types of alternative interventions seen in the drug CEA literature include the following: single drug therapy versus combination drug therapy (e.g., combined tetracycline and ampicillin vs. either drug alone for endocervical gonorrhea)[6]; drug therapy alone versus drug therapy plus other diagnostic or therapeutic modality[6,17,18]; inpatient versus outpatient drug therapy[19]; alternative formulations of the same drug (e.g., premixed admixtures vs. compounded doses)[20]; and different dosage regimens of the same drug.[14] With all of these alternatives, however, it should be recognized that during the course of treatment these interventions are not mutually exclusive. For example, a patient with acute otitis media may fail to improve after receiving the initial antibiotic selected (e.g., amoxicillin), and will require another antibiotic (e.g., cefaclor).

The most common pitfall in identifying alternatives arises when the analyst jumps directly to this stage of the analysis without having carefully defined the problem and objectives of the study. Under such circumstances, it is easy to identify the wrong alternatives. For example, an analyst might be interested at the outset in showing that a single dose of a new antibiotic is more cost-effective than multiple doses of an older antibiotic in reducing the rate of postsurgical infection. However, if the analyst had stepped back and really considered the problem objectively, additional relevant alternatives might be identified (e.g., a single dose of the older, and less expensive, drug).

DESCRIBING THE PRODUCTION RELATIONSHIPS

Defining the health problem, objective(s), and alternatives establishes the conceptual framework of a CEA. The next step in the analysis—describing the relationship between resource inputs, resource outcomes, and health outcomes—expands upon this framework. Describing the production relationship ultimately results in identification and measurement of resource use required to provide each intervention. It also provides the technical framework for the quantitative assessment and comparison of net costs with net effectiveness. There are several methods for characterizing these production relationships. All approaches involve development of a model that specifies how inputs are combined and how much output a given grouping of inputs will produce. An important aspect of these models is the assessment of marginal inputs and outputs. In brief, the tendency of many analysts is to rely on average inputs needed to produce a unit of output. There are several problems with this approach, among which is the overestimation of opportunity costs of an intervention by inclusion of its associated fixed inputs. The appropriate approach is to address the question: For each additional unit of input, how much additional output will be gained? This concept of marginal analysis is discussed in detail in Chapter 3.

The model may be as simple as a flow chart, identifying all inputs and their quantities at the points where they enter the production process or it may be a more complicated technique. Modeling techniques that can be used include Monte Carlo and Markov Chain models,[21] decision tree analysis (see Chapter 8), regression equations,[5] and life-table methods.[5]

Decision tree analysis has been the most commonly used modeling technique in drug therapy CEAs.[6,9,12,13,17]

IDENTIFYING AND MEASURING COSTS OF INTERVENTIONS

A resource utilization profile is developed that parallels the structure of a decision tree, but which delineates all health resources involved in each step of the decision tree. The amounts of resources used will later be converted to dollar amounts to estimate the costs of the intervention.

Production costs are costs associated with providing an intervention and are determined by first itemizing the resources used to actually provide the intervention. For each event represented in the corresponding decision tree, health resource use such as services by physicians and other health professionals, hospital services, diagnostic tests, and drug therapy must be identified. This information must be specific, detailing the exact quantities and types of resources needed. For services by professionals, the specific services and the type of professional providing them must be specified. Is the service provided by a physician, nurse, or pharmacist? Even more specifically, how specialized are these professionals? Is the nurse an LPN, RN, or nurse practitioner? One particular service provided by nurses that is especially relevant to drug therapy CEAs is drug administration. For pharmacists, time involved in traditional dispensing services (e.g., compounding, supervision of technicians) as well as pharmacists' cognitive services (e.g., pharmacokinetic monitoring) that are a part of the particular intervention should be itemized. The number of times each service is provided by each of these professionals and the time required per episode also is required. For hospital services, the type of unit on which the services are provided should be specified (e.g., intensive care unit, burn unit, emergency room). Furthermore, the number of days or hours spent in each type of unit is needed. Specific diagnostic tests and the number of times each is used must be identified. For drug therapy, the analyst must specify the specific drugs, their dose, dosing interval, duration of therapy, and route of administration.

The health resources discussed so far have all been direct production costs. Indirect production costs—resources used indirectly in the production process—also may be included, depending on the perspective of the analysis. An example of the latter is the amount of patient time required to participate in the intervention.

IDENTIFYING AND MEASURING OUTCOMES OF EACH INTERVENTION

There are two types of outcomes that result from an intervention: health outcomes and resource or economic outcomes. Health outcomes refer to changes in morbidity, mortality, and quality of life, whereas resource outcomes refer to induced resource savings on avoided costs of illness and induced resource losses due to adverse effects of the intervention. Resource outcomes (induced savings and losses) are distinguished from resource use (production costs) in that the latter are limited to resources used to produce the identified outcomes.

Analytically, measurement of health and resource outcomes is often performed indirectly by comparing them with a no-therapy alternative. In other words, differences in rates or magnitude of outcomes would first be measured between each intervention and no therapy. Then, the different interventions would be compared in terms of their relative savings and losses against the no-therapy alternative. For example, if drug A and drug B are both used to prevent coronary disease, the health and resource outcomes with drug A would be compared with no therapy at all and likewise for drug B. One reason for this practice is that this is the way that data are typically available (i.e., many drug efficacy studies compare a drug with placebo).

IDENTIFYING AND MEASURING HEALTH OUTCOMES

If the problem, objectives, and alternative interventions have been carefully developed, identification of relevant health outcomes will have been already accomplished. In fact, these must be identified to complete the decision trees linking inputs to outcomes. Health outcomes may occur as a result of both the beneficial and adverse effects of an intervention. Probabilities of the various events that may result from an intervention (e.g., cure, death, adverse reactions) will have been incorporated into these decision trees in the course of defining the production relationship. These probabilities are instrumental in measuring health outcomes.

Sources of Data About Health Outcomes. The actual values for the probabilities in the various branches of the decision tree can be obtained from a variety of sources. Primary data collection by the analyst is one source of these probabilities. The clinical literature and expert opinion are other sources. Estimates of required probabilities are often based on results of multiple studies of a similar topic. To derive a single probability estimate from these multiple sources, meta-analysis can be used. Cochran's[22] method of meta-analysis, which pools results by assigning weights to different studies to reflect their sample sizes and the similarity of their results, was used by Weinstein et al.[9] to estimate aminoglycoside toxicity rates. They conducted a search of the English-language journals published since 1969; data from the papers that met the minimum criteria of study design were combined using meta-analysis.

Critical Evaluation of Published Literature. Careful and discriminatory evaluation of published studies are essential to avoiding misinterpretation of study results. Polk and Hepler[23] reviewed the problems with design and statistical evaluation of clinical trials and made recommendations for evaluating study outcomes. A common conclusion of a randomized trial is that there is no significant difference between the two clinical regimens being compared. In fact, many drug therapy CEAs are based on such studies. Thus, an analyst will assume equal health effectiveness of two interventions and proceed to conduct a comparative cost analysis, concluding that the intervention with the lowest cost is, therefore, most cost-effective.

When a study reports that two therapies are equivalent, there are actually three possible reasons why "no significant difference" was reached.[23] First, the conclusion may be correct. This may be a proper interpretation if the sample size was sufficient and if the differences in outcome are clinically unimportant. However, a conclusion of equivalence may be reached even if there is a real difference between the two regimens. Such a difference may not be detected in a study for two reasons: (1) the study lacked sufficient power to detect clinically important differences (type II error), or (2) there are confounding factors or a flawed study design obscuring the difference. The likelihood of a type II error is higher when the sample size is small and differences are described between groups that could be clinically important. When two regimens are compared and both are expected to be highly effective, it is especially difficult to demonstrate that one regimen is better than the other. This is because the difference between the two, even if clinically meaningful, is likely to be small and the sample size required to achieve statistical significance may be quite large. Tables are available for estimating the probability that a clinically important difference was missed in a study because of insufficient sample size.[24]

Similarly, when a study reports that one regimen is significantly superior to another, there are three possible explanations for the finding. First, the author's conclusion may be correct. This is most likely when the observed differences are clinically important. However, there may be no real difference between regimens despite the detection of a "significant difference" (type I error). There are two reasons this can happen: (1) the difference was due to a type I error (i.e., the probability of finding a difference when there is actually no difference); or (2) confounding factors or poor study design produced an artificial difference. The best protection against committing a type I error is to seek independent confirmation of the finding through multiple studies. Thus, a conclusion of unequivalent effects in a single study should be considered cautiously, even if the study is well designed, until independent confirmation can be made from results of other studies. In summary, when conducting a CEA, the analyst must be as cautious in accepting the conclusion of differences between regimens as in accepting the conclusion of no difference. Either error can have tremendous impact on the resulting analysis.

The Randomized Controlled Trial: Efficacy versus Effectiveness. Most drug studies are randomized controlled trials (RCTs). Since RCTs occur under ideal conditions, the probabilities (e.g., of drug efficacy) obtained from them may not be representative of what can be expected when drugs are used under less than ideal conditions (the "real world"). Thus, it is desirable to distinguish between the concepts of efficacy (how well the drug works under ideal conditions) and effectiveness (how well it works under conditions of average use). Unfortunately, whereas estimates of drug efficacy are relatively easy to come by, estimates of effectiveness are not. However, results from RCTs regarding drug efficacy can be used and adjustments made to reflect expected conditions of actual use such as inaccuracies in diagnosis and prescriber and patient noncompliance with recommended regimens. These adjustments are often subjective in nature, as few data are available for most drugs regarding the relationship between degree of compliance and drug effect. The Lipid Research Clinics–Coronary Primary Prevention Trial (LRC–CPPT)[25] is a rare example of a study that was able to quantify the relationship between patient compliance and drug effect. A 1987 CEA of antihyperlipemic therapy in the prevention of coronary heart disease was able to use this observed relationship to estimate the expected degree of compliance and the resulting reduction in drug efficacy.[5]

Other Sources of Health Outcome Data. Observational studies provide information on the strength of associations between certain factors (e.g., an intervention, patient age, patient smoking history) and occurrence of disease or disease outcome. These studies may be either retrospective or prospective, but they usually lack the random allocation of subjects seen in RCTs. An advantage is that they may more accurately reflect conditions of actual drug use outside the ideal conditions of the RCT. Information required to estimate the decision-tree probabilities is sometimes not available in the medical literature. Other times, the data that are available are scant and their reliability questionable. Under such circumstances, probabilities may be arrived at by obtaining the judgments of panels of physicians based on their clinical experience.

Until recently, health outcomes have typically been expressed in terms of morbidity and mortality rates associated with a disease or intervention. However, much emphasis has been placed in recent years on improving the quality of life.[26] Because many current interventions, especially drug regimens, are aimed at alleviating disease conditions or relieving symptoms rather than at saving lives, the ability to measure quality of life is important. Given that this is a relatively new area of research, much controversy exists regarding the best methods for measuring quality-of-life effects, but the consensus is that performing this research is definitely feasible and highly desirable.[26] Even if the analyst chooses not to measure quality of life as a health outcome, the subject should at least be dealt with descriptively in the presentation of the results.

IDENTIFYING AND MEASURING RESOURCE OUTCOMES

As with health outcomes, resource outcomes derive both from the beneficial and the adverse effects of an intervention. Resource outcomes are the induced losses and savings associated with an intervention. Beneficial effects result in resource savings (induced savings), whereas adverse effects result in resource losses (induced losses). Both resource savings and losses can be either direct or indirect effects of the intervention in question.

Direct health resource savings refer to savings on direct medical costs of illness that would occur if the intervention were not present. Direct medical costs of illness have been defined and illustrated in Chapter 3. For example, in a CEA of antihyperlipemic therapy in the prevention of coronary heart disease,[5] the direct health resource savings associated with the intervention (antihyperlipemic therapy) would be the expected savings in lifetime medical care costs due to avoided coronary heart disease.

Direct health resource losses are direct medical costs associated with the adverse effects of an intervention. These can include the costs of diagnosing and treating adverse effects. In the above example, the direct health resource losses associated with antihyperlipemic therapy would be the expected cost of treating medication-related adverse effects over the course of therapy.

Indirect resource savings and losses (savings and losses on indirect costs of illness) can also be included in a CEA, depending on the perspective of the analysis. Illness has an impact on the time people work and their productivity while working, both of which affect overall work output. Indirect resource outcomes thus occur in the form of work productivity savings (e.g., those resulting from avoided illness) and losses (e.g., those resulting from adverse effects). Savings and losses in time spent by patients and families receiving medical care are examples of indirect resource outcomes that might be included in a CEA. Indirect savings and losses have not typically been included in healthcare CEAs.

The rationale for omission of indirect effects from CEAs of drug therapy has been that it is more consistent to include only the components of dollar costs that add to or subtract from the resources available for health care, since these net costs are being compared with net health effectiveness.[4] However, these time and productivity losses and gains may have substantial financial consequences for individuals and society. It would certainly be possible to estimate all resource savings and costs, including the value of time and productivity losses and gains. In such a case, the nonmonetary effectiveness measure could be judged against a more comprehensive assessment of economic impacts.

One of the most controversial aspects of CEA is the issue of whether to include healthcare costs occurring in the added years of life. Some believe that these costs, which include the costs of treating diseases that would not have occurred if the patient had not lived longer as a result of the original intervention, should be incorporated.[4,5] Others believe that these costs should not be included, since this overestimates the costs associated with life-saving interventions.[1,2] Furthermore, it seems inconsistent to include consumption of healthcare resources in added years without including productivity and other types of consumption that also come with prolonged life.[1,2]

VALUING ECONOMIC AND HEALTH VARIABLES

Valuation of Economic Variables. The valuation of economic variables entails conversion of production resource use, induced savings, and induced losses (measured in quantities of resources) into dollar values. This process has been discussed in detail in Chapter 3. One important point will be reiterated here, however. That is, uncritical use of market prices should be avoided because there are times (e.g., use of hospital charges to reflect cost of hospital care) when they may not reflect the true opportunity costs of resources. It should be mentioned, however, that although adjustment of market prices to represent true opportunity cost is important from a societal perspective, charges may be more relevant to analyses from an insurer's perspective.

Valuation of Health Variables. With CEA, the effectiveness of an intervention is not valued in monetary units. Although health status is multidimensional, we are often concerned with a single health measure and the most efficient means of reaching it. For example, which of two drugs will produce the greatest number of cures per dollar spent? In this case, the number of cures can serve as the single measure of health effectiveness. Similarly, a single measure for mortality could be the number of lives saved (or lost) by each intervention.

Another approach to measuring the health effectiveness of interventions is through the use of multiple health effectiveness measures. For example, rather than combine the beneficial and negative health effects of an intervention in a single nonmonetary unit of measure, each effect can be presented separately, often using different units of measure. For example, in a CEA of a topical versus a systemic agent for the treatment of papulopustular acne, the systemic agent had greater benefit (fewer weeks of morbidity from acne) and lower dollar cost; however, it was also associated with nearly double the risk of adverse effects from treatment.[6]

The approaches just described avoid valuation of effectiveness altogether and simply provide rates of various health outcomes for each intervention (e.g., mortality rates, cure rates, rates of adverse reactions). However, when there is more than one relevant health effect, it may be desirable to use some nonmonetary valuation method to provide a single unit of measure. One way of aggregating different health events into a common measure is to determine the number of years of life saved and/or lost due to an intervention's multiple health effects. For example, in a study of the cost-effectivenss of antimicrobial choices for nosocomial pneumonia, Weinstein et al.[9] combined each regimen's expected effects on mortality from infection with its expected effects on mortality from drug toxicity. These were combined to form the total expected loss in life expectancy for each regimen. The regimen with the lowest expected loss in life expectancy thus exhibited the highest net effectiveness. When interventions affect both quality and length of life, the two can be incorporated into a single unit of measure by calculating quality-adjusted life-years remaining.[27]

Discounting Costs and Effectiveness. Even if all economic variables, present and future, are adjusted for inflation, it is still necessary to discount future costs. The reasons are that a dollar not spent now can be invested to yield a larger number of dollars in the future and that society generally prefers the certainty of money in hand versus the uncertainty of having that money in the future.[3] The need to discount economic variables is unquestioned—only the choice of a discount rate is somewhat controversial. This and relevant issues have been discussed in Chapter 4.

Although the need to discount economic variables is accepted, controversy remains regarding the need to discount nonmonetary health outcomes. Some researchers advocate discounting effectiveness because people generally prefer to have additional life years sooner rather than later. These proponents further state that a sufficient reason to discount effectiveness is that it is being valued relative to discounted costs.[4] Those that disagree state that there is no trade-off between having additional life years sooner rather than later because you cannot have them later if you do not have them sooner.[1]

INTERPRETATION AND PRESENTATION OF RESULTS

In CEA, the economic impact of an intervention is summarized as a net cost. Net costs are calculated by aggregating the production costs (associated with delivering the intervention) and the economic outcomes (induced resource losses and savings) of an intervention. For example, in a study of an osteoporosis therapy, the costs of avoided fractures would be subtracted from the costs of the therapy to arrive at net cost. Negative net cost values mean that savings from avoided costs of illness outweigh the costs of the intervention itself. The manner in which results are displayed must be given serious consideration. The temptation is to rely solely on the cost-effectiveness ratio as an index of the relative merit of the alternative interventions. Using this ratio as a criterion, the most cost-effective intervention would be the one with the lowest net cost per unit of effectiveness.

Whenever one or more alternative intervention both costs more and is more effective, the simple cost-effectiveness ratio can be misleading. Under such circumstances, greater insight would be provided by analyzing incremental cost-effectiveness ratios: the additional cost of an alternative relative to its additional effectiveness.

SENSITIVITY ANALYSIS

Because many of the estimates used in CEA are uncertain, there is a strong need to test the sensitivity of the results to changes in these estimates. If the results of the analysis change little when these estimates are varied, confidence in the results is increased. On the other hand, if the results change substantially, then the analyst should be more concerned about the uncertainty of the particular estimate. Common sources of uncertainty are efficacy rates (especially comparative efficacy of the alternative interventions), adverse reaction rates, event rates in untreated individuals, estimates of cost components, and the selected discount rate. A useful approach to sensitivity analysis is the establishment of confidence intervals around the various estimates and then allowing the estimates to take on the upper and lower bounds of the interval. This is especially useful when the results of multiple studies provide varying estimates, as these multiple estimates can aid in establishing reasonable upper and lower bounds.

Extreme caution in interpretation and, ultimately, presentation of the results of the CEA is important. Readers of CEAs will rely heavily on the analyst's interpretation, since the reader of a CEA usually is privy only to the presented summary of the analysis. The presentation of results should clearly identify the critical uncertainties of the analysis along with discussion of the likely impact of these uncertainties on the results of the analysis. Furthermore, any relevant considerations that have not been addressed in the analysis should be discussed. For example, if health outcomes such as changes in quality of life were identified but not addressed quantitatively, these should be discussed along with their likely impact on the analysis.

Applications of CEA

The application of CEA techniques will be illustrated with the following three case studies. Each is derived from an actual CEA publication in the clinical literature. The accompanying critical appraisals of each study are intended to emphasize important CEA issues and not criticize the studies themselves. In fact, all three studies were selected because of their overall high quality.

CASE STUDY 1: ANTIBIOTIC PROPHYLAXIS AFTER CESAREAN SECTION

The cost-effectiveness of cefonicid sodium versus cefoxitin sodium for the prevention of postoperative infections after nonelective cesarean section was studied.[28] Using a double-blind, randomized, controlled trial design, 60 women received cefonicid 1 g iv at cord clamping followed by two intravenous placebo doses; another 60 women received cefoxitin 2 g iv at cord clamping followed by two similar doses at six-hour intervals. The outcomes measured were febrile morbidity (defined as an oral temperature of 38° C or greater occurring twice, at least six hours apart, within the first 10 postpartum days, excluding the first 24 hours) and occurrence of documented infections. Three types of infections were considered: endometritis, wound infection, and urinary tract infection. No significant differences in patient demographic characteristics or in risk factors for postoperative infection were found between the two groups. No significant differences were found between groups in occurrences of febrile morbidity or rates of documented infections. Adverse reactions occurred in only two patients. The only costs measured were drug acquisition costs. The difference between the acquisition cost for three doses of cefoxitin and one dose of cefonicid for 838 cesarean sections per year was estimated to be $29,975. The authors concluded that, in the dosage regimens used, cefonicid is more cost-effective than cefoxitin for preventing infection after delivery by cesarean section.

Critique. The implied perspective of the anlysis is that of the hospital. The authors perceived that the problem to be addressed was whether single-dose therapy would be more cost-effective than multiple-dose therapy. The objective of the study was clear: to prevent postoperative infections.

The authors' single- versus multiple-dose orientation when approaching the problem may have caused them to fail to identify relevant alternatives for analysis. If the goal was to determine the most cost-effective approach to antibiotic prophylaxis after cesarean section, other possible regimens might have been found even better if studied. Other alternatives that might have been included would be an older (therefore, less expensive) accepted drug in a multiple-dose regimen, single-dose cefoxitin, or any of a group of other antibiotics that are used in this therapeutic situation.

The only production cost identified and measured was drug acquisition cost. Although the authors identified nursing and pharmacy time as relevant concerns, neither was measured and included as production costs. Identification and measurement of most health outcomes was excellent. Because few adverse reactions were identified, they were assumed to occur equally between groups and were not included in the CEA. Similarly, because the two regimens appeared to be equal in efficacy and adverse effects, it was assumed that no resource savings or resource losses would be induced for either regimen. The major problem with these assumptions of equal efficacy and adverse effects is that, although none of the differences between the two groups were significant, the power of the study to detect a clinically meaningful halving of the infection rate was only 35%. To achieve 90% power, roughly 250 subjects per group would be required. If, in fact, differences did exist between groups in efficacy and/or adverse effects, the difference between groups in associated resource savings and losses could no longer be assumed to be zero.

The authors chose to present multiple effectiveness measures rather than attempt to use a combined measure. Neither costs nor effectiveness was discounted. This was probably appropriate as this was an acute situation in which neither costs nor benefits are likely to occur over a long period of time following therapy.

The uncertainty of various assumptions made in the analysis was not addressed. Assumptions that could have been subjected to sensitivity analysis were the assumptions of equal efficacy and adverse effects, which could be criticized because of low study power. In presenting their results, the authors did mention the possibility of a type II error; however, they did not discuss the implications of this for their analysis. One might justify the assumption of equal efficacy by saying that if a real difference in efficacy existed, it is likely to be in favor of cefonicid. In that case, the study results would not be changed; rather, the relative efficacy of cefonicid and, hence, associated resource savings would have been underestimated under this study's assumptions. This may be a reasonable argument since, although not statistically significant, the rates of all types of infectious morbidity were lower in the cefonicid group. The same argument cannot be made for adverse effects because the data are much too scarce.

A similar argument could be used for including only drug acquisition costs as production costs. Since the cefoxitin regimen requires multiple doses, the associated compounding and administration costs would be higher for that regimen. Thus, the study actually underestimates the production costs associated with cefoxitin, and inclusion of these other components would only increase the relative cost-effectiveness of the cefonicid regimen. The authors did not discuss these issues, however.

The authors concluded that, because efficacy and toxicity were demonstrated to be equivalent, the decision to select one antibiotic over the other should be based on cost. As cefonicid was the least costly in this study, it was therefore considered most cost-effective. These are valid conclusions but, because they rely on the assumptions of equal efficacy and toxicity, the potential effects of violating these assumptions should have been discussed.

CASE STUDY 2: TOPICAL VERSUS SYSTEMIC ACNE TREATMENT

CEA was used to compare two strategies for clearing papulopustular acne: topical therapy alone as initial therapy or initial treatment with a combination of systemic antibiotics and topical agents.[12] Each strategy was displayed in the form of a decision tree. Although the topical agent strategy initiates therapy with topical agents only, the decision tree allowed for the therapy to be switched to a systemic agent in patients in whom therapy with topical agents failed. As is common in CEA studies, no actual patients were involved in the study. Rather, two sources of data were used to determine the decision-tree probabilities: the literature and a survey of dermatologists (the latter was used to obtain probability estimates when data were not available in the literature). Costs were estimated using charges for physician visits plus drug costs necessary to achieve clearing of the acne. The outcomes assessed were weeks of morbidity from acne until clearing (or failure) and episodes of adverse effects. Clearing was defined as a decrease of at least 50% in lesion count or a good to excellent response based on clinical assessment.

The systemic agent strategy resulted in six fewer weeks of morbidity from acne per patient, lower costs of care (about $20 per patient), and twice the number of adverse effects as the topical agent strategy. When sensitivity analysis was conducted, the magnitude of these differences changed but the direction of the differences did not. The choice of topical therapy in a population of patients was estimated to cost an additional $764 to avoid one additional episode of adverse effects (most commonly gastrointestinal upset and vaginitis). Choice of the topical therapy also would cost an additional 4.6 years of morbidity (since topical therapy is less efficacious in achieving clearing) to avert one additional episode of adverse effects. The authors judged that neither price would be worth paying to reduce the risk of adverse effects and concluded that initial treatment with combined systemic antibiotics and topical agents was most cost-effective. The authors suggest that patients with an increased risk of vaginitis or gastrointestinal effects, however, might be willing to accept a longer period of morbidity from acne to avoid the development of an adverse effect.[12]

Critique. The implied perspective of the analysis is that of the patient and of the physician as patient advocate. The authors perceived the problem as a clinical dilemma: they observed that the clinical literature advocates initial treatment with topical therapy alone whereas practicing dermatologists frequently prescribe systemic agents as part of a patient's initial treatment regimen. Realizing that the use of systemic agents is associated with adverse effects that may add dollar costs, but also may save costs by speeding resolution and reducing the need for return visits, their objectives were clear: to measure time to clearing, episodes of adverse effects, and associated resource savings and losses. The authors' orientation toward deciding which of two interventions should be preferred may have lead them to omit another relevant regimen: systemic antibiotics alone. Such a strategy would have lower drug costs than the combined therapy and, if efficacy was not much less, the number of physician visits might be similar to that of the combined regimen.

The authors used the techniques of decision analysis to define the production relationship between production costs and health (and associated resource) outcomes. They appear to have included relevant direct production costs (medication costs and physician visits). However, indirect production costs were not included. Since the perspective of the analysis was that of the patient, it would have been reasonable to include the indirect costs of patient and family time involved in the treatment process. The specific dollar costs associated with each cost component were not itemized. This would have been helpful since, without this information, the reader is unable to evaluate the appropriateness of the estimated number of physician visits needed for follow-up and dollar values assigned to physician visits.

Relevant health and direct resource outcomes were identified and measured appropriately. Because the topical agent strategy allowed for adding systemic antibiotics for patients whose acne failed to improve, there was no difference between strategies in the number of patients whose acne was cleared. Thus, since there was no difference in this health outcome, there was no associated induced resource savings for either intervention. However, the difference in rates of clearing was reflected within the production relationship and was associated with substantially lower production costs for the systemic strategy. Because the strategies had different rates of adverse reactions, there was an associated induced resource loss resulting from treatment of adverse effects (medication costs and physician visits). Indirect resource outcomes were not included. Given that the implied perspective of the study was that of the patient, it would have been reasonable to include the indirect resource losses of patient and family time required for treatment of adverse effects.

Two effectiveness measures were used: weeks of morbidity from acne and episodes of adverse effects per 1000 patients. Estimates of efficacy, adverse effect rates, and medication costs were displayed along with the ranges used in the sensitivity analysis. As with case study 1, neither costs nor effectiveness were discounted; this was probably appropriate given the acute nature of the clinical question. One- and two-variable sensitivity analyses were conducted for all relevant variables. The presentation of results included a detailed discussion of the sensitivity analysis and implications for the study's conclusions. The authors acknowledged that their analysis was only designed to consider the relative costs and effectiveness up to the time a patient's condition clears or fails to clear. They recognized that acne is a chronic condition that requires maintenance therapy to keep a patient free of acne following clearing, but cost-effectiveness of alternative approaches of maintenance therapy was not within the scope of the study.

CASE STUDY 3: ANTIHYPERLIPEMIC THERAPY AND CORONARY HEART DISEASE

Using cholestyramine as a model, the cost-effectiveness of antihyperlipemic therapy in the primary prevention of coronary heart disease in men with increased concentrations of total plasma cholesterol (>6.85 mmol/L [>265 mg/dL]) was evaluated.[5] The perspective adopted was that of society as a whole. All data were obtained from the literature. The ratio of net change in medical care costs to the net increase in life expectancy was calculated:

$$C \div E = (dCRx + dCSE - dCMorb + dCRxdLE) \div dLE$$

where dCRx indicates the expected lifetime cost of drug therapy (based on a national survey of retail pharmacy prices for bulk cholestyramine); dCSE, the expected cost of treating medication-related adverse effects over the course of therapy; dCMorb, the expected savings in lifetime medical care costs as a result of a decreased incidence of cardiovascular disease; dCRxdLE, the expected cost of treating noncardiac diseases during the years of additional life conferred by treatment; and dLE, the increase in life expectancy that results from adherence to a specified regimen of drug therapy. All future costs and changes in life expectancy were discounted at a rate of 5%. Baseline estimates of cost-effectiveness were calculated assuming a dosage of 16 g/d, which was the mean daily intake in the LRC–CPPT.[24] These results also were used to determine the expected relationship between drug dose and decline in cholesterol concentration.

A multivariate logistic function from the 16-year follow-up of Framingham Heart Study[29] participants was used to estimate future annual probabilities of coronary heart disease for patients with given risk factors, including cholesterol concentration and age. Future coronary risk was estimated for various age groups. To estimate the reduction in coronary risk resulting from treatment, the expected reductions in cholesterol concentration from various initial concentrations were first calculated using LRC–CPPT data. The Framingham Heart Study logistic function then was used to estimate, for the different combinations of pre- and posttreatment concentrations, the maximum possible reduction in risk. The authors then assumed that patients would not benefit from treatment during the first two years—corresponding to the LRC–CPPT experience—but they would realize maximum possible benefit in succeeding years. These reductions in risk then were used to calculate changes in life expectancy and lifetime medical care costs as a result of therapy (dLE, dCMorb, and dCRxdLE). Cost-effectiveness was evaluated for varying lengths of therapy and for subgroups of patients defined by specific constellations of concomitant risk factors. Sensitivity analysis was conducted for several assumptions and parameter estimates.[5]

Cost-effectiveness of lifelong therapy varied from $56,100 to over $1 million per year of life saved, depending on age at initiation of therapy and pretreatment cholesterol concentrations. Costs per life-year gained were lower for younger patients and for those with higher pretreatment concentrations of cholesterol. Less-than-lifelong therapy was generally more cost-effective than lifelong therapy. The exception to this was that therapy lasting only a few years was less cost-effective than lifelong therapy, reflecting the assumed absence of benefit during the first two years of treatment. Cost-effectiveness varied according to concomitant risk factors, with cost per life-year gained declining as the number of coronary risk factors increased.[5]

Critique. The societal perspective was clearly stated. The authors' problem orientation was toward weighing the economic cost of antihyperlipemic therapy against its clinical benefit. The objectives were to reduce the number of life-years lost as a result of coronary heart disease.[5]

The perspective and objectives of the analysis were consistent with evaluation of a wide variety of alternative approaches to prevent or treat coronary heart disease. The authors evaluated only one of these. Other interventions to which cholesterol lowering might be compared are antihypertensive therapy, coronary bypass surgery, and beta-blockade in patients who have had an MI.[30] Thus, this study is useful from the standpoint of quantifying the expected costs and increased life expectancy resulting from cholesterol lowering and for assessing how the balance of costs and life-years saved varies according to duration of treatment and concomitant risk factors. It can only be used indirectly (through comparison with other cost-effectiveness studies) to assess the relative cost-effectiveness of cholesterol lowering compared with alternative interventions.

The production relationship was modeled using the dose–response relationship observed in the LRC–CPPT trial and a multivariate logistic function calibrated to the Framingham Heart Study. Direct resource use (dCRx) was appropriately evaluated using estimated retail price and expected mean daily drug intake. Indirect resource costs were not included, although their inclusion would have been consistent with the societal perspective.

The health outcomes identified and measured were: (1) coronary heart disease risk (measured as life expectancy), and (2) occurrence of gastrointestinal adverse effects. Associated direct resource outcomes were induced savings on expected lifetime medical care costs as a result of decreased incidence of cardiovascular disease (dCMorb), induced losses resulting from the treatment of adverse effects (dCSE), and treating noncardiac diseases that occur in added years of life (dCRxLE). Although controversial, it can be argued that inclusion of these costs occurring in added years of life overestimates the induced costs associated with antihyperlipemic therapy. Indirect resource savings and losses were not included. Although occurrence of adverse effects was measured, this information was used only in determining the induced resource losses that resulted from the treatment of adverse effects. The occurrence of adverse effects was not included in the measure of net health effectiveness, despite its likely effect on quality of life. Effectiveness was measured as the increase in life expectancy that results from antihyperlipemic therapy. Both costs and effectiveness were appropriately discounted since both costs and changes in life expectancy were projected years into the future.

The interpretation and presentation of results were extensive. Incremental cost-effectiveness of continuing treatment each additional five years was presented, expressed as the ratio of the increase in discounted cost of therapy divided by the resulting increase in life-years saved due to these additional years of treatment. Extensive discussion of the results of sensitivity analysis and their likely impact on the results of the analysis was provided. Finally, a complete presentation of the methodologic limitations of the study was included, with corresponding interpretation of their likely effects on the study results.

Summary

CEA is a means of identifying, measuring, and comparing the net costs and net health benefit of alternative healthcare practices. Net costs are calculated as production costs plus induced resource losses minus induced resource savings. Production costs are the costs of resources used to actually provide an intervention. Induced resource losses are the resources consumed in tests and treatments undertaken as a consequence of the initial intervention (e.g., to diagnose and treat adverse drug effects). Induced resource savings are resource expenditures that are averted as a consequence of improved health. Net health benefit includes the beneficial and adverse effects of an intervention and is measured using a nonmonetary approach. Single, combined, or multiple nonmonetary measures of health effects can be used.

Cost-effectiveness is used to imply value for money. If one drug costs less and is more effective than another, it is clearly the most cost-effective of the two. However, when one drug both costs more and is more effective than another, the decision of relative cost-effectiveness depends on whether the decision-maker believes the extra effectiveness is worth the extra costs.

In conducting a CEA, the perspective of the analysis, a well-defined problem statement, and concrete objectives provide boundaries on the variety of alternative interventions. Decision trees or other modeling techniques are important for identifying alternative interventions and for describing the production relationship between resource inputs and resource and health outcomes. These outcomes can be measured by primary data collection, or by obtaining information from published studies or from expert opinion. Critical evaluation of published studies is important for obtaining accurate estimates of health and resource outcomes. Discounting should be used to measure future costs and effectiveness and sensitivity analysis of important uncertainties should be conducted. The analyst's presentation and discussion of results is critical to appropriate interpretation by readers. Caution should be exercised when using the simple cost-effectiveness ratio to summarize results as there are conditions under which this will be misleading. Incremental cost-effectiveness ratios or presenting costs and effectiveness without constructing ratios is preferred in these situations.

References

1. Warner KE, Luce BR. Cost-benefit and cost-effectiveness analysis in health care: principles, practice, and potential. Ann Arbor, MI: Health Administration Press, 1982.

2. Dao TD. Cost-benefit and cost-effectiveness analysis of drug therapy. Am J Hosp Pharm 1985;42:791-802.

3. Drummond MF, Stoddart GL, Torrance GW. Methods for the economic evaluation of health care programmes. New York: Oxford University Press, 1987.

4. Weinstein MC, Stason WB. Foundations of cost-effectiveness analysis for health and medical practices. N Engl J Med 1977;296:716-21.

5. Oster G, Epstein AM. Cost-effectiveness of antihyperlipemic therapy in the prevention of coronary heart disease: the case of cholestyramine. JAMA 1987;258:2381-7.

6. Washington AE, Browner WS, Jorenbrot CC. Cost-effectiveness of combined treatment for endocervical gonorrhea considering co-infection with *Chlamydia trachomatis.* JAMA 1987;257:2056-60.

7. Rose DN, Schechter CB, Fahs MC, Silver AL. Tuberculosis prevention: cost-effectiveness analysis of isoniazid chemoprophylaxis. Am J Prev Med 1988;4:102-9.

8. Doubilet P, Weinstein MC, McNeil BJ. Use and misuse of the term "cost-effective" in medicine. N Engl J Med 1986;314:253-5.

9. Weinstein MC, Read JL, MacKay DN, Kresel JJ, Ashley H, Halvorsen KT, et al. Cost-effective choice of antimicrobial therapy for serious infections. J Gen Intern Med 1986; 1:351-63.

10. Warner KE, Hutton R. Cost-benefit and cost-effectiveness analysis in health care: growth and composition of the literature. Med Care 1980;18:1069-84.

11. Luft HS. Benefit cost analysis and public policy implementation: from normative to positive analysis. Public Policy 1976;24:437-61.

12. Stern RS, Pass RM, Komaroff AL. Topical versus systemic agent treatment for papulopustular acne: cost-effectiveness analysis. Arch Dermatol 1984;120:1571-8.

13. Holloway JJ, Smith CR, Moor RD, Feroli ER, Lietman PS. Comparative cost-effectiveness of gentamicin and tobramycin. Ann Intern Med 1984;101:764-9.

14. Hull RD, Raskob GE, Hirsh J, Sackett DL. A cost-effectiveness analysis of alternative approaches for long-term treatment of proximal venous thrombosis. JAMA 1984; 252: 235-9.

15. Willems JS, Sanders CR, Riddiough MA. Cost-effectiveness of vaccination against pneumococcal pneumonia. N Engl J Med 1980;303:553-9.

16. Gagnon JP, Osterhaus JT. Proposed drug-drug cost effectiveness methodology. Drug Intell Clin Pharm 1987;21:211-6.

17. Nettleman MD, Jones RB, Roberts SD, Katz BP, Washington E, Dittus RS, et al. Cost-effectiveness of culturing for *Chlamydia trachomatis:* a study in a clinic for sexually transmitted diseases. Ann Intern Med 1986;105:189-96.

18. Laffel GL, Fineberg HV, Braunwald E. A cost-effectiveness model for coronary thrombolysis/reperfusion therapy. J Am Coll Cardiol 1987;10:79B-90B.

19. Eisenberg JM, Kitz DS. Savings from outpatient antibiotic therapy for osteomyelitis: economic analysis of a therapeutic strategy. JAMA 1986;255:1585-8.

20. Zarowitz BJ, Owen H, Popovich J, Pancorbo S. Evaluation of gentamicin premixed admixtures: cost and clinical utility. Hosp Pharm 1987;22:257-60.

21. Beck JR, Pauker SG. The Markov process in medical prognosis. Med Decis Making 1983;3:419-58.

22. Cochran WG. The combination of estimates from different experiments. Biometrics 1954;10:101-29.

23. Polk RE, Hepler CD. Controversies in antimicrobial therapy: critical analysis of clinical trials. Am J Hosp Pharm 1986;43:630-40.

24. Desky AS, Sackett DL. When was a "negative" clinical trial big enough? How many patients you needed depends on what you found. Arch Intern Med 1985;145:709-12.

25. Lipid Research Clinics Program. Coronary primary prevention trial results, II: the relationship of reduction in incidence of coronary heart disease to cholesterol lowering. JAMA 1984;251:365-74.

26. Katz S, ed. The Portugal conference: measuring quality of life and functional status in clinical and epidemiological research. J Chron Dis 1987;40:459-650.

27. Weinstein MC, Fineberg HV. Clinical decision analysis. Philadelphia: WB Saunders, 1980:253-4.

28. Briggs GC, Moore BR, Bahado-Singh R, Lange S, Bogh P, Garite TJ. Cost-effectiveness of cefonicid sodium versus cefoxitin sodium for the prevention of post-operative infections after nonelective cesarean section. Clin Pharm 1987;6:718-21.

29. McGee DL. Probability of developing certain cardiovascular diseases in eight years at specified values of some characteristics. Section 28. In: Kannel WB, Gordon T, eds. The Framingham Study: an epidemiological investigation of cardiovascular disease. Department of Health, Education, and Welfare Publication (NIH) 74-610. Bethesda, MD: Public Health Service, 1977.

30. Weinstein MC, Stason WB. Cost-effectiveness of interventions to prevent or treat coronary heart disease. Ann Rev Public Health 1985;6:41-63.

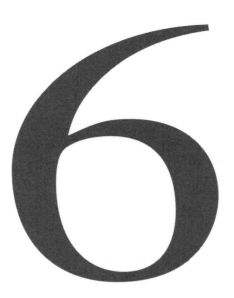

Cost-Utility Analysis

Stephen Joel Coons
Robert M. Kaplan

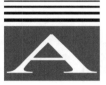s observed by Neumann and Weinstein,[1] the American public has a love–hate relationship with medical technology. Medical technologies are lauded for saving lives and improving the quality of medical care while, at the same time, they are condemned as the primary cause of the unchecked growth of medical care costs.

Our society's ambivalence stems, in part, from the lack of critical information as to what value is received for the tremendous amount of resources expended on medical care. As Maynard[2] has stated, it is commonplace in health care "for policy to be designed and executed in a data free environment!" Although the implicit objective of medical technology is to improve health outcomes, there is minimal evidence of the true effectiveness of many current healthcare practices.[3] In addition, measures of the overall quality of the US healthcare system, such as access to primary health care, health indicators (e.g., infant mortality, life expectancy), and public satisfaction in relation to costs, provide evidence that we trail other countries that spend significantly less than the US does on medical care.[4]

Earlier chapters have discussed the pressing need to maximize the net health benefit derived from the utilization of limited healthcare resources. Cost-effectiveness analysis (CEA) and cost-benefit analysis (CBA) have been presented as methods for assessing the costs and consequences of healthcare technologies, particularly pharmaceuticals. The purpose of this chapter is to discuss another method for evaluating the value obtained for the money spent: cost-utility analysis (CUA).

What Is Cost-Utility Analysis?

CUA is a formal economic technique for assessing the efficiency of healthcare interventions. It is considered by some to be a specific type of CEA[5] in which the measure of effectiveness is a utility- or preference-adjusted outcome. However, in this chapter, we will consider it as a separate and distinct economic technique.

CUA is one of the newest, and perhaps most controversial, types of economic evaluation. The controversy stems mainly from the measurement of utility. Utility is the value or worth placed on a level of health status, or improvement in health status, as measured by the preferences of individuals or society.[6] The measurement of utility is necessary for the calculation of the most commonly used outcome measure in this type of analysis: *quality-adjusted life-years* (*QALYs*) *gained.* There is no true consensus as to the most appropriate measurement approach. (The measurement of utility is discussed in greater depth later in the chapter.)

Nevertheless, CUA has some distinct advantages over CBA and CEA. CBA suffers from the difficulty of translating all costs and consequences into monetary terms.[7] It is especially difficult to translate patient-reported outcomes (e.g., quality of life) into dollars. In addition, CBA carries the potential for discrimination because it favors treatment for people who are working or those who are more wealthy. CEA is limited by the inability to simultaneously incorporate multiple outcomes from the same intervention or to compare interventions with different outcomes. In CEA, although the outcome measure is in natural units (e.g., life-years saved), no attempt is made to value the consequence or outcome in terms of quality or desirability. In contrast, CUA incorporates the quality of (or preference for) the health outcome achieved.[6] CUA, using QALYs gained as the outcome measure, is the most common approach to combining quantity and quality-of-life outcomes in economic evaluations.[8]

When Is Cost-Utility Analysis Appropriate?

Drummond et al.[6] enumerated several circumstances where CUA may be the most appropriate analytic approach:

1. When quality of life is *the* important outcome. For example, when comparing interventions that are not expected to have an impact on mortality, but a potential impact on patient function and well-being (e.g., treatments for arthritis).

2. When quality of life is *an* important outcome. For example, evaluation of the outcomes associated with the treatment of acute myocardial infarction. Not only is lives saved an important outcome measure, but also the quality of the lives saved (e.g., the impact of a treatment-induced stroke

in a survivor). Another example is the treatment of cancer. A chemotherapeutic agent may increase survival while it decreases the quality of the life being lived.

3. When the intervention affects both morbidity and mortality and a combined unit of outcome is desired. For example, evaluation of a therapy, such as estrogen use by postmenopausal women, that can improve quality of life, may reduce mortality from certain conditions (e.g., heart disease), but may increase mortality from other conditions (e.g., uterine cancer).

4. When the interventions being compared have a wide range of potential outcomes and there is a need to have a common unit of outcome for comparison. This is most commonly the case when a decision-maker must allocate limited resources among interventions that have different objectives and resultant benefits. For example, the choice between providing increased prenatal care or expanding a hypertension screening and treatment program.

5. When the objective is to compare an intervention with others that have already been evaluated in terms of cost per QALY (or equivalent) gained.

The identification, valuation, and measurement of costs is covered elsewhere in this book and will not be repeated here. In addition, Chapter 7 covers quality-of-life assessment. Health-related quality of life is an integral part of CUA; however, not all instruments measuring this component have outcome scores that can be incorporated into CUA. As stated by Hopkins,[9] quality of life measures:

> . . . have proved successful in tracking the effects of medical and surgical interventions and reflecting apparently more realistically the outcomes of these interventions. However, the multidimensional nature of these scales is perceived by some as a disadvantage, as it is difficult to compare outcomes between patients and across procedures. How can there be a 'trade-off,' for example, between reduction in pain and depression of mood? There is therefore considerable interest in attempting to value a health state in terms of a single number. Such valuations can then be integrated with the dimension of time in that state to allow comparisons of values achieved by different interventions in different clinical disorders. The best known of these integrated indices is the quality-adjusted life year . . .

QALYs integrate in a single summary score the net health improvement gains, in terms of both quantity and quality of life, experienced by a group of individuals. Although some economic evaluations reported in the literature have used disease-specific quality-of-life scales or general health profiles as outcome measures, most have incorporated valuations of health state preferences or utilities for the purpose of calculating QALYs.[8] This chapter focuses on assessing the health state utilities needed to calculate QALYs, the CUA ratio's most commonly used denominator.

However, before proceeding, we must clarify some terminology. The term "utilities" used in health state valuation literature does not correspond to the classical use of the same term by economists and philosophers of the 19th century. The current use of the term is derived from von Neumann and

Morgenstern's[10] theory of rational decision-making. Torrance and Feeny[11] suggested that to avoid confusion it would be preferable to call some of the valuations discussed in the following section health state "value preferences" rather than utilities; however, in this chapter, that distinction will not be made. This will be discussed in greater detail below.

Need for Health State Utility Assessment

Health care has different objectives. The objective of the care provided by a diabetologist might be a reduction in diabetic complications. Oncologists strive to keep their patients alive and may be satisfied with a short increase in survival time, whereas primary care providers often focus on shortening the cycle of acute illnesses for which mortality is not an immediate concern. All of these providers are attempting to improve the health of their patients. However, they each measure health in a different way. Comparing the productivity of a diabetologist to that of an oncologist may be like comparing apples to oranges. In other words, there is usually no way to directly compare the productivity of different providers when the intended outcomes are different.

The diversity of objectives and resulting outcomes in health care has led many analysts to focus on the simplest common ground. Typically, that is mortality or life expectancy. When mortality is studied, those who are alive are statistically coded as 1.0 and those who are dead are statistically coded as 0.0. Mortality allows the comparison between different diseases. For example, we can compare the years of life lost from heart disease to the years of life lost from cancer. The difficulty is that everyone who remains alive is given the same score. A person with endstage renal disease is given the same score as someone who is healthy. Utility assessment allows the quantification of levels of wellness on the continuum anchored by death and optimum function.

Conceptual Model

To evaluate health-related quality of life, we must consider all of the different ways that illness and its treatment affect outcomes. It can be said that there are only two central categories of outcomes: life duration and quality of life.[12] We are concerned about any illness or disability because it might make us live a shorter period of time. In addition, we are concerned about the impact of an illness or the effects of its treatment on quality of life. Assessment should consider three basic questions[13]: (1) Does the illness or its treatment shorten life? (2) Does the condition or its treatment make life less desirable and, if so, how much less desirable? (3) What are the duration effects; that is, how much life is lost or how long is the period of diminished quality of life?

Life duration, or quantity of life, as affected by an illness or its treatment is the easier of the concepts to measure. Actuarial mortality data allow for the determination or estimation of the shortened quantity of life. However, the impact of an illness or its treatment on the quality of life is less obvious or objective.

Health-related quality of life is a multidimensional construct. Its general measurement can result in a single outcome score (i.e., health index) or an array of scores for individual quality-of-life dimensions (i.e., health profile). The index and the profile represent the two complimentary approaches to quality-of-life assessment: the decision theory or utility approach and the psychometric approach, respectively.[14] Chapter 7 addresses quality-of-life assessment. This chapter's discussion of quality of life will focus on the incorporation of the utility approach in CUA.

Within the last few years there has been growing interest in using quality-of-life data to help evaluate the cost-effectiveness or cost-utility of healthcare programs. As touched upon earlier, CUA expresses the outcomes of health care in a common outcome unit that is equivalent to a well-year of life. The same outcome has been described as QALYs[15] or healthy years of life.[16] Since the term "QALY" has become most popular, we will use it in this chapter. QALYs integrate mortality, morbidity, and preferences into a comprehensive index number. If a man died of a stroke at age 50 and we would have expected him to live to age 75, it might be concluded that the disease was associated with 25 lost life-years. If 100 men died at age 50 (and also had a life expectancy of 75 years) we might conclude that 2500 life-years (100 men $\times$ 25 years) had been lost.

Death is not the only outcome of concern in stroke. For many adults the stroke results in disability over long periods of time. The quality-of-life loss can occur even when life expectancy is unaffected. Quality-of-life consequences of illnesses can be quantified and used to adjust length of life for its quality. For example, a disease that reduces quality of life by half will take away 0.5 QALYs over the course of one year. If it affects two people, it will take away 1.0 QALYs (2 $\times$ 0.5) over a one-year period. A medical treatment that improves quality of life by 0.2 for each of five individuals will result in the equivalent of 1.0 QALY if the benefit is maintained over a one-year period. This system has the advantage of considering both benefits and adverse effects of interventions in terms of the common QALY units.

Concept of Relative Importance of Dimensions

Nearly all health-related quality-of-life measures have multiple dimensions. The exact dimensions vary from measure to measure. There is considerable debate about which dimensions need to be included. For example, the most commonly included dimensions are physical functioning, role functioning, and mental health.

Different dimensions might be used to record treatment adverse effects as well as benefits. For example, a medication to control high blood pressure might be associated with low probabilities of dizziness, tiredness, impotence, and shortness of breath. The major challenge is in determining what it means when someone experiences an adverse effect. This requires the effect to be placed within the context of the total health outcome. For example, should a patient with insulin-dependent diabetes mellitus discontinue therapy because of skin irritation at the injection sites? Clearly, local irritation is an adverse effect of treatment. But, without treatment the patient would die. Often the issue is not whether treatment causes adverse effects, but how we should place these effects within the perspective of total health. Ultimately, we must decide whether treatment produces a net benefit or a net deficit in health status.

Many measures of health-related quality of life simply tabulate frequencies for different symptoms or represent health status using profiles of outcomes. Figure 1 is a representation of one such profile.[13] The figure represents three hypothetical treatment profiles. It is common in the presentation of these profiles to connect the points even though increments on the x axis are not meaningful. T-scores (y axis) are standardized scores with a mean of 50 and a standard deviation of 10. Treatment 1 may produce benefits for physical functioning but decrements for role functioning. Treatment 2 may produce decrements for physical functioning but increments for role functioning. This information may be valuable for diagnostic purposes. However, ultimately, clinicians make some general interpretations of the profile by applying a weighting system. They might decide that they are more concerned about physical than role functioning, or vice versa. We must recognize, however, that judgment about the relative importance of dimensions is common. Physicians may ignore a particular test result or a particular symptom because another one is more important to them. Typically, however, it is done arbitrarily. We suggest that the process by which relative importance is evaluated can and should be studied explicitly.

There are a variety of conceptual and technical issues relevant to preference or utility assessment.[17-20] For example, different approaches to preference assessment can yield different results. However, these differences might be expected because the different approaches are based on different underlying conceptual models. As a result, the preference assessment techniques ask different questions. The following sections attempt to elucidate some of these conflicts.

Concept of Utility

The concept of QALYs has been discussed in the literature for nearly 25 years. Perhaps the first application was suggested by Fanshel and

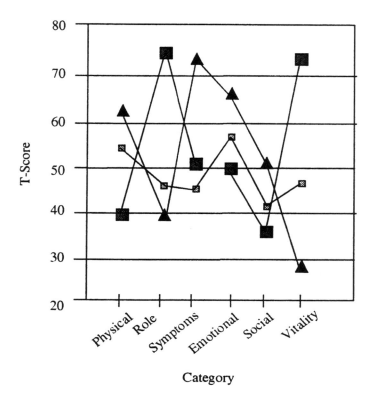

Figure 1. Comparison of profiles from three hypothetical treatments.[13] T-scores are standardized scores with a mean of 50 and a standard deviation of 10. ▲ = treatment 1; ▨ = treatment 2; ■ = treatment 3.

Bush.[21] Soon after, Torrance[22] introduced a conceptually similar model. Since then, a variety of applications have appeared. Although most of these models are conceptually alike, variations between the approaches have led to some inconsistent findings, some of which are highlighted later in the chapter.

Despite the differences in approach, some important assumptions are similar. For example, all of these approaches assume that one full healthy year of life is scored 1.0. Years of life in less than optimal health are scored as less than 1.0. The basic assumption is that two years scored as 0.5 add up to the equivalent of 1.0 year of complete wellness. Similarly, four years scored as 0.25 sum to the equivalent of 1.0 completely well-year of life. A treatment that moves a patient from 0.5 to 0.75 produces the equivalent of 0.25 QALYs. If applied to four individuals, and the duration of the treatment effect is one year, the effect of the treatment would be equivalent to

1.0 completely well-year of life. The disagreement among most researchers is not over the QALY concept but rather over how the weights for cases between 0.0 and 1.0 are obtained. However, that is not to say that there are no concerns about using QALYs in health policy decisions.[23-27] In addition Mehrez and Gafni[28,29] have proposed that the healthy-year equivalent (HYE) is a more appropriate outcome measure than the QALY. They assert that the HYE, like the QALY, combines both quality of life and quantity of life; however, HYEs more fully represent individuals' preferences in the calculation of the trade-offs between quality and quantity of life. A discussion of these concerns is beyond the scope of this chapter.

HISTORY OF THE UTILITY THEORY

The history of the utility theory and its applications to health outcomes assessment has been reviewed by Torrance and Feeny.[11] Health utility assessment has its roots in the work of von Neumann and Morgenstern[10] who published their classic work a half century ago. Their mathematical decision theory characterized how a rational individual should make decisions when faced with uncertain outcomes. They outlined axioms of choice that have been formally evaluated and have become basic foundations of decision analysis in business, government, and health care. Their work has been expanded upon by Raiffa[30] and others.[31,32] Torrance and Feeny[11] emphasized that the use of the term "utility theory" by von Neumann and Morgenstern was unfortunate. Their reference to utility differs from the more common uses by economists that emphasize consumer satisfaction with commodities that are received *with certainty*. Nineteenth century philosophers and economists assumed the existence of cardinal (or interval level) utilities for these functions. A characteristic of cardinal utilities is that they can be aggregated across individuals and used for utilitarian social policy.

By the turn of the century, Pareto challenged the value of cardinal utilities and demonstrated that ordinal utilities could represent consumer choice.[33] In a classic essay, this work was extended by Arrow and Debreu.[34] Arrow[35] had previously argued that there are inconsistencies in individual preferences under certainty and that meaningful cardinal preferences cannot be measured and may not even exist. As a result, most economists maintain that averaged or aggregate preferences have little meaning.

There are several reasons why Arrow's work may not be applicable to the aggregation of utilities in the assessment of QALYs. First, utility expressions for QALYs are expressions of consumer preference *under uncertainty*. The traditional criticisms of microeconomists are directed toward decisions under certainty rather than uncertainty.[11] A second issue is that Arrow assumed that the metric underlying utility was not meaningful and not standardized across individuals. Substantial psychometric evidence now suggests that preferences can be measured using scales that have meaningful interval or ratio properties. When cardinal (interval) utilities are used instead of rankings, many of the potential problems in the Impossibility Theorem are avoided.[36,37]

It is also important to recognize that different approaches to the calculations of QALYs are based on very different underlying assumptions. One approach considers the duration someone is in a particular health state as conceptually independent from the utility for the state.[12,15] The other approach merges duration and utility.[11] This distinction is central to the understanding of the difference in approaches and the required evidence for the validity of the utility assessment procedure.

In the approach advocated by Kaplan and Anderson[12] and Weinstein and Stason,[15] utilities for health states are obtained at a single point in time. For example, persons in a particular health state, such as confinement to wheelchair, who performed no major social role are asked to assess the utility of that health state. Suppose that this state is assigned a value of 0.5. Then, patients in this state are observed over the course of time to empirically determine their transitions to other states of wellness. If they remain in the state for one year, then they would lose the equivalent of 0.5 well-years of life. The key to this approach is that the preferences only concern a single point in time and that the transition is determined through observation or expert judgment. The alternative approach emphasized by Torrance and Feeny[11] and Nord[38] obtains preference for both health state and for duration. These approaches also consider the more complex problems of uncertainty. Thus, they are consistent with the von Neumann and Morgenstern's[10] notion of decision under uncertainty in which probabilities and trade-offs are considered explicitly by the judge.

Methods for Assessing Utility

CUA requires an assessment of utilities for health states. A variety of different techniques have been used to assess these utilities. These techniques will be summarized briefly. Then, comparisons between the techniques will be considered. Some analysts do not measure utilities directly. Instead, they evaluate health outcome by simply assigning a reasonable utility.[39] However, most current approaches have respondents assign weights to different health states on a scale ranging from 0 (for dead) to 1.0 (for wellness). The most common techniques include category rating scales, magnitude estimations, the standard gamble, the time trade-off, and the equivalence person trade-off. Each of these methods will be described briefly.

RATING SCALES

Rating scales require the respondent to assign a numeric value to objects. There are several methods for obtaining rating scale information. The category scale, exemplified by the familiar 10-point rating scale, is efficient, easy to use, and applicable in a large number of settings. Typically, the subjects read the description of a case and rate it on a 10-point scale ranging from 0 for dead to 10 for asymptomatic optimum function. The endpoints of the scale are typically well defined.

Another common rating scale method is the visual analog scale. The visual analog method shows a subject a line, typically 100 centimeters in length, with the endpoints well defined. The subject's task is to mark the line to indicate where their preference rests for one or more health states in relation to the two poles.

Appropriate applications of rating scales reflect contemporary developments in cognitive sciences. Judgment-decision theory has been dominated by the belief that human decisions follow principles of optimality and rationality. A considerable amount of research has challenged the normative models that have attempted to demonstrate rational choice. The development of cognitive theories, such as information integration theory,[40] provide better explanations of the cognitive process of judgment. Information integration theory includes two constructs: integration and valuation. A large body of evidence indicates that rating scales provide meaningful metrics for the expression of these subjective preferences.[40] Although there have been some challenges to the use of rating scales, most biases can be overcome with the use of just a few simple precautions, such as clear definitions of the endpoints and preliminary practice with cases that make the endpoints salient.[40]

MAGNITUDE ESTIMATION

Magnitude estimation is a common psychometric method that is believed by psychophysicists to yield ratio scale scores. In magnitude estimation, a specific case is selected as a standard and assigned a particular number. Then, other cases are rated in relation to the standard. Suppose, for example, the standard is assigned the number 10. If a case is regarded as half as desirable as the standard, it is given the number 5. If it is regarded as twice as desirable, it is given the number 20. Ratings across subjects are standardized to a common metric and aggregated using the geometric mean. Advocates for magnitude estimation argue that the method is meaningful because it provides a direct estimate of the subjective ratio. Thus, they believe, the magnitude estimate has the properties of a ratio scale. However, magnitude estimation has been challenged on several grounds. The method is not based on any specific theory of measurement and gains credibility only through face validity.[40] Further, the meaning of the scores has been challenged. For example, the values are not linked directly to any decision process. What does it mean if one case is rated as half as desirable as another? Does it mean that the respondent would be indifferent between a 50–50 chance of the higher valued outcome and a certainty of the alter-

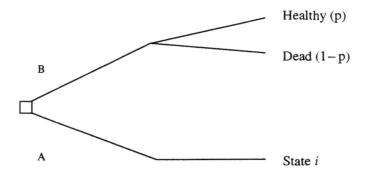

═══ **Figure 2.** Standard gamble for a chronic health state. i = chronic health state; p = probability
━━━ of achieving perfect health.

native valued as half as desirable? These issues have not been systematically addressed in the health status literature.

═══════ **STANDARD GAMBLE**

Category rating and magnitude estimation are methods commonly
used by psychometricians. Typically, the tasks emphasize wellness at a particular point in time and do not ask subjects to make trades or to consider
aspects of uncertainty. Several methods more explicitly consider decisions
under uncertainty. The standard gamble offers a choice between two alternatives: choice A—living in health state i (a chronic health state between
perfect health and death) with certainty, or choice B—taking a gamble on
a new treatment for which the outcome is uncertain. Figure 2 shows this
trade. The respondent is told that a hypothetical treatment will lead to perfect health with a probability of p or immediate death with a probability of
$1 - p$. They can choose between remaining in state i that is intermediate
between wellness and death or taking the gamble and trying the new treatment. The probability is varied until the subject is indifferent between
choices A and B. For example, if a subject is indifferent between choices
A and B when p = 0.65, the utility of state i is 0.65.

The standard gamble has been attractive because it is based on the
axioms of utility theory. The choice between a certain outcome and a gamble conforms to the exercises originally proposed by von Neumann and
Morgenstern.[10] Although the interval properties of the data obtained using
the gamble have been assumed, they have not been empirically demonstrated.[17] A variety of other problems with the gamble also have become
apparent. For example, it has often been stated that the standard gamble has
face validity because it approximates choices made by medical patients.[41]
However, treatment of most chronic diseases does not approximate the

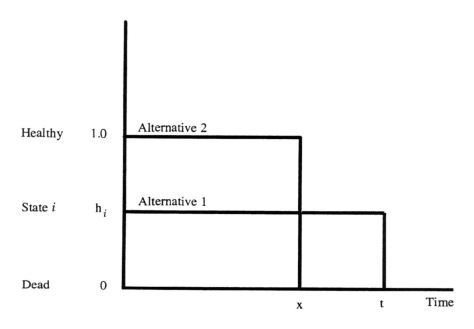

Figure 3. Time trade-off for a chronic health state. $h_i = x \div t$, where h_i = preference value or utility for state i; state i = chronic health state; t = life expectancy for an individual with chronic health state i; and x = time at which respondent is indifferent between alternatives 1 and 2.

gamble. There is no known product that will cure a patient with arthritis nor is there one that is likely to kill her. In other words, the decision-making experience of the patient is not likely to include an option that has a realistic gamble. Further, the cognitive demands of the task are high.

TIME TRADE-OFF

The concept of probability is difficult for most respondents and requires the use of visual aids or props to assist in the interview. Thus, an alternative to the standard gamble, which is also consistent with the von Neumann and Morgenstern[10] axioms of choice, uses a trade-off in time.[42] Figure 3 demonstrates the trade-off for a chronic disease state. Here, the subject is offered a choice of living in health state i (chronic health state considered better than death but less desirable than perfect health) for time t (life expectancy for an individual with chronic health state i) or perfect health for time x. Time x and t are followed by immediate death. Time x is varied until the respondent is indifferent between the two alternatives. Presumably, all subjects would choose a year of wellness versus a year with some health problem. However, by reducing the time of wellness and leaving the time in the suboptimal health state fixed (such as one year), an indifference point can be determined ($h_i = x \div t$) (h_i is the utility or preference value for chronic health state i). For example, a subject may rate being in a wheelchair for two years as equivalent to perfect wellness for one year ($1 \div 2 = 0.5$). The time trade-off is theoretically appealing because it is conceptually equivalent to a QALY.

PERSON TRADE-OFF

Finally, a person trade-off technique allows comparisons of the numbers of people helped in different states. For example, respondents might be asked to evaluate the equivalencies between the number of persons helped by different programs. They might be asked how many persons in state B must be helped to provide a benefit equivalent to helping one person in state A. From a policy perspective, the person trade-off also directly seeks information similar to that required as the basis for policy decisions.

Differences Between the Methods

Several papers in the literature have compared utilities for health states as captured by different methods. These differences have been reviewed by Nord.[43] In general, standard gamble and time trade-off methods give higher values than rating scales in most, but not all, studies. In about half of the studies reported, time trade-off yields lower utilities than standard gamble. In one of the earlier studies, Patrick et al.[44] found that person trade-off methods gave the same results as rating scales. However, these findings were not confirmed in more recent studies.[38] Magnitude estimation has produced results that are highly inconsistent across studies.[43]

The variability of health state utilities in comparisons of different studies is hardly surprising. The methods differ substantially in the questions posed to respondents. In summary, there is substantial debate about which technique should be used to acquire utility information. Results obtained from different methods do not correspond, although they typically have a high degree of similarity in the ranks they assign to outcomes. However, the differences in preferences yielded by different methods can result in different allocations of resources if the preferences are not obtained on a linear or interval response scale. For example, suppose that the difference between the effect of a drug and a placebo is 0.05 units of well-being as assessed by rating scales and 0.02 as measured by magnitude estimation. The benefit would have to last 20 years to produce 1.0 QALY if rating scale utilities were used, and 50 years if magnitude estimation utilities were used. Aggregation of benefits necessarily requires an underlying linear response scale in which equal differences at different points along the response scale are equally meaningful. For example, the differences between 0.2 and 0.3 (0.1 QALY if the duration is one year) must have the same meaning as the difference between 0.7 and 0.8. A treatment that improves a patient's condition from 0.2 to 0.3 must be considered of equal benefit to a treatment that improves it from 0.7 to 0.8. Confirmation of this scale property has been demonstrated for rating scales but not for other methods.[40,45]

Another difference between methods is the inclusion of information about uncertainty in the judgment process. Time trade-off, standard gamble, or person trade-off all theoretically include some judgment about duration of stay in health state. Magnitude estimation and rating scales typically separate utility at a point in time from probability. Considerably more theoretical and empirical work will be necessary to resolve these differences of approach.

Nord[46] recently argued for quality assurance standards for QALY calculations. These recommendations were based on a review that revealed inconsistency in the methods used to assess utilities. According to Nord, the utility assessment typically lacked a theoretical or empiric basis. Apparently, this refers to inattention to economic theories. However, others have noted that some utility assessment approaches are based on different theoretical models and empiric results. For example, advocates for the use of rating scales offer evidence that the methods found theoretically and empirically justified by economists fail to meet the basic requirements for an interval response scale.[47] Nord et al.[48] suggested that the person trade-off be used as the standard against which other methods are compared. However, they did not offer evidence that data obtained using the person trade-off meet standards of reliability, validity, and interval scale property. The person trade-off does not meet the face validity criterion of being a direct estimate of a QALY. However, it is not clear that subjects do not make other cognitive errors when applying the method. This is likely to remain an area of active debate into the near future.

Whose Utilities or Preferences Should be Used?

Choices between alternatives in health care necessarily involve preference judgment. For example, the inclusion of some services in a basic benefits package and the exclusion of others is an exercise in value, choice, or preference. There are many levels at which preference is expressed in the healthcare decision process. For example, an older woman may decide to cope with the symptoms of upset stomach in order to gain relief from the discomfort of osteoarthritis. A physician may order pelvic ultrasound to ensure against missing the very low probability that a 40-year-old woman has ovarian cancer. Or, an administrator may decide to put resources into prevention for large numbers of people instead of devoting the same resources to organ transplants for a smaller number.

In CUA, preferences are used to express the relative importance of various health outcomes. There is a subjective or qualitative component to health outcome. Whether we prefer a headache or an upset stomach caused by its treatment is a value judgment. Not all symptoms are of equal importance. Most patients would prefer mild fatigue (an adverse effect of treatment) to a severe headache (the symptom eradicated by treatment). Yet, providing a model of how well treatments work implicitly includes these judgments. Models require a precise numeric expression of this preference. CUA explicitly includes a preference component to represent these trade-offs.

Some models obtain preferences from random samples of the general population.[37] It is recognized that administrators ultimately choose between alternative programs. Community preferences may represent the will of the general public and not those of administrators. Yet there is considerable debate about technical aspects of preference assessment. Some of the debate has to do with whose preferences are considered.

In most areas of preference assessment, it is easy to identify differences between different groups or different individuals. It might be argued that judgments about net health benefits for white men should not be applied to Hispanic men who may give different weight to some symptoms. Preferences for movies, clothing, or political candidates differ for social and cultural groups; it is assumed that these same differences extend to health states. Allocation of resources to Medicaid recipients, for example, would be considered inappropriate when the preferences came from both Medicaid recipients and nonrecipients.[49] Other analysts have suggested that preference weights from the general population cannot be applied to any particular patient group. Rather, patient preferences from every individual group must be obtained.

Most studies do not support the common belief that preferences differ. Some small, but significant differences between demographic groups have been observed.[50] Studies have found little evidence for preference difference between patients and the general population. For example, Balaban et al.[51] compared preference weights obtained from patients with arthritis with those obtained from the general population in San Diego. They found a high degree of correspondence for ratings of cases involving patients with arthritis. Similar results were found by Hughes et al.[52] among HIV-infected patients. Studies of patients with cancer have had comparable findings (unpublished study: Nerenz DR, Golob K, Trump DL. Preference weights for the Quality of Well-Being Scale as obtained from oncology patients. Henry Ford Hospital, Detroit, MI, 1990). Studies also have shown a high degree of similarity in preferences provided by men versus women, the medically insured versus the uninsured, those ever in wheelchairs versus those never in wheelchairs, British versus Americans, citizens of Oregon versus those of California, and residents of three different European communities.[53]

It would be incorrect to say that there are never any mean differences in preference, since significant differences in preferences have been observed in several studies. However, these differences were typically small.[53] Further analysis will be required to determine whether these differences affect the conclusions of various analyses.

A related problem is the assumption that all people in the same health state should get the same score. Most approaches to utility assessment use the mean preference for a particular case to represent all individuals who meet a common definition. For example, suppose that the average utility for being in a wheelchair, limited in major activities, and having missing limbs is 0.50. The models would assign the same number to all individuals who occupy that state. However, there is substantial variability in how individuals view their own health. If individual preferences are used, there might be significant variation in scores across people with identical objective descriptions.[54] Despite the appeal of individualized preferences, they rarely lead to different treatment decisions than would be obtained from the use of aggregate preferences.[55]

Multiattribute Health Status Classification Systems

Although it is important to understand the various approaches to the measurement of health state utilities/preference values, some pharmacoeconomic researchers conducting a CUA will not measure health state utilities directly. They may use one of the existing multiattribute health status classification systems for which the utility functions have been empirically derived. Two such instruments developed in North America are the Quality of Well-Being Scale (QWB) developed at the University of California–San Diego, La Jolla, CA, and the Health Utilities Index (HUI) developed at McMaster University, Hamilton, Ontario, Canada.

The QWB is a general quality-of-life instrument that includes symptoms or problems plus three dimensions of functional health status: mobility, physical activity, and social activity. Standardized preference weights for the QWB have been measured (using the category rating scale method) and validated on a general population in San Diego.[56] Other investigators have reweighted the symptoms/problems and function levels of the QWB in specific populations, such as patients with arthritis[51] and HIV-infected subjects,[52] and have found the generalizability of the original weights to be very high.

The HUI is another general instrument that describes the health status of a person at a point in time in terms of ability to function on a set of attributes or dimensions of health status. The original version (Mark I) of the HUI consists of four attributes and a formula to calculate utilities.[57] The second version (Mark II) consists of seven attributes and formulas for the calculation of utilities and preference values.[58] The measurement of the preferences/utilities for the health status classification system were made with visual analog scales and the standard gamble technique. The most recent and potentially most useful version, Mark III, has eight attributes: vision, hearing, speech, ambulation, dexterity, cognition, pain and discomfort, and emotion.[59] The utility/preference functions are not yet available, but those for the Mark II can be used in the interim.[a]

Two additional potentially useful multiattribute health status systems in the latter stages of development in Europe are the EuroQol[60] and the Index of Health-Related Quality of Life.[61] The EuroQol was developed concurrently in five languages (Dutch, English, Finnish, Norwegian, and Swedish) by a multidisciplinary team of European researchers.[60] (Spanish and Catalan translations are now available and French, German, and Italian versions are in preparation.) The EuroQol instrument was designed to be self-administered and short enough to be used in conjunction with other measures. It has two parts: a visual analog scale on which patients rate their own health on a scale of 0 to 100, and a questionnaire that classifies subjects into one of 243 health states. The current EuroQol health status classification system has five dimensions: mobility, self-care, usual activities, pain/discomfort, and anxiety/depression. Each dimension has three levels. An earlier version of the instrument had six dimensions and classified individuals into three levels of mobility, self-care, and pain, and into two levels of main activity, family/leisure activity, and anxiety/depression.[62] The EuroQol is truly an instrument in development and a great deal of research is ongoing, and necessary, to demonstrate its use and usefulness.[63-65]

The Index of Health-Related Quality of Life is a measure of social, psychological, and physical functioning that is in development in the UK.[61] It is based on a five-level multidimensional classification system and provides a health profile as well as a unidimensional health index value (0 to 1). The health index value or global score is comprised of three primary dimensions: disability, physical discomfort, and emotional distress. The dimensions are further subdivided into attributes, then scales, then descriptors. The complex and multilevel valuation approach, which incorporated both standard gamble and category rating techniques, is addressed elsewhere.[66] The validity, reliability, and usefulness of the instrument is yet to be determined.

Cost-Utility Analysis and Healthcare Interventions

Figure 4 presents a graphic representation of a hypothetical case in which treatment has increased both the quantity and quality of life for a

[a]For further information on the QWB contact: Robert M. Kaplan, PhD, Division of Health Care Sciences, School of Medicine, 9500 Gilman Dr, University of California–San Diego, La Jolla, CA 92093. For further information on the HUI contact: George W. Torrance, PhD, Health Sciences Centre 3H1C, McMaster University, 1200 Main St West, Hamilton, Ontario, Canada L8N 3Z5.

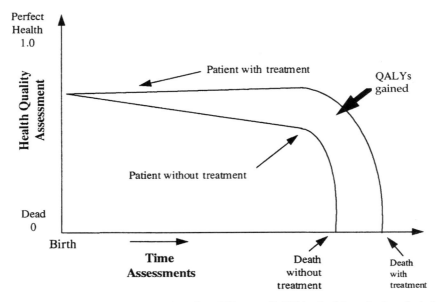

Figure 4. Representation of quality-adjusted life-years (QALYs) gained through a hypothetical treatment.

patient or group of patients. The area between the curves would be calculated to measure the QALYs gained. To complete the CUA, the incremental cost of providing the treatment would be measured and divided by the QALYs gained. Table 1, adapted from Detsky and Naglie,[67] illustrates the different elements that are needed to conduct CEA and CUA when comparing two alternative interventions. An assumption in the table is that quality of life (utility) remains constant over the full life expectancy.

Table 1. Economic Analysis of Two Alternative Treatment Interventions[67]

INTERVENTION	COST ($)	EFFECTIVENESS (LIFE EXPECTANCY) (y)	HEALTH STATE (UTILITY)	QALYs
Treatment A	20,000	4.5	0.60	2.7
Treatment B	10,000	3.5	0.72	2.5

$$\text{Incremental cost-effectiveness ratio} = \frac{\$20,000 - \$10,000}{4.5\,y - 3.5\,y} = \$10,000 \text{ per life-year gained}$$

$$\text{Incremental cost-utility ratio} = \frac{\$20,000 - \$10,000}{2.7\,QALYs - 2.5\,QALYs} = \$50,000 \text{ per QALY gained}$$

QALY = quality-adjusted life-year.

Table 2. Quality-Adjusted Life-Years Gained:
Some Tentative Estimates[2]

INTERVENTION	COST/QALY (£)[a]
Cholesterol testing and diet therapy only (all adults, aged 40-69 y)	220
Neurosurgical interventions for head surgery	240
General practitioner advice to stop smoking	270
Neurosurgical intervention for subarachnoid hemorrhage	490
Antihypertensive therapy to prevent stroke (ages 45-64 y)	940
Pacemaker implantation	1,100
Valve replacement for aortic stenosis	1,140
Hip replacement	1,180
Cholesterol testing and treatment	1,480
Coronary artery bypass graft (left main vessel disease, severe angina)	2,090
Kidney transplant	4,710
Breast cancer screening	5,780
Heart transplantation	7,840
Cholesterol testing and treatment (incrementally) of all adults 25-39 y	14,150
Home hemodialysis	17,260
Coronary artery bypass graft (one vessel disease, moderate angina)	18,830
Continuous ambulatory peritoneal dialysis	19,870
Hospital hemodialysis	21,970
Epoetin alfa therapy for anemia in patients undergoing dialysis (assuming a 10% reduction in mortality)	54,380
Neurosurgical intervention for malignant intracranial tumors	107,780
Epoetin alfa therapy for anemia in patients undergoing dialysis (assuming no reduction in mortality)	126,290

QALY = quality-adjusted life-year.
[a]British pounds as of August 1990.

A common method of summarizing and comparing the results of CUAs is in the form of a league table. Table 2 shows a league table compiled by Maynard.[2] There are many concerns regarding the manner in which league tables are constructed and applied.[68,69] As observed by Mason et al.[68] the source studies in league tables often use various means of calculating QALYs and different years of origin, discount rates, settings, and types of comparison programs. For example, a study by Hornberger et al.[70] compared six methods for deriving cost/QALY data for patients receiving in-center hemodialysis. Results from the 58 patients in their study demonstrated a range of $34,893 to $45,254 per QALY gained based on the Sickness Impact Profile[71] and standard gamble technique, respectively. Nevertheless, Mason et al.[68] concluded that although league tables have serious limitations, the systematic comparisons that league tables provide are preferable to the alternative: the reliance on the informal, unsystematic assessments made in the absence of data.

━━━━ **IMPACT OF PHARMACEUTICAL INTERVENTIONS**

For pharmaceuticals, as with most other healthcare interventions, the ultimate therapeutic endpoint or outcome is the enhancement of quality of life and/or length of life. Therefore, in theory, the most appropriate outcome measure would be QALYs. There are a number of published studies that have used QALYs and the cost-utility approach to evaluate the economic efficiency of healthcare programs/interventions.[72-74] However, there are very few published reports of the impact of pharmaceutical interventions in which QALYs were an outcome measure. In addition, those studies that have been published are limited by their methodologic approach to the measurement of QALYs. In some cases, QALYs are estimated/modeled from cross-sectional data rather than measured prospectively.

A number of examples of the use of CUA in the evaluation of cancer chemotherapy have appeared in the literature.[75-77] The study by Smith et al.[77] illustrates the importance of adjusting length of life/survival for quality. The authors compared the incremental costs per QALY for surgery plus adjuvant chemotherapy versus surgery alone in patients with colon cancer. They estimated that 2.4 unadjusted life-years were gained from the addition of chemotherapy; however, after adjusting for quality of life, only 0.4 QALYs were gained. The costs of surgery alone and surgery plus chemotherapy were $6000 and $13,000 per patient per 12 months of treatment, respectively. Since the incremental cost of adding the chemotherapy was $7000, the calculated cost per life-year gained was $2916 and the cost per QALY gained was $17,500. The findings are limited by the study's small sample size and other methodologic weaknesses (e.g., measurement of QALYs). However, it demonstrates the potential power of appropriately conducted CUAs in evaluating the outcomes of pharmaceutical interventions more comprehensively than through other approaches (e.g., CEA).

━━━━ **Summary**

In a society in which healthcare resources are limited, it is essential that the resources available are used efficiently and equitably. However, for this system to function effectively, data about costs and outcomes are essential. Resources should be used for programs that produce the greatest benefit for the greatest number of people. The lack of good information about input–output relationships in health care has lead to enormous variations in costs and clinical practice patterns.[5] There has been little consensus on what constitutes good clinical practice. The integration of data on the quality of life with corresponding data on life expectancy yields a single index of health benefit, expressed in terms of QALYs. Our interest in life expectancy and quality of life arises from the fact that health care can influence either or both of these.

It is likely that the use of CUA will increase as the need to evaluate the benefits derived from very different healthcare interventions increases. This type of analysis will assist in ensuring that resources are allocated as efficiently as possible to serve health outcome goals. Resources will never be sufficient to provide all the health care that might be given; there are finite resources and potentially infinite demands. CUA provides a systematic approach to comparing ways of using the resources most efficiently in the process of meeting those demands.

Pharmaceutical interventions are a critical component of health care. Pharmaceuticals can produce QALYs by lengthening life, improving the quality of life, or both. As seen in the cancer treatment example, chemotherapy can be a double-edged sword: it can lengthen life while decreasing its quality. However, it is more common for pharmaceuticals to be prescribed to improve the quality of life in people who have non–life-threatening but potentially debilitating conditions (e.g., arthritis, glaucoma). If conducted properly, CUA can be a powerful tool to more comprehensively evaluate the overall impact of pharmacotherapy. This type of research is needed to document the relative value of pharmaceuticals when compared with other medical interventions and to inform decisions as to the most efficient use of finite healthcare resources.

 References

1. Neumann PJ, Weinstein MC. The diffusion of new technology: costs and benefits to health care. In: Gelijns AC, Halm EA, eds. The changing economics of medical technology. Washington, DC: National Academy Press, 1991:21-34.

2. Maynard A. Developing the health care market. Econ J 1991;101(408):1277-86.

3. Roper WL, Winkenwerder W, Hackbarth GM, Krakauer H. Effectiveness in health care: an initiative to evaluate and improve medical practice. N Engl J Med 1988;319: 1197-202.

4. Starfield B. Primary care and health: a cross-national comparison. JAMA 1991;266: 2268-71.

5. Weinstein MC, Stason WB. Foundations of cost-effectiveness analysis for health and medical practice. N Engl J Med 1977;296:716-21.

6. Drummond MF, Stoddart GL, Torrance GW. Methods for the economic evaluation of health care programmes. New York: Oxford University Press, 1987.

7. Patrick DL, Erickson P. Health status and health policy: allocating resources to health care. New York: Oxford University Press, 1993.

8. Drummond M. The role and importance of quality of life measurements in economic evaluations. Br J Med Econ 1992;4:9-16.

9. Hopkins A. Editor's introduction. In: Measures of the quality of life and the uses to which such measures may be put. London: Royal College of Physicians of London, 1992:iii-iv.

10. von Neumann J, Morgenstern O. Theory of games and economic behavior. Princeton, NJ: Princeton University Press, 1944.

11. Torrance GW, Feeny D. Utilities in quality-adjusted life years. Int J Technol Assess Health Care 1989;5:559-75.

12. Kaplan RM, Anderson JP. The general health policy model: an integrated approach. In: Spilker B, ed. Quality of life assessments in clinical trials. New York: Raven Press, 1990:131-49.

13. Kaplan RM, Coons SJ. Relative importance of dimensions in the assessment of health-related quality of life for patients with hypertension. Prog Cardiovasc Nurs 1992; 7:29-36.

14. Coons SJ, Kaplan RM. Assessing health-related quality of life: application to drug therapy. Clin Ther 1992;14:850-8.

15. Weinstein MC, Stason WB. Hypertension: a policy perspective. Cambridge, MA: Harvard University Press, 1976.

16. Russell LB. Is prevention better than cure? Washington, DC: The Brookings Institution, 1986.

17. Froberg DG, Kane RL. Methodology for measuring health state preferences, II: scaling methods. J Clin Epidemiol 1989;42:459-71.

18. Froberg DG, Kane RL. Methodology for measuring health state preferences, III: population and context effects. J Clin Epidemiol 1989;42:585-92.

19. Froberg DG, Kane RL. Methodology for measuring health state preferences, IV: progress and a research agenda. J Clin Epidemiol 1989;42:675-85.

20. Froberg DG, Kane RL. Methodology for measuring health state preferences, I: measurement strategies. J Clin Epidemiol 1989;42:345-52.

21. Fanshel S, Bush JW. A health-status index and its applications to health-services outcomes. Operations Res 1970;18:1021-66.

22. Torrance GW. Social preferences for health states. An empirical evaluation of three measurement techniques. SocioEcon Plan Sci 1976;10:129-36.

23. Carr-Hill RA. Allocating resources to health care: is the QALY (quality adjusted life year) a technical solution to a political problem? Int J Health Serv 1991;21:351-63.

24. Coast J. Developing the QALY concept: exploring the problems of data acquisition. PharmacoEconomics 1993;4:240-6.

25. Harris J. Life: quality, value and justice. Health Policy 1988;10:259-66.

26. LaPuma J, Lawlor EF. Quality-adjusted life-years: ethical implications for physicians and policymakers. JAMA 1990;263:2917-21.

27. Loomes G, McKenzie L. The use of QALYs in health care decision making. Soc Sci Med 1989;28:299-308.

28. Mehrez A, Gafni A. Quality-adjusted life years, utility theory, and healthy-years equivalents. Med Decis Making 1989;9:142-9.

29. Mehrez A, Gafni A. The healthy-years equivalents: how to measure them using the standard gamble approach. Med Decis Making 1991;11:140-6.

30. Raiffa H. Decision analysis: introductory lectures on choices under uncertainty. Reading, MA: Addison-Wesley, 1968.

31. Bell DE, Farquhar PH. Perspectives on utility theory. Operations Res 1986;34:179-83.

32. Howard RA. Decision analysis: practice and promise. Manag Sci 1988;34:679-95.

33. Parsons T. The structure of social action. Vol. 1. New York, Free Press, 1937:241-9.

34. Arrow KJ, Debreu G. Existence of equilibrium for a competitive economy. Econometrica 1954;22:265-90.

35. Arrow KJ. Social choice and individual values. New York: Wiley, 1951.

36. Keeney RL. A group preference axiomatization with cardinal utility. Manag Sci 1976;23:140-5.

37. Kaplan RM, Anderson JP, Ganiats TG. The Quality of Well-Being Scale: rationale for a single quality of life index. In: Walker SR, Rosser RM, eds. Quality of life assessment: key issues in the 1990s. Lancaster, UK: Kluwer Academic Publishers, 1993:65-94.

38. Nord E. The validity of a visual analogue scale in determining social utility weights for health states. Int J Health Plan Manag 1991;6:234-42.
39. Weinstein MC, Stason WB. Cost-effectiveness of coronary artery bypass surgery. Circulation 1982;66(suppl 3):56-66.
40. Anderson NH. Contributions to information integration theory. Vol. 1–3. Hillsdale, NJ: Erlbaum Publishers, 1991.
41. Mulley AJ. Assessing patient's utilities: can the ends justify the means? Med Care 1989;27(suppl):S269-81.
42. Torrance GW, Thomas WH, Sackett DL. A utility maximization model for evaluation of health care programmes. Health Serv Res 1972;7:118-33.
43. Nord E. Methods for quality adjustment of life years. Soc Sci Med 1992;34:559-69.
44. Patrick DL, Bush JW, Chen MM. Methods for measuring levels of well-being for a health status index. Health Serv Res 1973;8:228-45.
45. Hughes TE, Coons SJ, Kaplan RM, Draugalis JR. Evaluation of linearity of the Quality of Well-Being Scale using functional measurement theory (abstract). Qual Life Res 1994;3:47-8.
46. Nord E. Toward quality assurance in QALY calculations. Int J Technol Assess Health Care 1993;9:37-45.
47. Kaplan RM, Feeny D, Revicki DA. Methods for assessing relative importance in preference based outcome measures. Qual Life Res 1993;2:467-75.
48. Nord E, Richardson J, Macarounas-Kirchmann K. Social evaluation of health care versus personal evaluation of health states. Int J Technol Assess Health Care 1993;9:463-78.
49. Daniels N. Is the Oregon rationing plan fair? JAMA 1991;265:2232-5.
50. Kaplan RM, Bush JW, Berry CW. The reliability, stability, and generalizability of a health status index. In: Proceedings of the American Statistical Association. Washington, DC: ASA Social Statistics Section, 1978:704-9.
51. Balaban DJ, Fagi PC, Goldfarb NI, Nettler S. Weights for scoring the quality of well-being instrument among rheumatoid arthritics. Med Care 1986;24:973-80.
52. Hughes TE, Coons SJ, Kaplan RM, Draugalis JR. Reweighting the Quality of Well-being Scale in HIV-infected subjects (abstract). Qual Life Res 1994;3:79-80.
53. Kaplan RM. The hippocratic predicament: affordability, access, and accountability in health care. San Diego: Academic Press, 1993.
54. O'Connor GT, Nease RF Jr. The descriptive epidemiology of health state values and utilities. Med Decision Making 1993;13:87-8.
55. Clancy C, Cebul R, Williams S. Guiding individual decisions. A randomized, control trial of decision analysis. Am J Med 1988;84:283-8.
56. Kaplan RM, Bush JW, Berry CC. Health status: types of validity and the index of well-being. Health Serv Res 1976;11:478-507.
57. Torrance GW, Boyle MH, Horwood SP. Application of multi-attribute utility theory to measure social preference for health states. Operations Res 1982;30:1043-69.
58. Feeny D, Furlong W, Boyle M, Torrance GW. Multi-attribute health classification systems: Health Utilities Index. PharmacoEconomics 1995;7:490-502.
59. Boyle MH, Furlong W, Feeny D, Torrance GW, Hatcher J. Reliability of the Health Utilities Index-Mark III used in the 1991 cycle 6 General Social Survey Health Questionnaire. Qual Life Res 1995;4:249-57.
60. The EuroQol Group. EuroQol: a new facility for the measurement of health-related quality of life. Health Policy 1990;16:199-208.
61. Rosser R, Cottee M, Rabin R, Selai C. Index of health-related quality of life. In: Hopkins A, ed. Measures of the quality of life and the uses to which such measures may be put. London: Royal College of Physicians of London, 1992:81-90.

62. Brazier J, Jones N, Kind P. Testing the validity of the EuroQol and comparing it with the SF-36 health survey questionnaire. Qual Life Res 1993;2:169-80.

63. Anderson RT, Aaronson NK, Wilkin D. Critical review of the international assessments of health-related quality of life. Qual Life Res 1993;2:369-95.

64. Essink-Bot ML, Stouthard MEA, Bonsel GJ. Generalizability of valuations on health states collected with the EuroQol-questionnaire. Health Econ 1993;2:237-46.

65. Rosser R, Sintonen H. The EuroQol quality of life project. In: Walker SR, Rosser RM, eds. Quality of life assessment: key issues in the 1990s. London: Kluwer Academic Publishers, 1993:197-9.

66. Rosser R, Allison R, Butler C, Cottee M, Rabin R, Selai C. The Index of Health-Related Quality of Life (IHQL): a new tool for audit and cost-per-QALY analysis. In: Walker SR, Rosser RM, eds. Quality of life assessment: key issues in the 1990s. London: Kluwer Academic Publishers, 1993:179-84.

67. Detsky AS, Naglie IG. A clinician's guide to cost-effectiveness analysis. Ann Intern Med 1990;113:147-54.

68. Mason J, Drummond M, Torrance G. Some guidelines on the use of cost effectiveness league tables. BMJ 1993;306:570-2.

69. Petrou S, Malek M, Davey PG. The reliability of cost-utility estimates in cost-per-QALY league tables. PharmacoEconomics 1993;3:345-53.

70. Hornberger JC, Redelmeier DA, Petersen J. Variability among methods to assess patients' well-being and consequent effect on a cost-effectiveness analysis. J Clin Epidemiol 1992;45:505-12.

71. Bergner M, Bobbitt RA, Carter WB, Gilson BS. The Sickness Impact Profile: development and final revision of a health status measure. Med Care 1981;19:787-805.

72. Boyle MH, Torrance GW, Sinclair JC, Horwood SP. Economic evaluation of neonatal intensive care of very-low-birthweight infants. N Engl J Med 1983;308:1330-7.

73. Oldridge N, Furlong W, Feeny D, Torrance G, Guyatt G, Crowe J, et al. Economic evaluation of cardiac rehabilitation soon after acute myocardial infarction. Am J Cardiol 1993;72:154-61.

74. Cook J, Richardson J, Street A. A cost utility analysis of treatment options for gallstone disease: methodological issues and results. Health Econ 1994;3:157-68.

75. Goodwin PJ, Feld R, Evans WK, Pater J. Cost-effectiveness of cancer chemotherapy: an economic evaluation of a randomized trial in small cell lung cancer. J Clin Oncol 1988; 6:1537-47.

76. Smith TJ, Hillner BE. The efficacy and cost-effectiveness of adjuvant therapy of early breast cancer in premenopausal women. J Clin Oncol 1993;11:771-6.

77. Smith RD, Hall J, Gurney H, Harnett PR. A cost-utility approach to the use of 5-fluorouracil and levamisole as adjuvant chemotherapy for Dukes' C colonic carcinoma. Med J Aust 1993;158:319-22.

7

Health-Related Quality of Life: An Overview

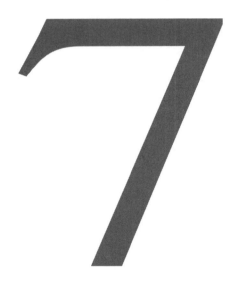

Kathleen M. Bungay
J. Gregory Boyer
A. Bruce Steinwald
John E. Ware, Jr.

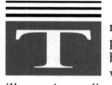raditionally, health has been considered from a medical point of view. From this perspective, discussions of health have been concerned with the activities associated with repairing injury, alleviating pain, and eliminating illness. As medical science has advanced and the conditions under which we live improve, this narrow view of health has become insufficient. Today's health professionals and their patients increasingly are faced with decisions that require a broader definition of health, a definition that considers the patient's entire life, not simply the biologic manifestations of the chronic or acute condition under treatment.

Although this more complete view of health has received much attention during the past decade, it is not a new concept. As long ago as 1948, the constitution of the World Health Organization defined health as more than freedom from disease; instead, it expanded the boundaries of health to include complete physical, mental, and social well-being.[1] Most contemporary health practitioners and health services researchers have adopted this expanded view of health and now strive to consider the impact a disease and its treatment have on patients' lives. The traditional medical approach is essential; however, patients, payers, and policy makers increasingly are demanding explanations as to how the medical care provides/promotes health. These explanations must encompass more than laboratory results and clinical opinions. Information about physical and social functioning and mental well-being are also required to answer the questions now being posed.

These nonclinically defined components of health are currently the focus of a number of studies. An entire area of research has evolved to capture and evaluate data necessary to provide insights into patient outcomes. This area of study is known as health-related quality of life (HRQOL) and is particularly relevant in the healthcare environment of the 1990s.

In the new era that we are entering, information about functional status, well-being, and other important health outcomes will be used both by policy analysts and managers of healthcare organizations. Policy analysts will compare the costs and benefits of competing ways of organizing and financing health cares to obtain the best value for each healthcare dollar spent. The information also will be used by clinician investigators evaluating new treatments and technologies as well as by healthcare practitioners trying to achieve the best possible patient outcomes. The primary source of new information on general health outcomes is standardized patient surveys. These tools are currently becoming accepted by clinicians, but have been serving researchers effectively during the past decade.

HRQOL is a specifically focused area of investigation within the larger field of health services research and/or quality-of-life research. Standardized questionnaires are used to capture HRQOL data in a variety of research settings, either by self-administration, telephone interview, personal interview, observation, or postal survey. In the jargon of this field of research, these standardized questionnaires are often called instruments, tools, surveys, scales, or measures; these terms are used interchangeably in the literature. Psychometrics, the science of testing questionnaires to measure attributes of individuals, is fundamental in the study of HRQOL.

While quality of life refers to an evaluation of all aspects of our lives, including such things as where we live, how we live, how we play, and how we work, HRQOL encompasses only those aspects of our lives that are dominated or significantly influenced by our personal health or activities performed to maintain or improve health.[2] Advances in medical science have encouraged this attention to HRQOL because medical care is no longer limited to providing only death-averting treatments. Today, maintaining or restoring quality of life is an important therapeutic goal for many medical conditions, among them arthritis and diabetes, conditions having no medical cure but for which medical treatment is targeted at controlling disease progression and symptoms. The use of HRQOL measures to capture appropriate data offers a way to monitor disease effects and treatment impacts in terms that are relevant to patients and that reflect the quality of their lives.

Historical View

The use of standardized surveys to assess functional status and well-being can be tracked back over 300 years. Methodologic interest, however, has been greatest during the last half of this century.[3] The psychometric techniques of scale construction, now more widely used in the healthcare field, have been available for most of the past century.[4-6] The study of methods to measure HRQOL began with physicians' attempts to measure patient functioning. The Karnofsky Functional Status Assessment[7] and the New York Heart Association Classification[8] were among the first instruments developed to capture data about a patient's level of physical activity. The first health status instruments sought to distinguish among patients' functional states and included symptoms, anatomic findings, occupational status, and activities of daily living. These early instruments were significant because they provided a standardized approach for physicians to document the consequences of patient care being provided. The early tools found application in inpatient studies designed to evaluate the functional status of patients with severe disabilities.

The first modern health status questionnaires appeared in the 1970s when social scientists and clinical experts came together with a common research agenda to answer questions about the consequences of the medical care provided. Most health measures prior to the 1970s were not based on methods of scale construction. The early tools were quite long, but the data they captured were valid, reproducible, and relevant. Their focus was multidimensional, providing assessments of physical, psychological, and social health.[9] The development, refinement, and use of the early instruments helped to establish the foundation for today's studies.[10] Many of these early measures are still popular today and will be familiar to many readers: Quality of Well-Being Scale,[11] Sickness Impact Profile,[12] the Health Perceptions Questionnaire,[13] and the OARS.[14] Tools of more recent origin include the Duke–UNC Health Profile,[15] the Nottingham Health Profile,[16] and the Medical Outcomes Study 36-Item Short Form Health Survey (MOS SF-36).[10]

Common to all of these assessment tools is a theoretical framework that views the measurement of biologic functioning as an essential but an inadequate component for comprehensively evaluating health. Beyond the documentation of organ system functioning, central to the traditional medical view of health, lies the need to assess general well-being and behavioral functioning. This broader assessment of health is necessary because the basic biologic abnormalities can extend into a person's behavioral functioning and sense of well-being, disrupting the person's HRQOL.[9] The analogy often given of the impact a disease can have on a person's life is that of a rock dropped into the center of a still pond, sending out ripples over the entire surface of the water. All of the variables detailed in Figure 1 must be addressed in an HRQOL assessment if a comprehensive understanding of the patient's condition is to be achieved.

The interest in HRQOL was greatly expanded in 1989 when the US Congress passed the Omnibus Budget Reconciliation Act.[17] This

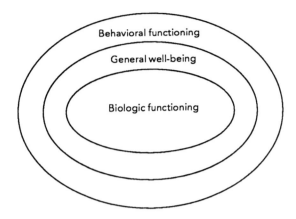

Figure 1. Health status concepts. The impact of a disease and its treatment often affects more than biologic functioning. Biologic abnormalities and imbalances can impact other important areas of a patient's life, including general well-being and behavioral functioning. This impact is comparable to that of a rock hitting the surface of a still pond, sending ripples over the entire water surface. Adapted from Ref. 13.

legislation required the Secretary of Health and Human Services to establish a broad-based, patient-centered outcomes research program, the Agency for Healthcare Policy and Research. Still an active research agenda, the objective of this initiative is to monitor the effectiveness of specific medical treatments by including assessments of patients' functional status, general well-being, and satisfaction with the medical care provided.[17] In addition to research, the Agency promotes clinical practice guidelines, database development, and information dissemination efforts.

Additionally, researchers in both academia and private industry interested in evaluating alternative medical, surgical, and pharmacologic treatments have adopted HRQOL assessments as a valid approach for documenting the consequences of using medications. These specialized researchers look forward to including HRQOL findings in their economic assessments of competing therapeutic options.

Components of Health-Related Quality of Life Measures

HRQOL focuses on those aspects of quality of life that are specifically related to personal health and activities to maintain or improve that level of health. Health is just one of the 12 domains of life identified by Campbell[18] to be considered when researching and evaluating overall quality of life. The other 11 domains are: community, education, family life, friendships, housing, marriage, nation, neighborhood, self, standard of living, and work. Thus, the term "health-related quality of life" has been adopted by researchers to set their research apart from the global concept of quality of life as identified by Campbell and to more accurately reflect the scope of their research.[19]

To provide an assessment of HRQOL one of three approaches is usually taken. Researchers can either select tools that focus on general health status, or they can choose tools that are more narrowly focused on specific aspects of the disease under study. For a comprehensive picture of a patients' HRQOL, it is often desirable to include both types of assessment tools, the general health and the disease-specific, in research projects having an HRQOL objective.

General Health Status Instruments

General health status instruments evaluate aspects of health relevant to all ages, races, sexes, and socioeconomic backgrounds. Questions in a general health status questionnaire are not defined by the disease or disorder under study. These questions have historically covered the full range of the state of disease or illness and have, therefore, emphasized the negative end of the health continuum. Increasingly, this limitation in older general health status instruments is being recognized and outcomes researchers are now constructing general health status tools that extend measurements into the well-being end of the health spectrum.[20]

General health status tools are by definition multidimensional, generally evaluating at least four key health concepts: physical functioning, social and role functioning, mental health, and general health perceptions.

PHYSICAL FUNCTIONING

Physical functioning as it relates to HRQOL assessment generally refers to the limitations or disability experienced by the patient over a defined period. The questions focus on observable and important physical limitations easily noticed and evaluated by the patient or observer. Among such limitations are difficulties in walking, eating, or dressing. In the past, questions concentrated on the negative end of the physical functioning continuum and provided no insight into the "well" range of physical functioning (e.g., playing sports, running).

To be comprehensive, measures of physical functioning should not be confined to limitations and disabilities; rather these measures should include questions covering activities of daily living, energy level, satisfaction with physical condition, and ability to perform all level of activities— from the most basic to the most vigorous. Without questions covering the entire continuum of this domain, only those persons with physical limitations or disabilities will be identified, evaluated, and segmented for

Table 1. General Health Concepts[21]

CONCEPT	DEFINITION
Physical functioning	
physical limitations	limitations in performance of self-care, mobility, and physical activities
physical abilities	ability to perform everyday activities
days in bed	confinement to bed because of health problems
bodily pain	ratings of the intensity, duration, and frequency of bodily pain and limitations in usual activities because of pain
Social and role functioning	
interpersonal contacts	frequency of visits with friends and relatives; frequency of telephone contacts with close friends or relatives during a specific period of time
social resources	quantity and quality of social network
role functioning	freedom from limitations due to health in the performance of usual role activities such as work, housework, school activities
Mental health	
anxiety/depression	feelings of anxiety, nervousness, tenseness, depression, moodiness, down-heartedness
psychological well-being	frequency and intensity of general positive affect
behavioral/emotional control	control of behavior, thoughts, and feelings during specific periods
cognitive functioning	orientation to time and place, memory, attention span, and alertness
General health perceptions	
current health	self-rating of health at present
health outlook	expectations regarding health in the future

research purposes; any differences among respondents without significant physical limitations or disabilities will be lost by assessments that do not include the well end of the range.

In addition to physical limitations, specific concepts often included in general health status questions are physical abilities, days in bed, bodily pain, and, more recently, physical well-being. Table 1 provides basic definitions of these components of the physical domain of general health assessments.[21]

SOCIAL AND ROLE FUNCTIONING

Although social and role functioning are often thought of as a single entity and used interchangeably, they are distinct concepts in terms of HRQOL. Social functioning addresses the extent a person participates in social interactions as well as the satisfaction derived from these interactions and the social network established. Role functioning questions are concerned with a patient's duties and responsibilities that are limited by health.

Social Functioning. Social functioning is defined as the ability to develop, maintain, and nurture mature social relationships. Social well-being is separated into two areas: (1) the frequency of social contacts, and (2) the nature of those contacts within the social network or community. Both of these areas must be considered together. Evaluating only the frequency of contacts in isolation from the nature of those contacts may offer no insight or the wrong insight into the person's state of social functioning; therefore, including a person's assessment of the adequacy of his or her social network is essential when evaluating social functioning in the context of HRQOL. It is known that belonging to a community, family, or neighborhood provides a strong sense of being wanted, loved, or valued[22] and has significant influence on assessments of mental as well as social health.[23]

Role Functioning. Role functioning is concerned with the impact health has on a person's ability to meet the demands of his or her normal life role. Work for pay, homemaking duties, and schoolwork all are covered by this concept. A role function assessment should identify everyday role situations or activities that can be directly affected or limited by disease, illness, or treatment. Although most role limitations are the result of physical health problems, role limitations have been observed both in the presence and in the absence of physical limitations.[24]

MENTAL HEALTH

Disease often affects behavioral as well as physical aspects of a person's life. General health status assessments therefore usually include questions covering aspects of psychological health. These questions typically focus on the frequency and intensity of symptoms of psychological distress. Anxiety and depression are common themes in mental health components of general health status instruments; however, scales focusing only on these two concepts do not adequately cover the full mental health continuum. Perceptions of psychological well-being, life satisfaction, and cognitive functioning also are needed if a comprehensive assessment of the mental health domain by an HRQOL instrument is to be achieved.[25] It is important to note that general health status questionnaires covering the mental health domain are not intended for use as diagnostic tools; however, some questions have been used as screens for certain disorders (e.g., depression).[21]

GENERAL HEALTH PERCEPTIONS

General health perceptions address overall beliefs and evaluations about health. Questions covered in this area focus on health preferences, values, needs, and attitudes. Assessments of general health perceptions are necessary because they allow consideration of individual differences in reactions to pain, perceptions of difficulty, the level of effort required, or the degree of worry or concern about health.[1]

Unlike questions that focus on measures of limitations, pain, or dysfunction used to assess other health domains, questions covering general health perceptions address positive feelings or can be positively framed, allowing the full spectrum of HRQOL to be evaluated.

Disease-Specific Health Status Instruments

Often it is necessary to focus on the particular impact that a certain disease has on patients. In such cases, general health status tools are inadequate for providing the information needed. To overcome this limitation, condition- or disease-specific measures often are used to supplement the general health status instrument. The more narrowly focused disease-specific measure requests detailed information on the patient's perspective on the impact of a disease and its treatment. Additionally, using disease-specific measures allows inclusion of domains of specific interest for the disease under study and the patients it affects. Among the specific areas previously investigated with disease-specific questionnaires are sexual and emotional functioning, nausea and vomiting, pain, anxiety and depression, asthma, and rhinitis.[26-31]

Psychometrics

The literature is ever expanding with reports of general health and disease-specific HRQOL research. As with any field of research, the studies being reported meet various levels of scientific rigor. Readers of these reports must have a basic understanding of psychometrics to draw appropriate conclusions from HRQOL findings.

Psychometrics is the science of using standardized tests or scales to evaluate attributes of an individual. It is used in the field of health assessment to translate people's behavior, feelings, and personal evaluations into quantifiable data. These data, once captured, must be both relevant and correct if they are to provide useful insights into HRQOL.

There are two psychometric properties that any measurement scale or instrument must possess: reliability and validity. Additionally, useful measuring scales must be sensitive to change and must be accepted by the investigators and respondents. Each of these properties will be discussed in turn.

RELIABILITY

When measuring reliability, the scientist is concerned with the relationship between true variation and random error.[32] Evaluations assess the consistency and repeatability of measurements. Reliability is expressed as decimal values between 0.0 and 1.0, with values closest to 1.0 indicating little chance variance. A reliability estimate of 0.85 reveals that 85% of the observed variance in the data is true variance and 15% of the observed variance is the result of chance. If there were no chance variance or random error in the measurement, the reliability estimate would be 1.0.

Reliability estimates are useful because they allow the researcher to examine the consistency of results from different measures thought to evaluate the same thing.[33] These estimates can be obtained by capturing data using the same tool on repeated administrations or by using alternative forms of a measure.

Stability of the responses is desired when evaluating reliability using the same tool on different occasions with the same study population. This approach is commonly called the test–retest procedure. It is, however, usually inadequate as the only determinant of an instrument's reliability. This method assumes that during the time interval between the two tests there will be : (a) no recall of the original response, (b) no change in the attribute being evaluated, and (c) no change in the respondent. Because health and disease are dynamic processes, ensuring that no change in the respondent occurs between the original assessment and the repeated assessment is particularly difficult. The time interval between administration of the tests is critical and must always be known before one can have any confidence in a test–retest of reliability. It has been noted that researchers relying on the test–retest method will most likely underestimate an instrument's reliability rather than overestimate it.[31]

The *alternative forms method* of estimating reliability avoids some of the problems inherent in the test–retest method. This approach requires that alternative, equivalent questionnaires be administered to the same individuals at the same time. The correlation between the scores provides an estimate of the reliability of the measure.

Rather than have equivalent forms of the same instrument (a difficult task certainly!), a useful approach is the *split-half method.* As its name implies, this method compares the score derived from half of the items with the score obtained from the other half. Convenient approaches to accomplish this are to compute a scale score using the even numbered items and a second score using the odd numbered items. If the original measure has been developed appropriately to measure a single health concept, the correlation between the two halves should be strong (i.e., close to 1.0).

An expansion of the split-half approach is the coefficient alpha estimate (often calculated using Cronbach's Coefficient Alpha). This estimate is essentially the average of all possible split-half correlations[34] and is known as the *internal consistency reliability estimate.*

It is important to note that reliability estimates are influenced by the number of items in the measure. Logically, the more questions asked about a particular subject, the more information will be gained from the inquiry. This trade-off between reliability and length of the measure is discussed in greater detail later in this chapter.

Acceptable reliability coefficients vary depending on what is being analyzed and to what end the findings will be used. Comparisons at the individual patient level require high reliability estimates (values greater than 0.90). For group comparisons, reliability estimates between 0.50 and 0.70 are considered acceptable.[35]

VALIDITY

A number of key questions must be answered if researchers are to have confidence in the data captured using HRQOL instruments. All are related to the validity of the assessment. Do the questions in the instrument really measure the concept under study? Do respondents understand the questions being asked? Are the response categories appropriate for the questions?

Validity refers to the extent to which differences in test scores reflect the true differences in individuals under study. Although it is the goal to elicit observed differences that are indeed true differences among respondents, factors such as how the measure is administered, who administers it, where it is administered, and when it is administered can affect responses across study participants; these factors can add a degree of uncertainty to the findings of an HRQOL assessment. There are no standard guidelines for validating health measures.

However, standards established by the American Psychological Association,[36] the American Educational Research Association, and the National Council on Measurement in Education have found application in evaluating measures.[37]

The types of validation necessary and most applicable to HRQOL measures are content, construct, and criterion.[27] Each of these three types of validity will be briefly covered below.

Content Validity. Researchers measuring content validity are concerned with how well the health concept is captured by the items in the measure. A scale with good content validity is one that covers all aspects of the concept being addressed. To establish content validity, a comparison is made between the items included in a scale and some definitional standard for which there is general acceptance. This type of validation assumes the researcher has confidence in the definitional standard. Additionally, the individual items included in the scale all must "appear" to measure the concept under study; this special type of content validity is commonly called face validity.

Construct Validity. The central question asked when determining construct validity is whether the health measure relates to other measures or variables in plausible ways. Evaluating scale scores in various patient groups known to differ in relevant ways (e.g., age, sex) is a frequent approach for determining construct validity. Validity is supported when scale scores for each patient group reflect the known group differences. Hypothesized relationships between relevant clinical parameters and scale scores often are evaluated to establish construct validity.

Convergent and discriminant validity are special types of construct validity. For convergent validity, correlations should be high between similar or related measures of the same health concept. For discriminant validity, correlations should be low between scales evaluating very different health concepts. Observing these expected or hypothesized relationships is evidence of construct validity. For example, if an instrument has construct validity, items designed to measure physical activity, mobility, and physical functioning should have high correlations with each other and should each have low correlations with measures of mental health such as anxiety or depression.

Criterion Validity. Criterion validity requires the comparison of a scale score with a known "gold standard." Unfortunately, there are no gold standards against which HRQOL measures can be evaluated. It is acceptable practice, however, to use longer, well-validated measures of HRQOL as criteria for evaluating the validity of shorter, newly developed measures. Because this approach uses a proxy as a criterion, it is more appropriately called criterion-related validity.[31]

For example, two external variables with known characteristics, such as resource use (dollars) and age (years), can be used to assess a relationship with physical and mental health concepts. An investigator would hypothesize and test that health status and resource use are negatively correlated; similarly, age and physical health should produce a negative correlation. Thus, resource use and age compared with patients' assessments of their physical and mental health are examples of useful ways to investigate the criterion-related validity.

A final word on validation is warranted. Without an understanding of the validity of an HRQOL scale, changes or differences in score are meaningless. Validation is, however, a continuous process. Each new use of an HRQOL scale provides new information about the interpretation and meaning of scores. Stewart notes that "there is no one point at which a measure is considered valid."[33] Certainly, a single study is inadequate to thoroughly provide validation of an HRQOL measure.

▬▬ SENSITIVITY

Perhaps the least well studied and documented aspect of HRQOL measures at this time is that of sensitivity.[33] Researchers evaluating sensitivity are concerned with detecting the true changes that occur in a health concept over time. It is important when assessing sensitivity that measures of change over time cover the entire range of a particular health concept. That is, they should extend from the severe limitations to well-being. This permits investigators a continuum of responses over which to detect changes. It has been suggested that sensitive measures should be stable in patients who do not change clinically and should shift in patients who do experience clinical changes.[38,39]

Sensitivity can be affected greatly by the simple choice of response options. Crude measures may use only the dichotomous yes/no response options. More advanced measures use graduated response categories, allowing respondents to record varying amounts of an attribute. An example of a frequently used graduated response option contrasted with a dichotomous yes/no response option is found in Table 2.

===== ACCEPTABILITY FOR USE

Both investigators and respondents will have valuable opinions about the acceptability of various HRQOL instruments. How easy the measure is to use, to score, and to interpret are all valid concerns. The completion rate, the extent of missing data, and the number and nature of complaints about the tool are all clues about the acceptability of the measure for use in a research or clinical setting. Acceptability also is expressed as respondent burden. Regardless of the administration format (self-administered, telephone interview, personal interview, observation, or postal survey), failure to consider respondent burden can doom any survey project.

Today's researchers strive to achieve a balance between an increase in reliability (achieved by asking more questions) and an increase in respondent burden (achieved with fewer questions). Some short-form multi-item scales derived from much longer measures are now in use. These short forms achieve an acceptably high level of precision when compared with their longer parent versions and are much less burdensome to both respondents and investigators. The MOS SF-36[40] and the 17-item Duke Health Profile[34,41] are two examples of short-form scales.

===== ## The Future of Health-Related Quality of Life Research

The agenda for the future of HRQOL research and its application is quite full. HRQOL measures appearing today are shorter and more user friendly than earlier versions. These shorter tools are gaining acceptance in clinical practice as well as industry and academic research. Future efforts require interpretation of patient scores and amalgamation of data from patient scores with traditional biologic markers of disease. Future research will test the use of these combinations in therapeutic decision-making as

Table 2. Example of Dichotomous and Graduated Response Options

Dichotomous

During the past 4 weeks, has nausea affected your daily functioning?

Yes [ ]

No [ ]

Graduated

How often during the past 4 weeks has nausea affected your daily functioning?

all of the time	[ ]
most of the time	[ ]
a good bit of the time	[ ]
some of the time	[ ]
a little of the time	[ ]
none of the time	[ ]

well as in monitoring therapy. Only through knowledge of the HRQOL of very healthy individuals, very disabled individuals and those in between, can findings from HRQOL research have meaning and find application. Establishing community norms and characteristic patterns within population segments also are important research objectives of many contemporary scientists.

The future research agenda focuses on the use of these instruments for three different, but interrelated purposes: (1) to continue to measure or define health states, (2) to assist with monitoring patient care, and (3) to be used as information with which to manage an individual patient's care.

Each of these three purposes is illustrated with examples. Findings from the MOS have been instrumental in measuring and defining health. Information gained from the use of these tools in clinical drug trials has assisted in furthering that mission and has enabled the exploration of how to use HRQOL assessments as monitoring parameters. Finally, the clinical application of HRQOL research is just now beginning to be realized. The routine use of this information as a management tool in making decisions about therapy has yet to be fully implemented.

THE MEDICAL OUTCOMES STUDY

Much has been and continues to be learned about measuring and defining health from the MOS.[42-44] (Tarlov, JAMA 1989, Stewart 1989, Wells 1989). In the MOS, a comprehensive approach to the assessment of health was first embraced. One of the major objectives of the MOS was to develop practical tools for monitoring patient outcomes and their determinants in routine medical practice. In particular, the study was designed to evaluate the impact of chronic disease on patient functioning and well-being and to determine if key features of medical care are associated with more favorable patient outcomes. Today, after eight years and baseline data on over

22,000 patients, information from approximately 2500 patients followed over four years continues to inform the research agendas.[45,46] This study is described more fully elsewhere.[47]

QUALITY OF LIFE RESEARCH IN CLINICAL TRIALS

Research on furthering the use of HRQOL instruments as a monitoring tool in clinical practice has been conducted in the context of clinical drug trials. However, clinical trial planning is driven largely by corporate needs to develop products and obtain regulatory approval to market them. With the recognition and demand for information about product attributes beyond traditional measures of safety and efficacy in the US and abroad, the only practical opportunity to conduct patient-based research on a product's attributes has been to integrate HRQOL components with Phase II, III, or IV studies. The results of this combination have been synergistic. Both clinical practice and the science of psychometrics has benefited from the resulting information of these combined studies.

Perspectives from which to Evaluate HRQOL Research from Clinical Trials. The current and future importance of the results from HRQOL studies depends, in large part, on how the information will be used as well as whose perspective is being considered. In the regulatory setting, HRQOL endpoints are included in clinical trials both to enhance product approval and to support promotional claims that will be made when the product is brought to market. To date, the Food and Drug Administration (FDA) has not published specific guidelines on when HRQOL endpoints are important for regulatory purposes. Yet, there is a clearly growing recognition within the FDA of the relevance of HRQOL data to establish product efficacy as well as a clear intention to regulate HRQOL claims.[48] Indicative of this intent was the distribution of the draft "Principles for the Review of Pharmacoeconomic Promotion" by FDA officials at a conference on treatment comparison studies in March 1995.

The results of these clinical trials with HRQOL data included are increasingly present in both the general medical literature and in medical specialty journals from which clinicians derive new information for patient care decisions. Another trend that has added relevance to the HRQOL data is the shift of the focus of decision-making away from individual practitioners to provider organizations, such as managed care and managed pharmacy benefit programs. These organizations systematically seek information on product attributes, including HRQOL data, to assist in decisions regarding which products to acquire or recommend to participating practitioners.

Payers also are using the results of HRQOL studies. In the world of increasing cost consciousness, it is tempting to assume that the payer concern is to minimize cost and the HRQOL benefits of a new product are not germane. Although clearly concerned with cost, payers are generally more interested in maximizing the value of healthcare purchases than in minimizing costs. The principal payers for health services in the US are employers, who act as advocates for their employees on many fronts. Employers generally will not withhold health services for covered indications from employees unless the costs are shown to exceed the value of the services. Moreover, employers have unions, courts of justice, and government regulations to contend with if they are seen to be sacrificing employee health in an effort to economize in healthcare costs.

Acceptance of the relevance of the results of HRQOL studies to payer coverage and related decisions has paralleled acceptance within the community of practitioners. Many of the specific decisions about product or technology coverage and payment are made by medical directors or technology advisory committees, who look to the same clinical journals for scientific, peer-reviewed evidence of HRQOL benefits. A final perspective is that of patients and organizations that represent patient interests. HRQOL results may become important support for disease areas where patient advocacy is strong, such as AIDS, cancer, and arthritis.

Strategic Considerations in Implementing HRQOL Assessments in Clinical Trials. The identification of potential uses for HQL data does not imply that an HRQOL assessment should be performed in every clinical trial. Deciding in which trials to include these assessments and which not to is an important strategic decision, especially in the case of complex, multinational clinical testing programs that involve many trials of the same product in varying formulations for different indications. Such decisions should be made with a clear idea of what purpose the HRQOL results will serve.

When recombinant epoetin alfa for treatment of anemia in endstage renal disease was examined in Phase III clinical trials, for example, the FDA was concerned about how the therapy would affect the lives of those treated.[49] The principal clinical endpoint, change in hematocrit concentration, was seen as insufficient to gauge the human impact, and a major quality-of-life component was integrated into this pivotal clinical trial. In this instance, there was clearly a regulatory need for quality-of-life information. Because the vast majority of persons with this disease in the US are covered by Medicare as part of the End-Stage Renal Disease Program, there was an important payer use for the data as well. Medicare program administrators were interested in the HRQOL benefits to the affected beneficiary population. This concern contributed to the decision to include HRQOL assessments in the Phase IV epoetin alfa studies.

Many HRQOL assessments focus on side effects rather than treatment effects. An example is the series of studies reported on the HRQOL of alternative antihypertensive therapies.[50,51] In this instance, the HRQOL consequences of side effects were highlighted in head-to-head comparisons of drugs with the same indications. The data reported could be useful for clinicians.

Another important strategic consideration for integrating HRQOL assessments in clinical trials is the compatibility between the clinical and HRQOL objectives. An example is a clinical study described to one of us (ABS) of a product indicated for treatment of skin ulcers. This is an area that generates considerable skepticism among payers. Thus, data showing improvement in HRQOL from a well-controlled study might have influenced payers to accept the product. The trial design specified that eligible patients would have wounds on opposing limbs, with one limb randomized to receive experimental treatment and the other conventional treatment. Although the design was created to reduce large variability introduced by outside factors in the clinical data analysis, the protocol was incompatible with designing a meaningful HRQOL assessment.

Although this is an extreme example, it illustrates that achieving compatibility between clinical and HRQOL study objectives is important when planning research. This is especially true when the purpose of collecting the information and reporting the results is to provide information to more than one party, such as regulatory agencies and payers or physicians.

Finally, real-world confirmation of findings from clinical trial results is becoming increasingly important among providers and payers charged with making cost-conscious decisions regarding the acquisition and financing of technology. To respond to this need, researchers will need to continue studies on HRQOL into Phase IV trials and independent effectiveness research to provide evidence of the durability of HRQOL benefits in clinical practice.

Using Health-Related Quality-of-Life Assessments in Routine Patient Care

Standardized measures capturing patient perspectives on their physical functioning, social and role functioning, mental health, and general health perceptions are likely to appear in routine patient records in the near future. Comparing an individual's scores with regional or national norms may provide clues to hidden health problems. A series of HRQOL assessments taken over time can provide the clinician with valuable information.

In a report of experiences using patient-based HRQOL assessments to monitor patient care in a busy dialysis clinic, Meyer et al.[52] related that HRQOL surveillance has provided more than a quantitative expression of the staff's intuition. The activity also reveals new information that is qualitatively different from the assessments that are otherwise made in the care of patients. The authors suggest that patient-based assessment can improve individual treatment regimens and can contribute to the epidemiology of treatment.

To the individual patient, HRQOL assessments offer a language in which to phrase experiences that may be difficult to express, are recognized only when prompted, or may not be remembered clearly later. It provides a thread along which to reconstruct those experiences. By objectifying the patient's subjective experience, HRQOL assessment makes that experience more consistently accessible to the staff who share responsibility for the patient's care. It puts the patient's experience on the agenda for discussion, regardless of whether the technical aspects of care need attention. Meyer et al.[52] argue that clinicians can make meaningful interpretations of an individual patient's score and that these interpretations enhance rather than simply summarize the collective understanding of a conscientious medical team.

It is important to note that if responses to health status assessments are understood as a form of speech, then by entering the results of HRQOL assessment into the medical record, the patient is being asked to make entries in the record. A health status database offers patients who wish to do so the opportunity to share their experiences over the course of illness and treatment with other patients who face similar clinical situations. Such a database could also be a valuable tool for clinicians trying to help patients make decisions.

Pharmacoeconomists, too, will find increasing use for HRQOL research. As the techniques for including patient preferences in economic assessments improve, pharmacoeconomists will be a primary user of HRQOL measures. Regardless of the final shape healthcare reform takes, patients, who can chose providers or healthcare programs, and payers, who can restrict or limit coverage, will continue to require answers to their questions about the outcomes of medical care options and will continue to demand high-quality outcomes. Providing these answers will remain a key objective of industry and academic researchers and clinical practitioners. It is feasible that the future will find HRQOL assessments remaining central to many research agendas and an accepted component of clinical practice.

Summary

The study of HRQOL requires a multidimensional approach. Assessments must include components that evaluate, at a minimum, the health concepts of physical functioning, social and role functioning, mental health, and perception of general health. Additionally, the full continuum of these concepts must be included, from the most limited to the most healthy. Approaches to capture HRQOL data include the self-administered questionnaire, personal interview, telephone interview, observation, and postal survey. The assessment instruments must possess acceptable reliability, validity, and sensitivity, and they must be accepted by the investigators as well as the participants. Psychometrics is an essential part of

HRQOL research, especially in today's research environment that requires shorter, more focused measures. Application of HRQOL research findings is just now beginning to be realized; however, as cost pressures continue to dominate health care, these research results will most certainly play an important role in documenting the outcomes of treatment and in justifying prescribed therapies.

References

1. World Health Organization. Basic documents: World Health Organization. Geneva, Switzerland: World Health Organization, 1948.

2. Bungay KM, Ware JE. Measuring and monitoring health-related quality of life. Kalamazoo, MI: Upjohn, 1993.

3. Katz S, Ford AB, Moskowitz RW, Jacobson BA, Jaffe MW. Studies of illness in the aged. The index of ADL: a standardized measure of biological and psychosocial function. JAMA 1963;185:914-9.

4. Guttman LA. A basis for rescaling qualitative data. Am Soc Rev 1944;9:139-50.

5. Likert R. A technique for the measurement of attitudes. Arch Psychol 1932;140:5-55.

6. Thrustone LL, Chage EJ. The measurement of attitude. Chicago: University of Chicago Press, 1929.

7. Karnofsky DA, Burchenal JH. The clinical evaluation of chemotherapeutic agents in cancer. In: Macleod CM, ed. Evaluation of chemotherapeutic agents. New York: Columbia Press, 1949:191-205.

8. Criteria Committee, New York Heart Association. Nomenclature and criteria for diagnosis of diseases of the heart and great vessels. 8th ed. Boston: Little Brown and Company, 1979.

9. Ware JE Jr. Scales for measuring general health perceptions. Health Serv Res 1976; 11:396-415.

10. Ware JE Jr, Sherbourne CD. The MOS 36-item short-form health survey (SF-36). Med Care 1992;30:473-82.

11. Fanshel S, Bush JW. A health-status index and its application to health-services outcomes. Operations Res 1970;18:1021-66.

12. Bergner M, Bobbitt RA, Kressel S, Pollard WE, Gilson BS, Morris JR. The sickness impact profile: conceptual formulation and methodology for the development of a health status measure. Int J Health Serv 1976;6:393-415.

13. Ware JE. Conceptualizing and measuring generic health outcomes. Cancer 1991; 67(suppl 3):774-9.

14. Pfeiffer E, ed. Multidimensional functional assessment: the OARS methodology. Durham, NC: Duke University Press, Center for the Study of Aging and Human Development, 1975.

15. Parkerson GR Jr, Gehlback SH, Wagner EH, James SA, Clapp NE, Muhlbaier LH. The Duke-UNC health profile: an adult health status instrument for primary care. Med Care 1981;19:806-28.

16. Hunt SM, McEwen J, McKenna SP. Measuring health status: a new tool for clinicians and epidemiologists. J R Coll Gen Pract 1985;35:185-8.

17. Omnibus Reconciliation Budget Act, 1989. Public Law 101-239. Washington, DC: Government Printing Office, 1989.

18. Campbell A. The sense of well-being in America: recent patterns and trends. New York: McGraw-Hill, 1981.

19. Patrick DL, Erickson P. Assessing health-related quality of life for clinical decision making. In: Walker SR, Rosser RM, eds. Quality of life: assessments and application. Lancaster, England: MTR Press, 1988:9-49.

20. Ware JE Jr. Measuring functioning, well-being and other generic health concepts. In: Osoba D, ed. Effect of cancer on quality of life. Boca Raton, FL: CRC Press, 1991:7-23.

21. Ware JE Jr. Standard for validating health measures: definition and content. J Chron Dis 1987;40:473-80.

22. Greenley JR. The measurement of social support. In: Donald CA, Ware JE Jr, eds. Research in community and mental health. Greenwich, CT: JAI Press, 1984;4:325-70.

23. Wortman CB. Social support and the cancer patient: conceptual and methodologic issues. Cancer 1984;53:2339-62.

24. Sherbourne CD, Stewart AL, Wells KB. Role functioning measures. In: Stewart AL, Ware JE Jr, eds. Measuring functioning and well being: the Medical Outcomes Study approach. Durham, NC: Duke University Press; 1992:205-19.

25. Veit CT, Ware JE Jr. The structure of psychological distress and well-being in general populations. J Consult Clin Psycol 1983;51:730-42.

26. Patrick DL, Deyo RA. Generic and disease-specific measures in assessing health status and quality of life. Med Care 1989;27(suppl):S217-32.

27. Wu AW, Rubin HR, Mathews WC, Ware JE, Brysk LT, Hardy WD, et al. A health status questionnaire using 30 items from the Medical Outcomes Study: preliminary validation in persons with early HIV infection. Med Care 1991;29:786-98.

28. Juniper EF, Guyatt GH. Development and testing of a new measure of health status for clinical trials in rhinoconjunctivitis. Clin Exp Allergy 1991;21:77-83.

29. Juniper EF, Guyatt GH, Ferrie PJ, Griffith LE. Measuring quality of life in asthma. Am Rev Respir Dis 1993;147:832-8.

30. Schipper H, Clinch A, McMurray A, Levitt M. Measuring the quality of life of cancer patients. The functional living index—cancer: development and validation. J Clin Oncol 1984;2:472-83.

31. Meenan RF. The AIMS approach to health status measurement: conceptual background and measurement properties. J Rheumatol 1982;9:785-8.

32. Selitiz C, Wrightsman LS, Cook SW. Research methods in social relations. 3rd ed. New York: Holt Rinehart and Winston, 1976:169-97.

33. Stewart AL. Psychometric considerations in functional status instruments. In: Functional status measurement in primary care. New York: Springer-Verlag, 1990:3-26.

34. Cronbach LJ, Warrington WG. Time-limit tests: estimating their reliability and degree of speeding. Psychometrika 1951;16:167-88.

35. Helmstadter GC. Principles of psychological measurement. New York: Appleton-Century-Crofts, 1964.

36. Standards for educational and psychological testing. Washington, DC: American Psychological Association, 1985.

37. Ware JE Jr. Measures for a new era of health assessment. In: Stewart AL, Ware JE, eds. Measuring functioning and well-being: the Medical Outcomes Study approach. Durham, NC: Duke University Press, 1992:3-11.

38. Deyo RA, Patrick D. Barriers to the use of health status measures in clinical investigation, patient care, and policy research. Med Care 1989;27(suppl);5254-68.

39. Launois R. Quality of life: overview and perspectives. Eurotext 1992;28:3-24.

40. McHorney CA, Ware JE, Rogers W, Raczek A, Lu JFR. The validity and relative precision of MOS short- and long-form health status scales and Dartmouth COOP charts. Med Care 1992;30(suppl 5):MS253-65.

41. Parkerson GR, Broadhead WE, Tse CK. Comparison of the Duke health profile and the MOS short-form in healthy young adults. Med Care 1991;29:679-83.

42. Tarlov A, Ware JE, Greenfield S, Nelson EC, Perrin E, Zubkoff M. The Medical Outcomes Study: an application of methods for monitoring the results of medical care. JAMA 1989;7:925-30.

43. Stewart AL, Greenfield S, Hays RD, Wells K, Rogers WH, Berry SD, et al. Functional status and well-being of patients with chronic conditions: results from the Medical Outcomes Study. JAMA 1989;7:907-13.

44. Wells KB, Stewart A, Hays RD, Burnam MA, Rogers W, Daniels M, et al. The functioning and well-being of depressed patients: results from the Medical Outcomes Study. JAMA 1989;7:914-9.

45. McHorney CA, Ware JE, Lu JFR, Sherbourne CD. The MOS 36-Item Short Form Health Survey (SF-36): III. Tests of data quality, scaling assumptions, and reliability across diverse patient groups. Med Care 1994;32:40-66.

46. Ware JE, Kosinski M, Keller SD. SF-12: how to score the SF-12 physical and mental health summary scales. Boston: The Health Institute, New England Medical Center, March 1995.

47. Stewart AL. The Medical Outcomes Study framework of health indicators. In: Stewart AL, Ware JE, eds. Measuring functioning and well-being: the Medical Outcomes Study approach. Durham, NC: Duke University Press, 1992:12-24.

48. Temple R. Quality of life assessment in the drug approval process. Drug Information Association Meeting, Washington, DC, January 18, 1994.

49. Evans RW, Rader B, Manninem DC. The quality of life of hemodialysis recipients treated with recombinant human erythropoetin. JAMA 1990;263:825-30.

50. Croog SH, Levine S, Testa MA, Brown B, Bulpitt CJ, Jenkins CD, et al. The effects of antihypertensive therapy on quality of life. N Engl J Med 1986;314:1657-64.

51. Testa MA, Anderson RB, Nackly JF, Hollenberg NK. Quality of life and antihypertensive therapy in men. N Engl J Med 1993;328:97-113.

52. Meyer KB, Espindle DM, De Giacomo JM, Jenuleson CS, Kurtin PS, Danes AR. Monitoring dialysis patient's health status. Am J Kidney Dis 1994;24:267-79.

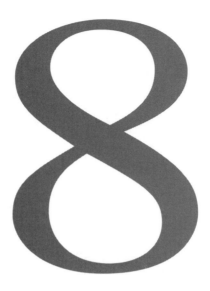

Decision Analysis and Pharmacoeconomic Evaluations

Judith T. Barr
Gerald E. Schumacher

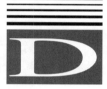ecisions. They are a fact of everyday life. Whether at home or in clinical practice, decisions must always be made. From a decision as mundane as whether to go to a movie or a concert to a clinical consideration of which antibiotic to select, decisions span a range of complexity. Using the techniques of reasoned guess, gut-reaction, or intuition in our decision-making process, our usual course of action is to implicitly consider the decision, its options, and possibly the near-term consequences. If other considerations are recognized, they are somehow factored into the process in an ad hoc juggling act. This chapter demonstrates that the decision process can be improved and that decision analysis can be an important tool in pharmacoeconomic evaluations.

 ## What Is Decision Analysis?

Our intuitive decision-making capabilities are limited, and we rarely attempt an explicit examination of all factors affecting a decision and its outcome. But, our decisions can be improved through the use of the explicit structure and quantitative techniques of decision analysis—a systematic approach to decision-making under conditions of uncertainty. Since few decisions are accompanied with absolute certainty of the consequences of their outcomes, decision analysis can be used to assist the decision-maker to (1) identify the available options when faced with a decision, (2) predict the consequences or outcomes of each option, (3) assess the likelihood or probability of the identified possible outcomes, (4) determine the value of each outcome, and (5) select the decision option that will yield the best payoff. Decision analysis not only forces an explicit, orderly, and careful consideration of a variety of important issues, but it provides insight into the process of decision making.

Decision analysis is explicit—it forces you to structure the decision you face as well as identify the consequences of the possible decision outcomes. It is quantitative—it forces you to assign numbers to probability estimates and outcome valuations. And, it is prescriptive—the analysis identifies the route to take to maximize the expected value of the decision.

The origins of decision analysis, as well as many of the techniques presented in this book, can be traced to the British during World War II when principles of game theory, systems analysis, and operations research were applied to decisions involving allocation of scarce resources. By the 1950s, these techniques were combined in the business world into the evolving field of decision analysis. The late 1950s saw the beginning of medical applications[1] and the approach reached the medical literature in the early and mid 1970s.[2-4] Cost-benefit, cost-effectiveness, and cost-utility are extensions of the decision analysis technology.[5]

Decision analysis is now an integral component of business school curricula as universities prepare future managers to make better allocative and strategic decisions. From Raiffa's classic lectures[6] to decision support computer packages, decision analysis is now central to modern business and economic decisions.

In healthcare fields, a review article identified nearly 200 decision analysis citations from the clinical literature that assist in decisions related to one or more of 13 categories of clinical problems.[5] In the medical community, decision analysis is being "institutionalized." The Society for Medical Decision Making was established in 1977 and publishes a quarterly journal, *Medical Decision Making;* clinical decision consultation services have been established to provide assistance with complex patient-specific decisions;[7] and the American Association of Medical Colleges has recommended the inclusion of clinical decision analysis in the undergraduate medical curriculum. In pharmacy several introductory articles have been published[8-10] and over 75 studies have used decision analysis to examine drug-related decisions with multiple options under conditions of uncertainty. Several of these studies are reviewed at the end of the chapter.

First, however, this chapter provides the opportunity to apply decision analysis to the process of combining the economic considerations of administrators with the associated health consequences of concern to clinicians. The steps and techniques of the decision analysis process are illustrated by their application to a decision facing a pharmacy and therapeutics (P&T) committee.

As you will see in the following case, decision analysis is a method with techniques to analyze situations. But perhaps more importantly, the use of decision analysis engenders an attitude toward the problem or decision—to think more analytically; to force the consideration of consequences of actions; to explicitly recognize that uncertainty is present, to estimate the degree of uncertainty, and to assess *your* attitude toward risk; to determine which are the relevant outcome measures; and to value *your* preferences for alternative outcomes.

The Case

Consider that alphazorin and omegazorin are the only Food and Drug Administration–approved members of a new (fictional) class of antibiotics. Both are effective against gram-negative bacteria that are resistant to multiple antibiotics, and both block the transfer of extrachromosomal resistance factors between bacterial cells. In clinical trials, 95% of the cases of gram-negative septicemia were susceptible to alphazorin; 87% were susceptible to omegazorin. Although omegazorin has a higher incidence of drug-associated toxicity, the concentrations of both must be maintained within a narrow therapeutic range. Toxic adverse effects for both include diarrhea and vomiting (gastrointestinal [GI] toxicity), hepatic enzyme alterations (hepatotoxicity), and megakaryocyte suppression (hematotoxicity).

The initial expenses of a 10-day course of intravenous alphazorin q8h are $1100 for the direct and indirect costs associated with drug acquisition and storage and $360 for dispensing and administration ($12/dose); for intravenous omegazorin q6h, the respective costs are $700 and $480 ($12/dose). Although alphazorin has the higher costs, it also has the higher percentage of successfully treated cases of gram-negative bacteremia and a lower incidence of drug-associated toxicity. Important characteristics for each antibiotic are summarized in Table 1.

The P&T committee has decided to approve the addition of at least one of these antibiotics to its formulary, but which one? How can it combine all the factors necessary to reach its decision—the cost of the antibiotics, the difference in susceptibility/resistance rates, the varying toxicity and subtherapeutic response rates, and the classification accuracy of the serum drug concentrations (SDCs)?

The application of decision analysis involves six major steps:

1. Identify the decision, including the selection of the decision options to be studied. Bound the timeframe of the decision and determine from which perspective the decision is to be made.
2. Structure the decision and the consequences of each decision option over time.

Table 1. Characteristics of Alphazorin and Omegazorin

CHARACTERISTIC	ALPHAZORIN	OMEGAZORIN
Cost of 10-day course of therapy	$1100	$700
Dosage regimen	q8h	q6h
Resistance rate	5%	12%
Drug-related toxicities		
gastrointestinal symptoms	7%	10%
hepatotoxicity	1.5%	3.5%
hematotoxocity	0.4%	1.5%
Subtherapeutic response rate	10%	15%
Characteristics of SDC at COL_t		
predictive value positive	80%	90%
predictive value negative	90%	85%
Characteristics of SDC at COL_s		
predictive value positive	90%	87.5%
predictive value negative	80%	90%

COL_s = subtherapeutic cut-off level; COL_t = toxic cut-off level; and SDC = serum drug concentration.

3. Assess the probability that each consequence will occur.
4. Determine the value of each outcome (e.g., in dollars, quality-adjusted life-years saved, utilities).
5. Select the option with the highest expected outcome.
6. Determine the robustness of the decision by conducting a sensitivity analysis and varying the values of probabilities and outcomes over a range of likely values.

The definitions and conventions of clinical decision analysis as presented by Weinstein and Fineberg[11] will be used throughout the chapter.

Identify and Bound the Decision

The ground rules of the decision are set at this stage. Who will be the decision-maker and what perspective will be considered? What is the decision and what options will be considered? Over what time span will the consequences be analyzed? The answers to these questions are necessary to properly structure the decision and to collect the appropriate data.

WHO WILL BE THE DECISION-MAKER?

This question is asked primarily to determine from what perspective the analysis is to be conducted. Is it from the point of view of the pharmacy department, the hospital, an insurance company, or a health maintenance organization? If we are considering the decision's impact on the financial resources of a unit, the type of unit will make a difference as to whether to measure costs or charges, which costs or charges to include, and over what time period they should be collected. For example, if the decision is being considered based on the financial impact to the pharmacy department, only the drug acquisition costs and the pharmacy-associated direct and indirect costs of the drug's storage, dispensing, administration, and monitoring would be included. On the other hand, a health maintenance organization would consider all inpatient and outpatient charges and costs related to the entire episode of care; an insurance company would be most interested in the episode-of-care charges covered under the terms of the insurance policy.

In this hypothetical case, the analysis will be conducted from the hospital's perspective. Therefore, in addition to the drug-related costs, the costs of all hospital goods and services during the hospitalization period generally are included in the study. However, since the P&T committee already has decided to add at least one of the drugs to the hospital formulary, it is not necessary to calculate the non–drug-related costs of an uncomplicated, 10-day hospital stay for intravenous treatment of similar gram-negative infections because they are the same for both alphazorin and omegazorin. Rather, the additional direct and indirect costs associated with the drugs and the consequences of their respective therapies will be included: drug acquisition, storage, and dispensing; drug administration; and additional monitoring and laboratory costs, hospital stay, and pharmacokinetic and infectious disease consultations due to bacterial resistance, adverse toxic or subtherapeutic consequences of the antibiotic, or of misclassification errors of the SDCs.

WHAT IS THE DECISION, ITS OPTIONS, AND THE DECISION CRITERIA?

The P&T committee has decided to add one member of the new antibiotic class to its formulary. Therefore, the decision is, Which of the two antibiotics will be added to the formulary?; this is the decision for which the decision tree will be constructed and the analysis performed. The decision options are alphazorin and omegazorin.

What decision criterion is to be used to select between the two antibiotics? The criterion is linked to the type of analysis to be performed. If cost and lives saved are selected, it would be a cost-effectiveness study; if cost and utilities are measured, it would be a cost-utility assessment. All of the previously described pharmacoeconomic analyses can use the steps and structure of clinical decision analysis; only the unit of outcome measurement would differ.

For this illustrative example, we will simplify the decision analysis process by considering only one form of outcome—economic costs. We can justify this approach, because in our fictional example, prior research documented that although the efficacy of the two drugs differed, the overall episode of care survival rates were equal. When an organism was resistant to either alphazorin or omegazorin, the course of therapy was switched to a restricted antibiotic, betasporin, resulting in equal effectiveness in the overall episode of care. Therefore, because the committee's two selected measures of outcome effectiveness (i.e., infections resolved and lives saved) were equal, this analysis is a cost minimization study[12] and only financial costs will be considered as the outcome measure. If noneconomic outcomes were not equal, then outcomes expressed in units of effectiveness or utilities also would need to be measured.

To standardize the analysis, the committee selected gram-negative septicemia as the base case since it is representative of the type of infections to be treated with these antibiotics. Now the decision criterion is clarified: the analysis will direct the decision-maker to the antibiotic that results in the lower expected cost for treatment of this representative infection.

Decision analysis uses the structure of a decision tree to organize the elements involved in the decision. A decision tree starts with the choice alternatives. In the "scientific notation" of decision analysis, a choice node (a square) indicates a point in time when the decision-maker can select one of several options or actions. The initial choice node is placed at the far left and designates the beginning of the decision tree; the possible options (alphazorin and omegazorin) then originate as branches to the right of this initial choice node. This tree will provide an explicit structure for this cost study. The start of the decision tree is displayed in Figure 1.

Following the selected decision criterion, the branch option with the lower expected cost will be the antibiotic selected for addition to the formulary.

OVER WHAT TIME SPAN WILL THE ANALYSIS APPLY?

The time period will begin with the initiation of either antibiotic to treat gram-negative septicemia (analysis limited to culture-confirmed cases) and end with the resolution of the infection.

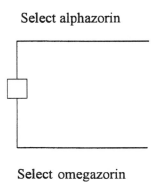

Figure 1. Initial choice node of decision tree to select addition to formulary.

☰ Develop a Decision Tree-Structure the Decision and Its Consequences Over Time

This is one of the most powerful features of decision analysis. The decision-maker is forced to explicitly structure the situation, thus changing the unexamined, intuitive process into one in which the thought process is clearly articulated. Laying out the tree prods the decision-maker to identify the relationships that exist between the decision options and the consequences of selecting each alternative. The tree becomes a tool to assist in thinking through a decision as well as to assist in communication among individuals and departments working on the same analysis. With a decision tree, coworkers can identify where they agree or disagree in the considered alternatives and consequences, suggest additional consequences that must be included in the tree, or recommend that a branch be trimmed.

Given the decision options originating from the initial choice node, the consequences of each action must be determined. These consequences are chronologically structured over time in a decision tree by asking a series of "what if" questions. This section will structure the decision tree and detail the consequences of the actions. The next section examines how likely each of these consequences is to occur, and the section after that determines the cost implications of each option.

What if patients with septicemia are given alphazorin? As the consequences are described, follow the alphazorin branch of the decision tree in Figure 2 and the omegazorin portion of the tree in Figure 3. In this section we will develop the structure for the decision tree. Later in this case, you can use this structure as a template to insert probabilities converted from results of a clinical trial, to assign cost outcomes to each consequence, and then to calculate the preferred course of action.

First, the outcome at this branch is no longer under the control of the decision-maker; some of the patients will respond and some will not. A chance node, indicated by a circle inserted in the appropriate branch, notes the point in time when the decision-maker loses control of the decision process, when future events are beyond the control of the decision-maker, and the outcome is uncertain. To assist you as the tree is developed, all chance nodes are indicated by a letter. In this case, the chance node is inserted in both the alphazorin and omegazorin branches, and the responding/nonresponding consequences are identified (nodes A and M, respectively).

In the "responding" branch of the alphazorin tree, if the fever recedes and the laboratory results indicate response to the antibiotic, the balance of the 10-day course of therapy may continue uneventfully or the patient may develop toxicity (node B). Three principal types of toxic reactions occur (node C): (1) GI effects, such as nausea, vomiting, and diarrhea, which usually occur on day 3 of therapy, (2) hepatotoxicity with elevated liver

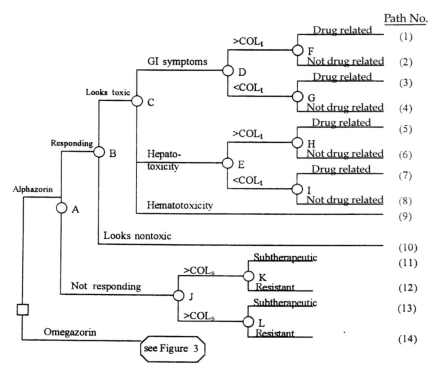

Figure 2. Alphazorin portion of decision tree showing initial decision selection, consequences of selecting alphazorin, chance nodes identified, and decision paths numbered. COL_s = subtherapeutic cut-off level; COL_t = toxic cut-off level; GI = gastrointestinal.

function enzymes and reduced liver function (day 5), and (3) hematotoxicity (day 6).

However, not all toxic symptoms in these patients are related to the antibiotic; rather, they can be associated with other medications or related to the nature of the patient's underlying illness. SDCs are used to determine if the toxicity is drug related. Therefore, a chance node with two branches follows each of the indicated toxicities—either the concentration is above or below the toxic cut-off level (COL_t). This occurs at nodes D and E in Figure 2 for alphazorin and nodes P and Q in Figure 3 for omegazorin.

It is rare when a test clearly separates one patient population from another; generally, there are areas of overlap.[13] As shown in Figure 4, three patient classifications are associated with SDCs: the patients' responses are either subtherapeutic, therapeutic, or toxic. However, setting a COL_t or a subtherapeutic cut-off level (COL_s) does not clearly separate these three classifications, and classification errors will occur. Referring to the COL_t, most of the SDCs above it are associated with drug-related toxicities (true

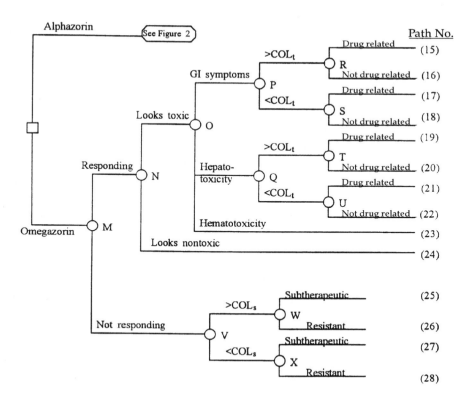

Figure 3. Omegazorin portion of decision tree showing initial decision, consequences of selecting omegazorin, chance nodes identified, and decision paths numbered. COL_s = subtherapeutic cut-off level; COL_t = toxic cut-off level; GI = gastrointestinal.

positive, "a" in Figure 4), but some patients with non–drug-related toxic symptoms also have high concentrations (false positive, "b"). And, for concentrations below the COL_t, most are associated with a therapeutic response (true negative, "d"), but there are some patients who have concentrations below the COL_t who do have drug-related toxicities (false negative, "c"). The same overlap, and resultant misclassification errors, also occurs between the subtherapeutic and therapeutic classifications.

Therefore, to display both the correct and incorrect classifications based on the COL_t, a chance node with drug- and non–drug-related toxicity branches follow all greater than COL_t (nodes F, H, R, and T) and less than COL_t (nodes G, I, S, and U). At this point, we are developing only the structure of the tree; in the next section we will incorporate information concerning the ability to separate toxic from nontoxic conditions related to alphazorin and omegazorin dosing based on the SDC.

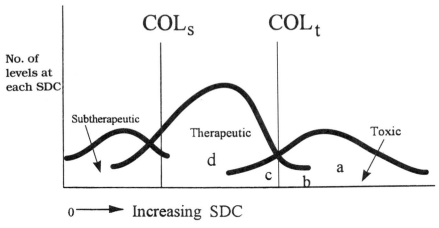

Figure 4. Frequency of patients whose response is subtherapeutic, therapeutic, and toxic at increasing serum drug concentration. a = patients with concentrations above the COL_t who have drug-related toxicities (true positive); b = patients with concentrations above the COL_t whose toxic symptoms are not drug related; c = patients with concentrations below COL_t who have drug-related toxicities (false negative); d = patients with concentrations below COL_t who have a therapeutic response with no toxic symptoms (true negative).

Additional consequences occur at many of these branches; for example, the misclassification of concentration below the COL_t as non–drug-related when the symptoms really are associated with drug toxicity, can lead to continuation of the antibiotic, the development of more serious adverse effects, and longer hospital stays. To simplify the decision tree, such additional consequences are not further detailed as additional branches in this tree, but are considered explicitly in the cost implication section.

In the "not responding" branch, SDCs are used to distinguish between two patient populations: (1) those with bacterial infections that are susceptible to the antibiotic but who are receiving inadequate dosages resulting in subtherapeutic concentrations; and (2) those with bacterial infections that are resistant to the antibiotic. Again, the SDC is used to differentiate between the two populations, but misclassification errors occur when the COL_s is applied.

Most SDCs that are above the COL_s are from nonresponding patients with resistant organisms; however, some are from patients who, while the concentration is above the COL_s, have subtherapeutic responses (node K). Rather than receiving the needed dosage adjustment, the antibiotic will be changed unnecessarily, thereby inducing additional hospital charges. On the other hand, most patients with concentrations below the COL_s, have susceptible infections and the dosage needs to be increased (node L). However, patients with low concentrations and resistant organisms are placed at risk because, rather than switching to a more appropriate antibiotic, the dosage is increased in response to the low SDC, and the course of ineffective therapy is lengthened.

The alphazorin and omegazorin sections of the decision tree, with all decision options and drug selection consequences chronologically arranged from left to right, is now complete. All decisions under the control of the decision-maker are indicated by choice nodes; all outcomes left to chance and beyond the control of the decision-maker are indicated by chance nodes. There are 14 possible outcomes for each drug selection (indicated by a number on the right side of each decision path in Figures 2 and 3). A decision path is a sequence of actions and events beginning with the decision at the initial choice node and following the consequences of that decision in a unique line from left to right through subsequent chance and/or choice nodes.

Although the inclusion of SDCs and the interpretation of whether the results indicate drug or non–drug-related toxicities add to the complexity of this decision tree, they explicitly must be recognized as elements of the complete decision process. To assume that all toxic symptoms are drug related or that all SDCs above the COL_t are toxic introduces error into the pharmacoeconomic analysis. It is important to recognize that clinical decision analyses that incorporate diagnostic tests also must include the possibility that the test results do not cleanly separate those with from those without disease. A good exercise is to examine a published pharmacoeconomic assessment and translate it into the decision tree format. It is very likely that you will find that the consequences of the decision are not completely specified, and if diagnostic tests are included in the management of the disease, the uncertainty associated with them is not factored into the decision process.

Note that the consequences of selecting alphazorin or omegazorin are represented by the same structure. If the consequences are the same, why are the two antibiotics not considered equal? First, the likelihood or probability of occurrence of each of the consequences differs between the two drugs; and second, the cost of the antibiotics as well as the cost of each decision path also differs. These are examined in the following two sections.

Assess Probabilities

The probabilities associated with the various consequences for each antibiotic have been calculated from a large randomized study of patients with possible gram-negative septicemia: half of them received alphazorin and the other half omegazorin. The first 1000 patients receiving alphazorin with gram-negative bacteria confirmed by culture comprise the alphazorin probability data set. The same method was used for the omegazorin probability estimates. The P&T committee has determined that the patient conditions and consequences in the clinical trial are representative of the patients at the hospital. The outcome results of the 2000 patients are summarized in Table 2.

The sum of the probabilities of all consequences originating from a chance node must be 1.0; therefore, it is essential that all possible consequences be identified at each chance node. Because there is a 100% certainty that something will happen at each chance node, nodes with probabilities totaling less than 1.0 do not have all consequences identified and, thus, have been incompletely specified. The probabilities associated with each branch originating from a chance node are displayed adjacent to the respective branch in Figures 5 and 6. They have been calculated as follows.

Of the 1000 patients receiving alphazorin, 850 (85%) responded with a reduction in temperature and change in the hematologic parameters and 150 (15%) did not respond. The probability of response/nonresponse are entered in the decision tree on the two branches originating from the alphazorin branch at the initial choice node (node A). Of the 850 responding patients, 680 (80%) had no toxic symptoms and 170 (20%) had possible drug-related toxicities (node B). Of the 170 patients with toxic symptoms, 131 (77%) experienced GI toxicity, 35 (20.6%) had elevated liver function enzymes suggestive of drug-related hepatotoxicity, and 4 (2.4%) had a marked reduction in platelet numbers and function (node C).

Serum alphazorin concentrations were determined in all patients with toxic symptoms. Eighty-one of 131 patients (62%) with GI symptoms had SDCs above the COL_t (node D). At node E, 16 of 35 patients (45.7%) with hepatotoxicity had SDCs above the COL_t, and 4 of 4 patients (100%) with hematotoxicity had SDCs above that level. However, as discussed earlier, the COL_t cannot be used to clearly identify those with and those without drug-related toxicities.

Measures of a test's predictive ability, predictive value-positive (PV+) and predictive value-negative (PV−) can be helpful. PV+ answers the question: Given a positive test result, what is the probability that the patient has the disease? For tests involving therapeutic drug monitoring, the question translates to: Given a concentration above the COL_t, what is the probability that the concentration is from a patient who has drug-related toxicity? For serum alphazorin concentrations, the PV+ is 80% (nodes F and H). Conversely, the probability that a concentration above the COL_t is from a patient whose toxicity is not drug-related is presented by the mathematical expression 1 − PV+, or 20% for alphazorin.

Similarly, the PV− answers the question: Given a negative test result, what is the probability that the patient does not have the disease. For therapeutic drug monitoring, that question translates to: Given a concentration below the COL_t, what is the probability that the concentration is from a patient who does not have drug-related toxicity? For serum alphazorin concentrations, the PV− is 90%. The probability that a concentration below the COL_t is from a patient with a drug-related toxicity is 1 − PV−, or 10% (nodes G and I).

Table 2. Outcomes of Patients Receiving Alphazorin and Omegazorin

OUTCOME	NO. OF PATIENTS					PATH NO.
Alphazorin (n = 1000)						
Responding					850	
symptoms resembling toxicity				170		
gastrointestinal toxicity			131			
$>COL_t$		81				
drug related	65					1
not drug related	16					2
$<COL_t$		50				
drug related	5					3
not drug related	45					4
hepatotoxicity			35			
$>COL_t$		16				
Drug related	13					5
Not drug-related	3					6
$<COL_t$		19				
Drug related	2					7
Not drug-related	17					8
hematotoxicity			4			9
no toxic symptoms				680		10
Not responding					150	
$>COL_s$				50		
subtherapeutic			10			11
resistant			40			12
$<COL_s$				100		
subtherapeutic			90			13
resistant			10			14
Omegazorin (n = 1000)						
Responding					730	
symptoms resembling toxicity				235		
gastrointestinal toxicity			164			
$>COL_t$		102				
drug related	91					15
not drug related	11					16
$<COL_t$		62				
drug related	11					17
not drug related	51					18
hepatotoxicity			56			
$>COL_t$		36				
drug related	32					19
not drug related	4					20
$<COL_t$		20				
drug related	3					21
not drug related	17					22
hematotoxicity			15			23
no toxic symptoms				495		24
Not responding					270	
$>COL_s$				110		
subtherapeutic			10			25
resistant			100			26
$<COL_s$				160		
subtherapeutic			140			27
resistant			20			28

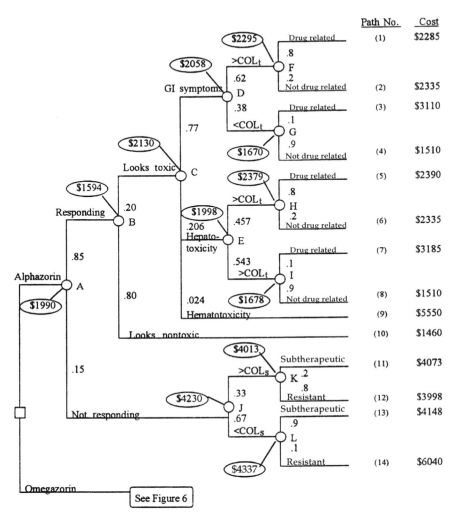

	Path No.	Cost

Figure 5. Alphazorin portion of structured decision tree including probabilities, outcome valuations in dollars, and expected cost of the alphazorin option. COL_s = subtherapeutic cut off level; COL_t = toxic cut-off level; GI = gastrointestinal.

In the nonresponding population, 100 of 150 patients (67%) had SDCs below the COL_s; the remaining 50 (33%) had results above the COL_s (node J). At this lower cut-off level, the PV+ is the proportion of concentrations below the COL_s that are from patients receiving a therapeutic dosage but who have a subtherapeutic response, or 90% for alphazorin. Ten percent of results below the COL_s are associated with resistant organisms (node L). PV− is the proportion of concentrations above the COL_s that are from pa-

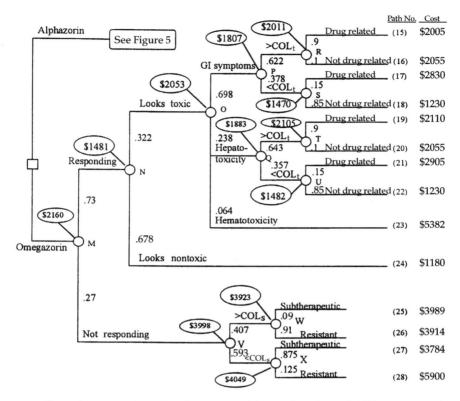

Figure 6. Omegazorin portion of structured decision tree including probabilities, outcome valuations in dollars, and expected cost of the alphazorin option. COL$_s$ = subtherapeutic cut off level; COL$_t$ = toxic cut-off level; GI = gastrointestinal.

tients with resistant organisms, or 80% for alphazorin. The remaining 20% are from patients whose concentrations are above the COL$_s$ but who need a higher dosage to obtain a therapeutic response (node K).

Different probabilities are associated with the population receiving omegazorin. Fewer of the causative organisms were susceptible to this drug (88% vs. 95%), and there was a higher incidence of drug-related toxicity (15% vs. 8.9%). Of the 1000 patients receiving this medication, 730 (73%) responded to the medication (node M); 495 of these (67.8%) had no toxic symptoms, while 235 (32.2%) did (node N). Of the patients with possible toxicity, 164 (69.8%) had GI symptoms, 56 (23.8%) had elevated liver function enzymes, and 15 (6.4%) had marked platelet dysfunction (node O).

At nodes R and T, 90% of the results above omegazorin's COL$_t$ are from patients with drug-related toxicities (PV$^+$ = 0.90), and at nodes S and

U, 85% of results below the COL_t are from patients without drug-related toxicities ($PV^- = 0.85$). In the nonresponding population, of the 59.3% with results below COL_s 140 of 160 patients (87.5%) are receiving an insufficient dosage and 12.5% have resistant organisms (node X). Of the 110 patients (40.7%) with results above the COL_s, 100 (91%) are associated with resistant organisms and 9% with subtherapeutic responses (node W).

To practice translating clinical data into probabilities for various chance nodes, we suggest you use the information in Table 2 to determine and insert probabilities into Figures 2 and 3. As you now can see, although the structures of the alphazorin and omegazorin tree are the same, the probabilities assigned to each chance node are not because of differences in outcomes of the clinical trials.

It must be noted that this is an ideal database, one rarely found in the clinical literature. As more clinical decisions are based on the cost and consequences of effective rather than efficacious care, it is essential that the collection of this type of patient outcome probability information become routine practice. An accurate cost impact assessment is not possible unless it is linked to the probabilities of clinical consequences. Until the pharmacoepidemiologic data are available, probability estimates can be generated using expert opinions, Delphi techniques, and meta-analysis of reports in the literature. The reader is referred to other sources for a critique of probability estimates resulting from methods other than direct clinical studies.[14,15]

Value Outcomes

The P&T committee has decided to value the outcomes by determining the monetary value of drug, drug-related, and drug-induced costs per case of septicemia. The drug costs include the direct and indirect expenses of drug acquisition and storage: a 10-day course costs $1100 for alphazorin and $700 for omegazorin. Drug-related costs consist of a $12 direct and indirect cost each time either drug is administrated. Alphazorin is administered every eight hours, resulting in a cost of $360 for 10 days of therapy; omegazorin is administered every six hours, costing $480 for the same length of therapy. When a change of therapy is indicated because of suspected bacterial resistance, a 10-day course of intravenous betasporin is initiated costing $1200 in drug and $240 in drug-related costs.

Drug-induced costs are those expenses incurred from the follow-up created by less-than-optimal response to either alphazorin or omegazorin. These costs, calculated by the input component method and incorporating direct and indirect expenses, include $650 per extra day of hospital stay, additional laboratory tests ($50/SDC, $35/liver function enzyme concentration, $40/platelet count), component therapy ($200/packed red blood cell transfusion and platelet concentrate), $75 per pharmacokinetic consult, and $250 per infectious disease and hematology consultation.

The costs of drug, drug-related, and drug-induced inputs required for each decision path in the alphazorin section of the decision tree are summarized in Table 3, and for the omegazorin tree in Table 4. The path costs are entered at the right of each path on the decision trees in Figures 5 and 6.

Choose the Preferred Course of Action—Calculate the Expected Cost for Each Decision Outcome

How does one combine the various decision options, probability estimates, and outcome valuations to choose the preferred course of action? How does one "solve" a decision tree?

First, it is necessary to break the decision tree into its component parts and analyze smaller sections. This is done in reverse order of the tree's development, starting from the right and working back to the initial decision or choice node on the left. The process is called "averaging out and folding back" since each path's outcome value is weighted by its probability of occurrence (averaging out) working from right to left, from outcomes to options (folding back).

At each chance node, outcome values (costs) are combined with, and weighted by, their respective probability of occurring. This yields an expected cost at each chance node. For illustration, a section of the alphazorin limb of the decision tree is reproduced in Figure 7. Starting on the top right with those patients who have GI symptoms and have SDCs above the COL_t, 80% will have alphazorin-related toxicity with an associated average cost of treatment of $2,285. However, 20% of the patients with high SDCs will not have drug-related toxicity; their dosage will be reduced unnecessarily and will result in an average cost of $2,335 for path 2. To calculate the expected cost of patients with GI symptoms and with alphazorin concentrations above the COL_t (node F), the cost of each outcome is weighted by the probability of its occurrence and then added to the weighted costs of all other outcomes originating from the same chance node. The expected cost at each chance node appears in a bubble attached to the respective node in the tree.

$$(80\% \times \$2285) + (20\% \times \$2335) = \$2295$$

For patients with GI symptoms and concentrations below the COL_t, 90% of the symptoms were non–drug-related at a cost of $1510. However, 10% of these concentrations will be from patients with drug-related toxicity. Their dosage will be continued, leading to additional toxicity and extended hospitalizations at an average cost of $1670. The expected costs of patients with GI symptoms whose concentrations are below the COL_t (node G) are calculated as follows:

$$(10\% \times \$3110) + (90\% \times \$1510) = \$1670$$

Table 3. Outcome Costs ($) Associated with Consequences of Alphazorin-Treated Septicemia

PATH NO.	CLINICAL CONDITION AND TREATMENT	DRUG	DRUG-RELATED	DRUG-INDUCED					TOTAL
				1[a]	2[b]	3[c]	4[d]	5[e]	
1	Drug-related GI symptoms, >COL_t, dosage adjusted	1100	360	650	100		75		2285
2	Non–drug-related GI symptoms, >COL_t, dosage reduced unnecessarily	1100	360	650	150		75		2335
3	Drug-related GI symptoms, <COL_t, delay in dosage adjustment	1100	360	1300	200		150		3110
4	Non–drug-related GI symptoms, <COL_t, therapy continued	1100	360		50				1510
5	Drug-related liver toxicity, >COL_t, dosage adjusted	1100	360	650	100	105	75		2390
6	Non–drug-related liver toxicity, >COL_t, dosage reduced unnecessarily	1100	360	650	150		75		2335
7	Drug-related liver toxicity, <COL_t, delay in dosage adjustment	1100	360	1300	100	175	150		3185
8	Non–drug-related liver toxicity, <COL_t, therapy continued	1100	360		50				1510
9	Drug-related hematotoxicity, drug switched (6 d alphazorin, 4 d betasporin)	1140	360	2600		800	150	500	5550
10	Uncomplicated response	1100	360						1460
11	Subtherapeutic response, >COL_s (3 d alphazorin, 10 d betasporin)	1530	468	1950	50		75		4073
12	Resistant, >COL_s (3 d alphazorin, 10 d betasporin)	1530	468	1950	50		150		3998
13	Subtherapeutic response, <COL_s, dosage adjusted, 13 d	1430	468	1950	150		150		4148
14	Resistant, <COL_s, adjust dosage (5 d); switch to betasporin (10 d)	1750	540	3250	100		150	250	6040

COL_s = subtherapeutic cut-off level;
COL_t = toxic cut-off level; GI = gastrointestinal.
[a] Extra hospital day, $650/day.
[b] Drug concentration determination, $50 each.
[c] Extra laboratory costs including component therapy.
[d] Pharmacokinetic consultation, $75 each.
[e] Hematology or infectious disease consultation, $250 each.

Table 4. Outcome Costs ($) Associated with Consequences of Omegazorin-Treated Septicemia

PATH NO.	CLINICAL CONDITION AND TREATMENT	DRUG	DRUG-RELATED	DRUG-INDUCED					TOTAL
				1[a]	2[b]	3[c]	4[d]	5[e]	
15	Drug-related GI symptoms, >COL_t, dosage adjusted	700	480	650	100		75		2005
16	Non–drug-related GI symptoms, >COL_t, dosage reduced unnecessarily	700	480	650	150		75		2055
17	Drug-related GI symptoms, <COL_t, delay in dosage adjustment	700	480	1300	200		150		2830
18	Non–drug-related GI symptoms, <COL_t, therapy continued	700	480		50				1230
19	Drug-related liver toxicity, >COL_t, dosage adjusted	700	480	650	100	105	75		2110
20	Non–drug-related liver toxicity, >COL_t, dosage unnecessarily reduced	700	480	650	150		75		2055
21	Drug-related liver toxicity, <COL_t, delay in dosage adjustment	700	480	1300	100	175	150		2905
22	Non–drug-related liver toxicity, <COL_t, therapy continued	700	480		50				1230
23	Drug-related hematotoxicity, drug switched (6 d omegazorin, 4 d betasporin)	900	432	2600		800	150	500	5382
24	Uncomplicated response	700	480						1180
25	Subtherapeutic response, >COL_s (3 d omegazorin, 10 d betasporin)	1410	504	1950	50		75		3989
26	Resistant, >COL_s, (3 d omegazorin, 10 d betasporin)	1410	504	1950	50				3914
27	Subtherapeutic response, <COL_s dosage adjusted, 13 d	910	624	1950	150		150		3784
28	Resistant, <COL_s, adjust dosage (5 d); switch to betasporin (10 d)	1550	600	3250	100		150	250	5900

COL_s = subtherapeutic cut-off level;
COL_t = toxic cut-off level; GI = gastrointestinal.
[a]Extra hospital day, $650/day.
[b]Drug concentration determination, $50 each.
[c]Extra laboratory costs including component therapy.
[d]Pharmacokinetic consultation, $75 each.
[e]Hematology or infectious disease consultation, $250 each.

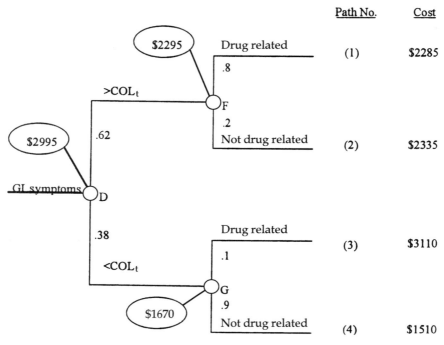

Figure 7. Section of alphazorin portion of decision tree. COL$_t$ = toxic cut-off level, GI = gastrointestinal.

The next step back to the origin, or left, of the tree requires determination of the average expected cost of all patients with GI symptoms. At the next chance node, the expected costs of patients with SDCs above and below the COL$_t$ are combined with their respective probability of occurring. There is a 62% probability that the concentration will be above the COL$_t$: that condition has an expected cost of $2295. There also is a 38% probability that the concentration will be below the COL$_t$, with an expected cost of $1670. Therefore, the expected cost of all patients with GI symptoms (node D) is:

$$(62\% \times \$2295) + (38\% \times \$1670) = \$2058$$

The averaging out and folding back process continues until the expected costs are determined for the two branches originating from the initial choice node. These have been calculated and appear in Figures 5 and 6. The expected cost of the alphazorin option is $1990 and the omegazorin option, $2160.

Thus, although the acquisition price of omegazorin is $400 lower than that of alphazorin, the institutional costs associated with omegazorin's higher resistance rate and increased drug-related toxicities increase omega-zorin's total septicemia treatment costs to be more than those of alphazorin. If the P&T committee had based its decision on the lower acquisition cost, it would have selected omegazorin, the selection with the higher overall treatment cost. That decision would have reduced the cost impact on the pharmacy budget, but would have created higher overall costs for the hospital. By using decision analysis and adopting an institutional perspective that included the cost consequences, not just acquisition costs, of the two antibiotics, the P&T committee arrived at a drug selection decision that will reduce the impact on institutional expenses. This analysis should be used to argue that, in this treatment decision, an increase in the pharmacy's drug acquisition budget will result in a savings to the institution.

From the identification of the decision options, the time frame, the decision criteria, and the objectives of the decision-maker; through the structuring of the decision and the identification of all consequences; to probability assessment and outcome valuation; the selection now has had an explicit, structured, analytic, and quantitative assessment with a preferred action course identified—only alphazorin should be added to the formulary.

Literature Examples of Clinical Decision Analysis in Drug-Related Studies

In a review of articles published from 1979 to 1990, Elixhauser et al.[16] identified 3,206 studies that used either cost-benefit or cost-effectiveness analysis. From that compendium, we attempted to identify and analyze the pharmaceutical-related publications that incorporated decision analysis as the underlying structure. To these we added other, more recent, investigations that examined prophylaxis, treatment, or interpretation options using decision analysis.

Three published case studies apply decision analysis to therapeutic selection and/or action.[17-19] Not only are these articles valuable examples of clinical applications of decision analysis, they also provide good discussions of the sources and quality of data used in the decision analysis process.

Gottlieb and Pauker[17] described a patient with acute myelogenous leukemia who likely has candidal esophagitis and, quite possibly, a disseminated fungal infection. But, without a confirmation of systemic mycosis, do the known risks of systemic amphotericin therapy outweigh the possible benefits? A tree was constructed, probabilities were estimated from the literature and then modified by expert opinion, and the outcome of each action consequence was measured as quality-adjusted life-months, a metric to combine quality and quantity of life. Based on this analysis and the assessment that the patient had a least a 30% probability of having systemic mycosis, the amphotericin action option was estimated to yield the highest number of quality-adjusted life-months.

Plante and Pauker[18] used a computer program, Decision Maker, to construct a decision tree with 773 paths (!) to consider whether a patient with enterococcal endocarditis, but with a possible history of penicillin hypersensitivity, should receive penicillin. Probabilities were determined from the literature and outcomes were valued using a complex morbidity and mortality utility scale. The article has an extensive discussion of data sources and data quality. The analysis indicated that penicillin is the preferred course of therapy based on this patient's clinical condition and other data sources.

Cuchural et al.[19] examined whether immunosuppression should be continued in a transplant patient with malignant melanoma. Probabilities were estimated from the literature and outcome expressed in quality-adjusted life-expectancy. This outcome unit uses the patient's preferences to determine the quality adjustment for the various outcome states. Based on the patient's preferences, his medical history, and probabilities from the literature, the decrease in life expectancy associated with an additional melanoma did not warrant discontinuation of the immunosuppressive drugs.

Examples of decision analysis applied to drug-related prophylaxis decisions include the cost-effectiveness of whether infants should be universally vaccinated against hepatitis B,[20] whether BCG vaccine should be used in homeless shelters,[21] the cost effectiveness of whether newborns should be screened for sickle cell disease and prophylactic penicillin given to infants who test positive to prevent pneumococcal sepsis,[22] whether chemoprophylaxis for tuberculosis in patients with diabetes will increase the years of life expectancy,[23] the cost effectiveness of whether patients with artificial joints[24] or mitral-valve prolapse[25] should receive antibiotic prophylaxis for dental procedures, the benefit-cost analysis of whether antimicrobial prophylaxis should be used in abdominal and vaginal hysterectomy,[26] the cost effectiveness of which prophylaxis method should be used to prevent deep vein thrombosis during major orthopedic surgery,[27] whether anticoagulant prophylaxis in heart disease reduces the rate of thromboembolism,[28] whether estrogen replacement therapy extends life-expectancy in menopausal women,[29-31] and the economic implications of whether misoprostol should be used to prevent gastric ulcers in patients taking nonsteroidal antiinflammatory drugs.[32-35]

Decision analysis studies also have been used to select among treatment options: whether to biopsy, treat, or wait in suspected herpes encephalitis[36] and selection among therapeutic strategies for treatment of streptococcal pharyngitis,[37,38] otitis media,[39] papulopustular acne,[40] chloroquine-resistant malaria,[41] Kawasaki syndrome,[42] endocervical gonorrhea coinfected with *Chlamydia trachomatis*,[43] and serious infections.[44-46] Hillner et al. used a decision analysis model to examine the cost-effectiveness of adjuvant chemotherapy in women with node-negative breast cancer[47,48] and in cancer treatment in general.[49]

In a series of articles, Schumacher and Barr[13,50-54] applied decision analysis techniques to the interpretation and characterization of SDCs, therapeutic ranges, and threshold probabilities to guide appropriate ordering of tests to monitor drug concentrations. They have asked such questions as: How can the patient's prior probabilities be incorporated with the information provided by a SDC to produce a patient-specific interpretation of the meaning of a patient's drug concentration? What are the inherent misclassification errors of serum drug testing for such drugs as digoxin, theophylline, aminoglycosides, and phenytoin? What are the implications of this information for the usefulness of the therapeutic range?

Decision analysis also has been used in administrative decisions. Schechter[55] and Kresel et al.[56] have applied decision analysis to selecting drugs to add to the formulary. In a health policy application, Oster et al.[57] used the techniques of decision analysis to assess the value and risks to consumers of switching histamine$_2$-blockers from a prescription to over-the-counter products.

And lastly, not all articles with decision analysis in the title are decision analysis studies. Unfortunately, the number of cost-effectiveness and decision analysis articles submitted to clinical journals can exceed the capacity of the editors to obtain expert reviews. Therefore, articles occasionally are published that do not meet the criteria of the claimed analysis. For example, a 1985 article applied "decision analysis" to the purchase of frozen premixed intravenous admixtures.[58] While this was a structured decision process, a decision tree was not created, consequences were not identified, and probabilites were not estimated. The analytic process used in the study was not decision analysis; however, it was similar to another form of structured decision-making, multiattribute utility theory (MAUT).

When this type of error occurs, it is likely to recur. Individuals planning studies use published research designs as models for their future investigations. Now the original error gets compounded. In this case, the MAUT-like decision analysis design was replicated in two published formulary evaluations.[59,60] Because decision makers rely on pharmacoeconomic studies to guide resource allocations and treatment decisions, journal reviewers and editors must critically evaluate the structure and content of the analyses. To the consumer of these studies, to paraphrase a warning from economics, "let the reader beware."

Decision Analysis Computer Support

Decision support systems provide the computational power to conduct complex analyses with multiple branches and a range of probabilities and outcome assessments. Several were originally developed for medical application: Decision maker (Stephen Pauker, 617/956-5910)[61] CE Tree

(T. Pass, Boston, MA), and SMLTREE (James Hollenberg, 526/625-4332).[62] Others were designed for a generic audience and can be adapted for clinical applications: Arborist: Decision Tree Software (Texas Instruments, Dallas, TX); SMaL TREE: The All Purpose Decision Tree Builder (Pratt Medical Group, Boston); Supertree (Strategic Decisions Group, Menlo Park, CA), and Decision Analysis by TreeAge (DATA; TreeAge Software, PO Box 990207, Boston, MA 02199-0207, 617/536-2128). DATA 2.5 is available for Macintosh computers. All others, as well as DATA 2.6 are available in MS-DOS versions.

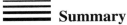

Summary

As you learn the principles of pharmacoeconomics, remember that decision analysis can be used to structure the considerations and identify the elements of any type of economic study. But also appreciate that decision analysis is more than a collection of mathematical calculations, probability estimates, and outcome valuations. It engenders an attitude toward a decision—an attitude to think more analytically, to force the consideration of consequences of actions, to recognize explicitly that uncertainty is present, to estimate the degree of that uncertainty, to assess your attitude toward risk, to determine the relevant outcome measures, and to value your preferences for alternative outcomes. Your completed decision tree gives you more than the answer to your question: it gives you the underlying structure and assumptions behind your decision. If additional information becomes available that changes the consequences, probabilities, or outcomes of your question, the new information can be incorporated and the decision recalculated. Although structured, the decision analysis approach is flexible and offers many opportunities to improve the decision-making process.

References

1. Ledley RS, Lusted LB. Reasoning foundations of medical diagnosis. Science 1959; 130:9-21.

2. Lusted LB. Decision making in patient management. N Engl J Med 1971;284:416-24.

3. McNeil BJ, Keeler E, Adelstein SJ. Primer on certain elements of medical decision making. N Engl J Med 1975;293:211-5.

4. Kassirer JP. The principles of clinical decision making: an introduction to decision analysis. Yale J Biol Med 1976;49:149-64.

5. Kassirer JP, Moskowitz AJ, Lau J, Pauker SG. Decision analysis: a progress report. Ann Intern Med 1987;106:275-91.

6. Raiffa H. Decision analysis: introductory lectures under uncertainty. Reading, MA: Addison-Wesley Publishing, 1968.

7. Plante DA, Kassirer JP, Zarin DA, Pauker SG. Clinical decision consultation service. Am J Med 1986;80:1169-76.

8. Einarson TR, McGhan WF, Bootman JL. Decision analysis applied to pharmacy practice. Am J Hosp Pharm 1985;42:364-71.

9. Crane VS, Holbein ME. Introduction to clinical decision analysis. Research Triangle Park, NC, Glaxo, 1988.

10. Barr JT, Schumacher GE. Applying decision analysis to pharmacy management and practice decisions. Top Hosp Pharm Manage 1994;13:61-71.

11. Weinstein MC, Fineberg HV, eds. Clinical decision analysis. Philadelphia: WB Saunders, 1980.

12. Drummond MF, Stoddart GL, Torrance GW. Methods for the economic evaluation of health care programmes. New York: Oxford Medical Publications, 1987.

13. Barr JT, Schumacher GE. Applying decision analysis in therapeutic drug monitoring: using the receiver-operating characteristic curves in comparative evolutions. Clin Pharm 1986;5:239-46.

14. Tversky A, Kahneman D. Judgment under uncertainty; heuristics and biases. Science 1974;185:1124-31.

15. Weinstein MC, Fineberg FV. Source of probability. In: Clinical decision analysis. Philadelphia: WB Saunders, 1980:37-74.

16. Elixhauser A, Luce BR, Taylor WR, Reblando J. Health care CBA/CEA: an update on the growth and composition of the literature. Med Care 1993;31(suppl):JS1-11.

17. Gottlieb JE, Pauker SG. Whether or not to administer amphotericin to an immunosuppressed patient with hematologic malignancy and undiagnosed fever. Med Decis Making 1981;1:75-93.

18. Plante DA, Pauker SG. Enterococcal endocarditis and penicillin allergy: which drug for the bug? Med Decis Making 1983;3:81-109.

19. Cuchural GJ, Levey AS, Pauker SG. Kidney failure or cancer: should immunosuppression be continued in a transplant patient with malignant melanoma? Med Decis Making 1984;4:83-107.

20. Krahn M, Detsky AS. Should Canada and the United States universally vaccinate infants against hepatitis B? Med Decis Making 1993;13:4-20.

21. Nettleman MD. Use of BCG vaccine in shelters for the homeless: a decision analysis. Chest 1993;103:1087-90.

22. Tsevat J, Wong JB, Pauker SG, Steinberg MH. Neonatal screening for sickle cell disease: a cost-effectiveness analysis. J Pediatr 1991;118:546-54.

23. Rose DN, Silver AL, Schechter CB. Tuberculosis chemoprophylaxis for diabetics: are the benefits of isoniazid worth the risk. Mt Sinai J Med 1985;52:253-8.

24. Tsevat J, Durand-Zaleski I, Pauker SG. Cost-effectiveness of antibiotic prophylaxis for dental procedures in patients with artificial joints. Am J Public Health 1989;79:739-43.

25. Clemens JD,Ransohoff DF. A quantitative assessment of pre-dental antibiotic prophylaxis for patients with mitral-valve prolapse. J Chronic Dis 1984;37:531-44.

26. Shapiro M, Schoenbaum SC, Tager IB, Munoz A, Polk BF. Benefit-cost analysis of antimicrobial prophylaxis in abdominal and vaginal hysterectomy. JAMA 1983;249:1290-4.

27. Oster G, Tuden RL, Colditz GA. Cost-effectiveness analysis of prophylaxis against deep-vein thrombosis in major orthopedic surgery. JAMA 1987;257:203-8.

28. Pauker SG, Eckman MH, Levine HJ. A decision analytic view of anticoagulant prophylaxis for thromboembolism in heart disease. Chest 1989;95(suppl):161S-9S.

29. Elstein AS, Holzman GB, Ravitch MM, Holmes MM, Hoppe RB, Rothert ML, et al. Comparison of physicians; decisions regarding estrogen replacement therapy for menopausal women and decisions derived from a decision analytic model. Am J Med 1989; 80:246-58.

30. Hillner BE, Hollenberg JP, Pauker SG. Postmenopausal estrogens in prevention of osteoporosis: benefit virtually without risk if cardiovascular effects are considered. Am J Med 1986;80:1115-27.

31. Zubialde JP, Lawler F, Clemenson N. Estimated gains in life expectancy with use of postmenopausal estrogen therapy: a decision analysis. J Fam Pract 1993;36:271-80.

32. Hillman AL, Bloom BS. Economic effects of prophylactic use of misoprostol to prevent ulcer in patients taking nonsteroidal anti-inflammatory drugs. Arch Intern Med 1989;149:2061-5.

33. Knill-Jones R, Drummond M, Kohil H, Davies L. Economic evaluation of gastric ulcer prophylaxis in patients with arthritis receiving non-steroidal anti-inflammatory drugs. Postgrad Med J 1990;66:639-48.

34. Carrin GJ, Torfs KE. Economic evaluation of prophylactic treatment with misoprostol in osteoarthritic patients treated with NSAIDs. The case of Belgium. Rev Epidemiol Sante Publique 1990;38:187-99.

35. Gabrel SE, Jaakkimainen RL, Bombardier C. The cost-effectiveness of misoprostol for nonsteroidal antiinflammatory drug-associated adverse gastrointestinal events. Arthritis Rheum 1993;36:447-59.

36. Barza M, Pauker SG. The decision to biopsy, treat, or wait in suspected herpes encephalitis. Ann Intern Med 1980;92:641-9.

37. Hedges JR, Lowe RA. Streptococcal pharyngitis in the emergency department: analysis of therapeutic strategies. Am J Emerg Med 1986;4:107-15.

38. Hillner BE, Centor RM. What a difference a day makes: a decision analysis of adult streptococcal pharyngitis. J Gen Intern Med 1987;2:242-8.

39. Callahan CW. Cost effectiveness of antibiotic therapy for otitis media in a military pediatric clinic. Pediatr Infect Dis J 1988;7:622-5.

40. Stern RS, Pass TM, Komaroff AL. Topical versus systemic agent treatment for papulopustular acne: a cost-effectiveness analysis. Arch Dermatol 1984;120:1571-8.

41. Sudre P, Breman JG, McFarland D, Koplan JP. Treatment of chloroquine-resistant malaria in African children: a cost-effectiveness analysis. Int J Epidemiol 1992;21:146-54.

42. Klassen TP, Rowe PC, Gafni A. Economic evaluation of intravenous immune globulin therapy for Kawasaki syndrome. J Pediatr 1993;122:538-42.

43. Washington AE, Browner WS, Korenbrot CC. Cost-effectiveness of combined treatment for endocervical gonorrhea: considering co-infection with *Chlamydia trachomatis*. JAMA 1987;257:2056-60.

44. Holloway JJ, Smith CR, Moore RD, Feroli R, Lietman PS. Comparative cost effectiveness of gentamicin and tobramycin. Ann Intern Med 1984;101:764-9.

45. Weinstein MC, Read JL, MacKay DN, Kresel JJ, Ashley H, Halvorsen KT, et al. Cost-effective choice of antimicrobial therapy for serious infections. J Gen Intern Med 1986;1:351-63.

46. Chalfin DB, Blair Holbein ME, Fein AM, Carlon GC. Cost-effectiveness of monoclonal antibodies to gram-negative endotoxin in the treatment of gram-negative sepsis in ICU patients. JAMA 1993;269:249-54.

47. Hillner BE, Smith TJ. Efficacy and cost effectiveness of adjuvant chemotherapy in women with node-negative breast cancer. N Engl J Med 1991;324:160-8.

48. Hillner BE, Smith TJ, Desch CE. Assessing the cost effectiveness of adjuvant therapies in early breast cancer using a decision analysis model. Breast Cancer Res Treat 1993;25:97-105.

49. Smith TJ, Hillner BE, Desch CE. Efficacy and cost-effectiveness of cancer treatment: rational allocation of resources based on decision analysis. J Natl Cancer Inst 1993;85:1460-74.

50. Schumacher GE, Barr JT. Applying decision analysis in therapeutic drug monitoring: using decision trees to interpret serum theophylline concentrations. Clin Pharm 1986; 5:325-33.
51. Schumacher GE, Barr JT. Making serum levels more meaningful. Ther Drug Monit 1989;11:580-4.
52. Schumacher GE, Barr JT. Using population-based serum drug concentration cutoff values to predict toxicity: test performance and limitations compared with Bayesian interpretation. Clin Pharm 1990;9:788-96.
53. Schumacher GE, Barr JT, Browne TR, Collins JF, Veterans Administration Epilepsy Cooperative Study Group. Test performance characteristics of the serum phenytoin concentration (SPC): the relationship between SPC and patient response. Ther Drug Monit 1991;13:318-24.
54. Schumacher GE, Barr JT. Bayesian and threshold probabilities in therapeutic drug monitoring: when can serum drug concentrations alter clinical decisions? Am J Hosp Pharm 1994;51:321-7.
55. Schechter CB. Decision analysis in formulary decision making. PharmacoEconomics 1993;3:454-61.
56. Kresel JJ, Hutchings HC, MacKay DN, Weinstein MC, Read JL, Taylor-Halvorsen K, et al. Application of decision analysis to drug selection for formulary addition. Hosp Formul 1987;22:658-76.
57. Oster G, Huse DM, Delea TE, Colditz GA, Richter JM. The risks and benefits of an Rx-to-OTC switch: the case of over-the-counter H$_2$-blockers. Med Care 1990;28:834-52.
58. Witte KW, Eck TA, Vogel DP. Decision analysis applied to the purchase of frozen premixed intravenous admixtures. Am J Hosp Pharm 1985;42:835-9.
59. Cano SB, Fujita NK. Formulary evaluation of third-generation cephalosporins using decision analysis. Am J Hosp Pharm 1988;45:566-9.
60. Barriere SL. Formulary evaluation of second-generation cephamycin derivatives using decision analysis. Am J Hosp Pharm 1991;48:2146-50.
61. Lau J, Kassirer JP, Pauker SG. DECISION MAKER 3.0. Improved decision analysis by personal computer. Med Decis Making 1983;3:39-43.
62. Siegel JE, Keaney KM. Introduction to SMLTREE. Med Decis Making 1993;13: 74-84.

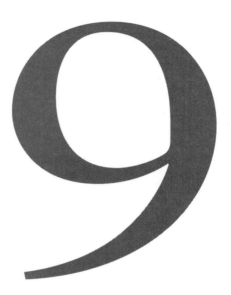

Epidemiology and Pharmacoeconomic Research

Paul E. Stang
Jacqueline Gardner

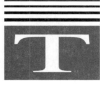he last few years have seen an explosion of interest in the methods used to examine questions of cost and outcome of diseases. Most of the momentum for this field has been an interest in systematically examining the cost of disease versus the cost of therapy to derive comparisons on which public policy and appropriations decisions can be based. Regulatory imperatives have now emerged in at least three countries (France, Australia, and Canada) that mandate economic analyses to justify pricing of pharmaceuticals. Explicit in these mandates are the conduct of epidemiologic investigations to determine economic modeling, market size estimation, and source population parameters. Particularly interesting among these efforts are those that examine the economic spectrum of medicinal therapy, as the approval of these therapies is based on proof of safety and efficacy with relatively little attention to issues of access or cost. Given the wide availability of pharmaceutical products and the potential for their use in a wide range of disease indications (some of which may be outside of the intended patient population), and the new regulatory initiatives, it is important that the researcher understand the basic characteristics of the disease and of those affected by it before developing research plans to examine costs associated with and affected by drug therapy. Further, concise descriptions of the existing therapy, the way the therapy is used in the population, and its effects on the target diseases are critical in analyzing the cost of both current and new therapies.

Epidemiology is a relatively old science and discipline that has enjoyed renewed enthusiasm in its application for determining the baseline and current state of diseases within populations, describing characteristics

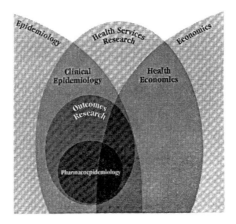

Figure 1. The relationship between economics and epidemiology. Reprinted with permission of H. Guess.

of patients with particular diseases, and identifying exposures that have a positive or negative impact on the occurrence and outcome of the diseases. The role of epidemiology is complimentary to that of economics; it encompasses rubrics ranging from health services research to pharmacoepidemiology, outcomes research, and clinical epidemiology (Figure 1). The resulting information is useful not only to the economist, but often has broader public health and policy implications.[1] The impact of interventions on cost also must be effectively linked to their impact on health.[2] As has been effectively demonstrated in macroeconomics, supplementing economic analyses with population-based epidemiology effectively addresses the benefits and risks of alternative approaches while placing these impacts into a public health perspective.[3]

This chapter examines the basic tools of epidemiology and how they contribute to our general understanding of the economics of disease. Specifically, this chapter will show how epidemiology can and should effectively be used in studies evaluating the economic impact of medicinal therapy. As part of the broad aegis of epidemiology, pharmacoepidemiology, or the study of the effects of drugs within populations, is discussed with respect to its role in pharmacoeconomic studies.

Basic Principles of Epidemiology

Epidemiology is a discipline whose goal is to describe the distribution of diseases and exposures in populations and draw conclusions regarding associations between the exposures and the diseases. Epidemiologists use a range of methods, from systematic surveillance and simple descriptive

The Epidemiology/Pharmacoeconomics Data Exchange

EPIDEMIOLOGIC DATA	EXAMPLES	MAJOR PHARMACO-ECONOMIC APPLICATIONS
Disease frequency	incidence, prevalence, demographics	new cases arising for intervention, magnitude of affected population, identification of high-risk groups and potential payer burden, quality-of-life parameters
Comorbidities, confounders, and effect modifiers	comorbid diseases, lifestyle factors (e.g., smoking, alcohol)	spectrum of disease and additional sources of potential costs, additional risk factors or consequences of disease, identification of high-risk groups, quality-of-life parameters, economic risk, and medical decision modeling
Disease natural history	outcomes including survival, changes in disease over time, changes in use of services over time, distribution of risk factors	course of disease and costs over time, trends in ascertainment and technology used, referral patterns, length and outcomes of illness, QALYs, DALYs, risk assessment of outcomes, quality-of-life parameters, economic risk, and medical decision modeling
Utilization of services	healthcare-seeking behavior and predictors, disease-specific and total usage, type (site, specialist) of services	proportion of those who do not seek care but may still be impacted by disease, predictors of healthcare-seeking behavior, interventions and therapies used, referral patterns
Therapy	effectiveness and adverse effects of current therapies, observational study of new drug over time in a population	adverse effect risk/cost data; utilization under current therapies; adverse effects on comorbid conditions; naturalistic usage and disease data on new therapy as it enters population; risk of using inappropriate, addictive, or dangerous medications due to lack of effective therapies; quality-of-life parameters; estimate long-term outcomes; identify comparators for economic studies
Diagnostic issues	diagnostic criteria, severity, accuracy of ascertainment, trends over time in coding	ability to look at increased costs due to missed diagnosis, issues of severity of disease and relationship to costs, severity as a marker for utilization, extent of under-ascertainment of disease
Risk assessment	rate of outcomes attributable to disease (attributable risk data), modeling of outcomes based on disease natural history	modeling of outcomes and their costs and consequences, economic risk and medical decision modeling, link manifestation of disease to outcome

reporting to rigorous multivariate analyses, to determine whether a particular characteristic or cluster of characteristics are associated with or predictive of a given outcome. Epidemiologic studies can be observational (no active exposure manipulation by the investigator) or interventional (the exposure is manipulated, as in clinical trials). Often, data collected for another purpose can be used. Interventional studies, in particular clinical trials, use random allocation of treatment to control for the effects of known and unknown covariates. Observational studies must systematically collect these data to examine and control their effects in the analysis. Clinical trials also are noteworthy for their short duration and unrealistically standardized monitoring, which often limits their generalizability and usefulness in examining issues related to decreased utilization of services, changes in quality of life, or detection of effects from long-term use.[4] Clinical trial sample sizes also are based on power necessary to detect efficacy differences and may not be large enough or cover populations broad enough to robustly address economic questions. These data can possibly be obtained through retrospective observational studies, as these studies often involve much larger, more diverse populations for longer periods of observation. This gives the economist a mechanism to compensate for the power lost in clinical trial data. However, observational studies will be limited to those products already marketed.

One of the roles of epidemiology is to protect economic studies from biases.[5] Pharmacoeconomics must assume a cause–effect relationship between drug treatment and disease indication. It is important to understand all of the phenomena that are related to the disease and the therapy prior to assessing baseline costs and eventual changes with therapy. For instance, patients with headache may be using a very small amount of resources directly related to the headache pain, but may be tremendous users of other medical services for associated diseases or symptoms resulting from their chronic disease or its therapy. In the case of headache, the patient may be seeking treatment from internal medicine for their gastrointestinal symptoms resulting from stress and chronic nonsteroidal antiinflammatory drug use, and from psychiatry for their comorbid depression and anxiety. It would be important to examine the changes in utilization and costs of these associated services with the introduction of a new therapy, as they may contribute substantial burden to the patient and the cost of the disease. Economic models become more robust by using realistic epidemiology data on risk factors, treatment alternatives, and outcomes.

EPIDEMIOLOGY NOMENCLATURE

It is important to understand the nomenclature used in epidemiology. Prevalence is a measure that reflects the number of people at a given point in time who have a particular disease or exposure of interest. Prevalence can be based on a particular day, previous week, previous month, previous year, or lifetime prevalence, which reflects whether or not the subject has ever had the condition in question. Prevalence estimates are usually obtained from cross-sectional or one-time sampling techniques, such as interviews administered either by telephone or in person, by self-administered questionnaire as in a mail survey, or by review of records or databases for the number of cases of a condition on record at any point in time. Prevalence in a broad sense represents the current disease burden from a population perspective.

Incidence, on the other hand, reflects the number of new cases arising in a population in a given period of time. Incidence estimates are much more difficult to obtain because they necessitate observing a population over a period of time to identify new cases that arise, or performing repeated prevalence estimates in the same population over a given period of time to differentiate between existing cases and cases of new onset. Incidence is a very powerful measure because it allows one to project population estimates into the future. Incidence also is not dependent on survival, as a case is identified and counted at the time it becomes a case. Incidence reflects the emerging disease burden.

Prevalence is survival-dependent, as the patient must be able to be sampled at the given time point of prevalence. Prevalence estimates for a disease with varying lengths of survival will include only those patients who have survived long enough to become a prevalent case. It is this "survival of the fittest" that may present a problem in using prevalence figures, as these cases do not represent all patients who have contracted the disease and certainly do not carry with them the total economic burden that the disease exacts on the population. The denominator in both prevalence and incidence estimates is the population at risk for experiencing the outcome of interest. If we are interested in outcomes among people taking a particular drug, we would want to assure ourselves that the denominator consists only of those people exposed to the drug for a given period of time. Hence, our prevalence or incidence estimate will have meaning and will be generalizable back to a known target population.

Case fatality rate is important only insofar as it affects the ability to identify cases, since those who die may not be captured in a prevalence-based study. Incident cases in contrast provide a realistic starting point from which to follow patients and the course of their disease and will not be affected by case-fatality. This is especially important when looking at health service utilization over time or in establishing temporal trends, as utilization of services may vary across the duration of the disease or when constructing quality-adjusted or disability-adjusted life years (QALYs and DALYs).

Inherent in the denominator of incidence is the concept of time, expressed as person-time, as each person may contribute a different amount to the length of observation. This allows us to include the contribution of each patient in the incidence estimate, regardless of how long they remain under observation. This concept is important in the quantification of utilization of services and eventual calculation of cost associated with a disease and is the key strength of disease natural history studies.

STUDY DESIGNS

A discussion of epidemiologic study designs, complete with their advantages and disadvantages, is beyond the scope of this chapter. Most commonly used are ecologic, cross-sectional (prevalence), cohort, and case-control study designs. The data derived from studies using each design offer unique advantages in given situations. Less often addressed is the way in which the data are presented and interpreted. Nonetheless, discussions about analytic techniques also will be deferred. For economic studies, the cohort design is favored for several reasons: cohorts are good observational approximations of real life and the natural course of disease that clearly define the temporal relationship between exposures and outcomes. They resemble clinical trials in their direction but they tend to be much larger and, as such, able to detect smaller differences between groups. Case-control studies have been used in economic analysis with some modest success. These studies are of limited utility as they are capable of exploring only a single outcome; however, they may be useful in examining the economic impact of adverse drug effects.[6]

Disease Natural History

Disease natural history implies the ability to give a "cradle-to-grave" characterization of a population. This includes changes in the disease over time, modifiers of disease outcomes, comorbidities, use of services, determination of severity indices, and the effect of treatment. These data are crucial in the determination of DALYs and QALYs. Such a longitudinal picture is very difficult to obtain; however, with the advent of computerized medical data, structured medical record systems, and the plethora of longitudinal cohort studies, it is often possible to follow affected people for several years. When using these secondary datasets, one must remember that they represent specific populations, often linked by a common health insurance payer, that may reflect socioeconomic status, geographic region, or employment status. These characteristics may limit the generalizability of findings to the broad population base. However, if one is interested in payer-specific data (e.g., Medicaid, health maintenance organization), it is appropriate to limit the scope of the project to a dataset derived from that payer. Longitudinal studies also facilitate the capture of total utilization of healthcare services in addition to identifying those services that are disease-specific. These studies are often instrumental in identifying marginal cost differences.

ASCERTAINMENT

It is important for the epidemiologist to provide some insight into how well patients are captured or identified in the medical care system. The extent to which a given disease is identified in a population and the likelihood of an individual being correctly identified once they enter the healthcare system bear directly on disease burden, direct and indirect costs, and perhaps the effectiveness of therapy. Sensitivity, specificity, and predictive value analyses of existing diagnostic systems are helpful not only in determining issues of disease frequency and recognition, but in providing a basis for confidence in future work in automated data and some guidance in the interpretability of patient-reported symptoms and diagnoses. Such efforts also may draw attention to the need for public health screening, clinician/patient education programs, or impact on the development of clinical guidelines. A diagnostic algorithm may need to be constructed to identify cases or may dictate the necessity for more stringent diagnostic criteria based on symptom cluster analyses. This is especially important in primary care diseases as evidenced by recent data on migraine headache where over 50% of those presenting with migraine symptoms were misdiagnosed.[7] The authors also presented an analysis of those symptoms most likely to improve or hinder the likelihood of a correct diagnosis.

Patient motivations for seeking medical attention, their satisfaction with their medical care, and their longevity in the medical care system also should be captured while examining ascertainment issues. Ascertainment data can be used in developing medical decision models, as patients who are missed (false-negatives) may be subject to a different treatment and utilization pathway. Similarly, quality of life may be impacted by misdiagnosis resulting in perhaps inappropriate therapy and poor outcome.

EXPOSURE AND DISEASE COMORBIDITY

A key by-product of a well-developed epidemiologic study is the identification of relationships among diseases or comorbid events. Chronic diseases rarely occur in isolation and are often manifestations of more diffuse disease processes. It is important to elucidate the relationship between the disease or risk factor under study and any comorbid conditions (consequent, concomitant, antecedent). Comorbidities are important when deciding on relevant quality-of-life measurements, as many chronic diseases carry some additional comorbid psychiatric disease or have substantive impact on nonphysical complaints. Comorbidities also impact medical decision and economic models as the constellation of risks, therapies, and outcomes are defined and their impact on the burden of the disease become apparent. Comorbidities, as a feature of disease natural history are particularly important data when defining drug effects. Adverse events often will be attributed to a drug when the event is actually part of the natural course of comorbid conditions occurring in people with the disease. The cost implications of comorbid conditions can be elucidated by examining the patient's total healthcare utilization rather than disease-specific utilization (this is essentially the way marginal costs are derived). For example, many diseases carry associated risks of comorbid psychiatric disease that may completely drive the patient's utilization of health care. This, for example, has been shown to be the case in functional bowel disease.[8] These psychiatric comorbidities are often poorly ascertained in clinical practice and hence poorly reflected in diagnostic codes. Similarly, it may be the comorbidities that affect patient quality of life or productivity, critical components of any economic analysis.

DISEASE AND RISK FACTOR TRENDS

It is also important for an epidemiologist to characterize trends in risk factors and outcomes, because as therapies change, the frequency and course of risks and diseases in populations change. Secular trends in our ability to diagnose and treat will affect any baseline estimates of disease cost, especially if the diagnosis is one of exclusion. Migraine headache, for example, has a high direct cost during the initial visits to the doctor, as many expensive tests are ordered to rule-out more life-threatening causes of headache.[9] Environmental triggers of the disease and the prevailing risk factor trends also should be studied, as these data are crucial for predicting trends in prevalence. Many costs also are being shifted within the system as new technologies become part of the natural course of disease: balloon angioplasty, outpatient/day surgery, endoscopy, and lithotripsy are a few examples of how technologies are affecting cost of disease and use of services over time. Disease frequency in populations, especially if there are susceptible populations or preferential distributions of diseases in populations (e.g., high-risk populations), can affect both aggregate estimates of costs of the disease as well as estimated costs to the patient. These trends can be measured as true prevalence or incidence of disease in the population, or as distributions of outpatient or inpatient treatments in a population. However, as with any of these data, ability to effectively and reliably identify people with the disease or disorder is critically important.

DISEASE SEVERITY

Disease severity is a particularly important issue in defining populations and ascribing costs (both fiscal and humanistic) to disease states. Severity has become synonymous with intensity of symptoms or, in the case of arthritis and neoplasia, a staged classification of pathophysiologic signs or objective evidence from radiographic or laboratory results. Although symptom intensity is an important component of disease severity, it often fails to discriminate the features and disability of those with higher levels of dysfunction. A well-constructed severity/impact index may become an effective link among physiology, clinical diagnosis, economics, and patient outcome as well as a guide for interventions. There are many desirable features of a useful classification of severity: (1) ordered categories that are mutually exclusive and exhaustive corresponding to qualitative differences in severity; (2) biologic relevance; (3) based on simple measurements that can be obtained in a variety of settings; (4) defined to yield homogenous groups; and (5) precise, reliable, and valid construction reflecting cross-sectional association with severity measures and predictive of patient outcomes.[10] Item response theory provides the methodologic framework for the development of these scoring systems; however, the challenge is in determining what constitutes the various levels of severity and how well it reflects outcomes. Von Korff et al.[10] include several applications of a well-constructed chronic severity index (Table 1) and apply some of these principles to the construction of a chronic disease score from automated pharmacy data.[11] It is generally assumed that people with more severe forms of disease are different than those with less severe disease, although there is rarely consensus on how severity levels are to be defined. The differences may be in intensity of symptoms or level of dysfunction that the patient experiences as a result of the disease. Level of dysfunction is a difficult parameter to measure because it may involve issues of humanistic impact and psychological well-being (e.g., quality of life), consumption of health care (both disease-specific and general), and impact on work and play. Severity differences are not consistently reflected in

Table 1. Applications of Severity Classification[10]

STUDY TYPE	APPLICATION
Epidemiologic field survey	more complete and reproducible differential of global severity among cases; ability to segment population by level of dysfunction
Clinical trial	improvement in qualitative description of patients at baseline and enhancement of qualitative changes at follow-up between groups
Observational/natural history	case-mix adjustment at baseline and assessment of outcomes over time
Meta-analysis	aid in the classification of studies and assessment of results by providing standardized criteria for patient outcomes
Clinical practice	improve prognostic advice and provide substantiation for treatment decisions and patient education
Clinical information and tracking system	ability to track patient progress over time with limited information

healthcare costs since when the disease is fatal, those with more severe (and rapidly fatal) disease may have lower direct and indirect costs over a period of time. The ability to chart disease progression over time, control for severity in analyses, identify homogeneous patient groups, and target those patients who could benefit most from intervention heighten the importance of severity assessment. The interplay between the epidemiologist and the pharmacoeconomist is particularly crucial in this arena, as severity may be the issue upon which all subsequent work and analyses are based and assessment of disease cost can be segmented. Hence, the measures should be complimentary to both and useful to the practicing clinician and clinical trialist alike. If costs are related to severity, then trials may be able to directly translate the effect of a therapy that reduces severity from one level to another or prevents a disease from advancing to a more severe stage. Burden of illness measures should reflect both disease severity and frequency. Using this paradigm, statistics can be employed that reflect the impact of an intervention in a population reflecting both severity reduction and prevention of outcome.[12]

Quantification of Risk

The epidemiologic concept of quantification of risk is very important to economic analysis. The magnitude of risk, that is, of an association between exposure and disease, is often represented as a ratio. For instance, people with hypertension may have a relative risk of 3.1 for experiencing a stroke. This means that they are three times as likely to experience a stroke as are people without hypertension. (Interestingly, Naylor et al.[13] showed that clinicians respond more favorably to data presented in relative terms.) However, people without hypertension also experience stroke, and this incidence of stroke among people without hypertension is known as the "background rate." What may be of most interest to economists is the proportion of strokes attributable to hypertension. This measure, called an "attributable risk proportion" (Figure 2), reflects the amount of disease outcome (stroke) in the population that could be prevented if the exposure (hypertension) were eliminated. Hence, determining both the background rate and the attributable risk proportion through epidemiologic studies becomes important. The economist can then begin the daunting task of translating this information into the economic benefits of intervening and preventing the costly outcome of stroke.

The relative risk and attributable risk approach also can be applied to interpretation of adverse events that may be attributed to a drug therapy, but that are actually part of the clinical sequelae of the disease for which the drug was prescribed. This misattribution of adverse drug effects is known as confounding by indication. For example, among depressed people, there is a given risk of suicide or violent behavior. If these people

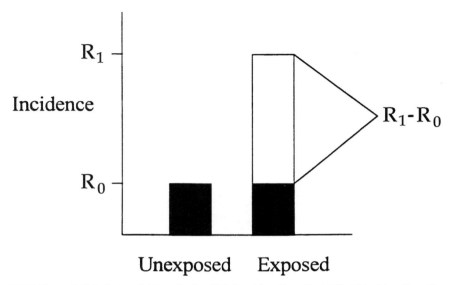

Figure 2. Calculation of risk attribution. Relative risk = $R_1 \div R_0$. Attributable risk = $R_1 - R_0$. Attributable risk proportion = $(R_1 - R_0) \div R_1$. R_0 = incidence of outcome in the unexpected; R_1 = incidence of outcome in those exposed.

are given a drug for depression, any observed incidence of this adverse behavior is often attributed to the drug, when it may in fact be a predictable part of the disease process. Similarly, a drug given to women during pregnancy may be identified as causing adverse birth outcomes, although there is a background rate of adverse birth outcomes independent of drug exposure. Anticipating these questions and determining the background rate of disease outcomes will provide valuable data for calculations of relative risk and attributable risk. This information may help either to defend or to indict a drug exposure, and will assist the economist in identifying disease features that add economic burden to the disease and perhaps to measure direct, indirect, or humanistic cost. Furthermore, these epidemiologic studies can be used to provide realistic data for predicting the outcomes of clinical and economic trials.

OUTCOMES, MODELING, AND DECISION ANALYSIS

A key part of the evaluation of the impact of a new therapy is the determination of the full impact of the disease, the possible clinical decisions associated with it, and the expectation of various outcomes. If the disease under study is part of a constellation of related diseases, trials may be able to show that effective early detection and intervention can prevent other deleterious outcomes and offset their associated economic and humanistic toll. Similarly, the unexpected positive effects of drug therapy[14] can be realized and quantified through epidemiologic studies, thereby providing a more balanced picture of a particular therapy and a new therapeutic avenue. Because disease severity may greatly influence outcomes and clinical decision-making, appreciation of severity levels must be achieved and integrated into this process. Hence, the judicious application of epidemiologic data can be used in a number of decision-intensive settings, which help to guide further research and arrive at informed decisions regarding disease and economic impact. These are the data used to make public policy decisions and, increasingly, new drug approvals. Modeling exercises rely on observational data to estimate the long-term effects, costs, and benefits of a new intervention in an unrestricted (i.e., nonclinical trial) population. Sound population data are crucial as the product of these models may guide future decisions on pricing, further clinical and economic research, and determinations of the impact of therapy. Decision analysis models, including those used in utility analysis and medical decision-making, need reality-based data on risks, treatment alternatives, and outcomes. These can easily be obtained from good-quality epidemiology studies. Development of data that provide probabilities and risks of outcomes also can be powerful in the early planning phases of clinical trials as they can be designed to capture some of these outcomes in the face of comparison to other therapies. These data also may be used to assess the feasibility of continuing development of a new compound or determining necessary sample sizes.

Resources for Epidemiologic Data

Epidemiology studies are designed to capture and characterize a population at a given point in time or over a designated period of time. For these data to be of maximum utility in assessing change due to a new therapy or technology, they should reflect the status prior to the availability of the new product or reimbursement scheme. In the case of new medicinal therapies, epidemiology studies should be undertaken when the compound is early in the development process. De novo prospective studies are the most expensive, logistically complicated, and time-intensive studies to undertake. Often, synthesis of the available literature may be sufficient to address many early data needs and opportunities to estimate the effects of therapy on long-term clinical outcomes may be available through clinical trials and ongoing larger cohort studies (e.g., longitudinal studies of aging) to capture information directly or through the addition of questions. Ongoing trials (e.g., Framingham Heart Study) also have the advantage of bringing you and your research interests and concerns to the attention of other researchers who, on their next research expedition, may perpetuate your data as a matter of course. Nonautomated alternatives exist, including the Rochester Epidemiology Project.[15,16] The researchers involved in this project have been performing population-based studies for years using a structured medical record system. Their ability to capture all healthcare encounters for the entire population of Olmsted County, Minnesota, has resulted in over 650 studies.

AUTOMATED DATA SOURCES

With the explosion in the computerization of data, especially medical and health service utilization data, vast amounts of information have become temptingly available to anyone clever enough to extract it from computerized files. Most of these data were created for reasons other than epidemiologic research; most commonly they were created by fiscal officers in healthcare settings to track charge data within their accounting systems. Whereas 20 years ago it was necessary to laboriously sift through reams of medical records data manually, the essence of those data can now be captured on computerized tape. This convenience comes at a price, however, as there are ever-present coding errors, difficulties in substantiating diagnoses, and problems linking patients between databases (often diagnostic codes appear in one database, medication codes on another, and hospitalization data on yet another), and so on. Furthermore, drug exposures indicated in such databases constitute evidence only of prescriptions dispensed or orders filled; they do not necessarily correspond to either evidence of drug consumption or the circumstances (e.g., timing, dosage, route of administration) that might have occurred. Finally, tantamount to the logistical problems are the problems of confidentiality, as data source managers are becoming more and more reluctant to allow access to interested parties outside of their own systems, a question that has now attracted some attention from ethicists.[17]

An extensive discussion of the advantages and shortcomings of the individual computerized databases is beyond the scope of this chapter. However, methods of conducting valid epidemiologic analysis using these datasets are being improved and are evolving as the advantage of computerized data is its capture of a unique payer perspective on the disease in question. These databases capture a relatively large population and facilitate the collection of utilization data. One could examine trends in the use of medical services and medications over time, the relationships between interventions and outcomes, indirect measures of compliance with therapy, and patterns of prescribed and administered care. In general, these data provide strong and relatively comprehensive capture of the direct cost of disease. They also provide the opportunity to assemble matched controls from which marginal costs and utilization ("attributable costs") can be derived. Furthermore, issues pertaining to adverse drug reactions, treatment failures, and therapeutic interchanges can be addressed and appropriately quantified in such data. Additionally, exclusively through observational methods and computerized data, the impact of a new therapy can be monitored as it penetrates a market. This provides additional data, under real-world circumstances, for documenting the impact of new therapy on direct costs, indirect costs, and humanistic parameters.

Caution is warranted, however, as the allure of the computerized system carries with it some risks. Recall that most systems were created by fiscal officers interested in streamlining the billing process and facilitating budget review. Several caveats govern epidemiologic studies using computerized administrative datasets. First, enrollee or eligible patient turnover may be high, thus compromising the potential for tracking individuals over long periods of time. For example, Ray and Griffin[18] found that in Medicaid data, only 79% of their original cohort had no lapses in eligibility over a one-year follow-up period; this proportion was further reduced to 38% over five years. The reason for dropping-out may not be as obvious or adverse-event related as is found in clinical trials because the eligibility criteria for that subject being carried on the database may have changed (e.g., lost eligibility for Medicaid, left job so is dropped from health maintenance organization rolls).

Secondly, data quality and comprehensiveness may affect the ability to accurately capture disease information. Because only diagnostic codes are recorded, it will be unclear how the diagnosis was made and how accurately it reflects the patient's true disease state.[7] Coded diagnoses lack detail on severity and chronicity and, in many databases, the number of diagnoses available for any given episode may be restricted. Hence, information on comorbidities may be unavailable. Source record validation is essential to assure accuracy of coding and perhaps to capture some of the additional data. Often the rigors of diagnostic ascertainment in a given disease are not apparent without access to source documents. This becomes a particularly important problem when data span changes in disease definition, therapeutic practices, or technologic advances. It is important to keep in mind that for most purposes, one would like to obtain the current status of knowledge or state-of-the-art of the disease and its therapies rather than capture a historic perspective that may no longer be relevant. Additionally, in conducting studies within computerized databases, one assumes that the temporal relationship between drug dispensing and subsequent events is causal; however, this is pure conjecture. Paradigms can be created to estimate compliance by looking at refill patterns, but at the end of the day, it remains unclear whether or how effectively patients took the medication. This may be especially true of device-delivered medications, such as inhalers or injections whose effectiveness depend not only on the patient attempting administration of the drug but also on their effectiveness in operating the device.

Finally, difficulties may arise when trying to attribute resource use because of the limitations in coding for administrative purposes. Similar problems arise when attribution of diagnostic tests or drug therapy is attempted, as the motivation for these tests and medications may be unclear or one test or visit may cover more than one medical problem. Misclassification in this respect can be minimized by making a priori decisions about which resources would potentially be affected by the disease or the therapy under study.

The federal government also conducts regular research on the US populous and makes the raw data available to the public. Notable among these government efforts are the National Health Interview Survey, an annual representative sample of the US (over 40,000 households) with data on chronic diseases, healthcare utilization, and demographics (including days spent in bed or days of restricted activity due to particular chronic diseases). Government prevalence estimates are derived from these data. The National Health and Nutrition Examination Surveys, the National Medical Expenditure Survey, and several site-specific surveys can all be accessed through the federal government at a modest price. Analysis of these datasets is somewhat complex because they are large and the weighting schemes are somewhat complicated necessitating sophisticated software packages for analysis. A fairly thorough accounting of these government data sources has appeared elsewhere,[19] as has a good commentary on their quality and appropriate use.[20]

Summary

Healthcare decisions are based primarily on a consideration of risk and benefit. Epidemiologic techniques of examining frequency and distribution of exposures and outcomes in the population provide a good foundation from which to project disease and therapeutic costs to the broader population. It is important to understand the total spectrum of the disease, comorbidities, severity issues, current treatment and service utilization patterns, and effectiveness and consequences of current therapies in order to gauge the potential impact of a new treatment. Policy-makers base most of their decisions on epidemiologic outcomes data in large part because they provide a realistic assessment of the population at large. Epidemiology also offers the opportunity to elucidate particular issues in disease ascertainment and therapeutic alternatives and how these may affect specific payer systems as well as the population at large. Specifically, issues relating to primary care of medical disorders may provide some clues to the initial cost and capture of diseases in populations. Epidemiology data are crucial in quantifying the burden of illness, identification of risks and outcomes, providing the basis for economic and medical decision models, and aiding in the prediction of outcomes in clinical trial populations. With the computerization of medical care data and the ability to observe large populations, sophisticated sampling and modeling techniques become important in ascertaining and attributing disease and utilization relationships within these populations and enabling high-quality observational data to form the basis of more risk and economic decisions. Finally, prior to declaring any effective change in cost, one must thoroughly understand the baseline state from which that change occurred. This is clearly the realm of the epidemiologist, and it presents a wonderful opportunity to merge the sciences of epidemiology and pharmacoeconomics to determine the impact of therapeutic innovation on the diseases that burden modern society.

References

1. Guess HA, Stephenson WP, Sacks S, Gardner JS. Beyond pharmacoepidemiology: the larger role of epidemiology in drug development. J Clin Epidemiol 1988;41:995-6.

2. Spitzer WO. Drugs as determinants of health and disease in the population. J Clin Epidemiol 1991;44:823-30.

3. Sen A. The economics of life and death. Sci Am 1993;268:40-7.

4. Simon G, Wagner E, Von Korff M. Cost-effectiveness comparisons using 'real world' randomized trials: the case of new antidepressant drugs. J Clin Epidemiol 1995;48:363-73.

5. Chrischilles EA. The contribution of epidemiology to pharmacoeconomic research. Drug Info J 1992;26:219-29.

6. Eisenberg JM, Koffer H, Glick HA, et al. What is the cost of nephrotoxicity associated with aminoglycosides? Ann Intern Med 1987;107:900-9.

7. Stang P, Von Korff M. The diagnosis of headache in primary care: factors in the agreement of clinical and standardized diagnoses. Headache 1994;34:138-42.

8. Whitehead WE, Bosmajian L, Zonderman AD, et al. Symptoms of psychological distress. A multivariate study of patients and non-patients with irritable bowel syndrome. Gastroenterology 1988;95:709-14.

9. Osterhaus JT, Stang PE, Yanagihara T, Swanson JW, Guess HA, O'Fallon WM, et al. Use of diagnostic procedures associated with incident migraine headaches among Olmsted County, MN (abstract). Proceedings of the 8th Annual Meeting of the International Society of Technology Assessment in Health Care, Vancouver, BC, September 1992.

10. Von Korff M, Ormel J, Keefe FJ, Dworkin SF. Grading the severity of chronic pain. Pain 1992;50:133-49.

11. Von Korff M, Wagner EH, Saunders K. A chronic disease score from automated pharmacy data. J Clin Epidemiol 1992;45:197-203.

12. Chang MN, Guess HA, Heyse JF. Reduction in burden of illness: a new efficacy measure for prevention trials. Stat Med 1994;13:1807-14.

13. Naylor CD, Chen E, Strauss B. Measured enthusiasm: does the method of reporting trial results alter perceptions of therapeutic effectiveness? Ann Intern Med 1992;117:916-21.

14. Lasagna L. Are drug benefits also part of pharmacoepidemiology? J Clin Epidemiol 1990;43:849-50.

15. Kurland LT, Molgaard CA. The patient record in epidemiology. Sci Am 1981;245:54-63.

16. Kurland LT, Molgaard CA, Schoenberg BS. Mayo Clinic records linkage system: contributions to neuroepidemiology. Neuroepidemiology 1982;1:102-14.

17. Westrin CG. Ethical, legal and political problems affecting epidemiology in European countries. IRB: A Review of Human Subjects Research (Hastings Center) 1993;15:6-8.

18. Ray WA, Griffin MR. Use of Medicaid data for pharmacoepidemiology. Am J Epidemiol 1989;129:837-49.

19. Gable CB. A compendium of public health data sources. Am J Epidemiol 1990;131: 381-94.

20. Hierholzer WJ. Health care data: the epidemiolgist's sand—comments on the quantity and quality of data. Am J Med 1991;91(suppl 3B):S21-6.

10

Incorporating Pharmacoeconomic Research into Clinical Trials

Jane T. Osterhaus
Raymond J. Townsend

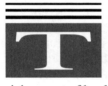he US healthcare model is undergoing a significant paradigm shift. This shift is occurring as a result of patient, provider, and payer frustration with the current healthcare system. These frustrations are being driven by the rising cost of health care and the lack of benchmarks as to what value is being obtained for the investment in healthcare resources relative to other societal investment opportunities. It is possible to replace or repair nearly every organ in the human body. But, what is the value of these interventions? Are they worth the resources invested? What is their "return"? The ability to measure these interventions will help lead to a more successful paradigm shift.

Many factors contribute to costs of health care, but drug costs often are scrutinized more than other components. Drug costs are more visible to consumers because more than 55% of prescription expenditures are paid for out-of-pocket, whereas only 3.4% of hospital care is directly paid for by consumers.[1] This method of payment creates disincentives to patients to use prescription medications, although their use may be very cost-effective from the perspective of total healthcare resource use. Changing the insurance system may reduce these disincentives, but it will not obviate the need to understand the value of pharmaceuticals and pharmacy services.

The most appropriate time to begin gathering data regarding the value a pharmaceutical product will bring to the healthcare setting is during clinical drug development. Pharmaceutical companies are increasingly being called on to document the value of their products, not only clinically, but also in terms of economic and humanistic value. This value can be measured via appropriate data collection and analysis techniques. Information collected early in clinical trials regarding the impact of a new product on the healthcare system can help to determine its price and provide initial information to prospective purchasers regarding the value this new product will have versus current therapy. Once a product is on the market, its value must be continually assessed relative to its role in providing comprehensive pharmaceutical care.

Pharmacoeconomic Research versus Traditional Research

Pharmacoeconomic research methods can be used to place value on therapies by identifying and measuring variables expected to be affected by healthcare interventions. Such research asks, What happened to the patient after an intervention? and What impact did it have on the use of other healthcare resources? What were the outcomes? Was the patient relieved of symptoms, was a condition cured, an illness prevented, or functional status restored? Until recently, such outcomes of medical care received little research attention. There is a paucity of data regarding the outcomes of medical care, surgical procedures, and behavioral interventions. Even diets generally are not thoroughly evaluated before they are incorporated into medical practice. In fact, drugs are considered to be the best paradigm for clinical outcomes in the US because of the rigorous testing required for approval of new drugs in the US marketplace.[2]

In order for a drug to be approved for marketing in the US, safety and efficacy must be demonstrated, usually by presenting evidence from two adequate and well-controlled clinical studies. This experimental model is well established; safety and efficacy are critical factors to address, but that model, in outcomes terms, is incomplete. To obtain a complete assessment of the outcomes of healthcare procedures and treatments requires scientific evaluation in three dimensions: clinical, economic, and humanistic. Although economic and humanistic measures are not currently required for the approval of a drug by the Food and Drug Administration (FDA), because of their mandate to regulate the promotion of pharmaceutical products the FDA has recently stated its intention to develop guidelines for standards of research to support pharmacoeconomic promotional claims.[3] Additionally, committees making decisions of whether or not to include a drug in a health maintenance organization, hospital, or other formulary are gaining an appreciation for the importance of evaluating all three dimensions. Increasingly, these formulary committees and other purchasing groups are expecting pharmacoeconomic issues to be addressed in a standard fashion prior to approval or inclusion on the formulary.

How are the three dimensions (clinical, economic, and humanistic) of outcomes from pharmacotherapy measured? The clinical dimensions of safety and efficacy are evaluated during the drug development process in clinical trials. The economic and humanistic dimensions of outcomes are measured using emerging pharmacoeconomic research methodologies and data collection techniques within and alongside the traditional drug development process. Although the process of drug development has been described elsewhere,[4] a brief overview of the process will provide a better understanding of how and where pharmacoeconomic research fits into the process.

Clinical Research: The Drug Development Process

After basic animal research has been conducted and the preclinical studies have shown that a compound warrants further testing, a pharmaceutical candidate is then tested in humans. This process is divided into three study phases. In Phase I studies, the drug is tested in small numbers of normal, healthy volunteers to evaluate safety. If the drug appears safe, Phase II studies begin in patients who have the disease for which the drug is expected to be indicated. Phase II studies are designed to define initial efficacy parameters and optimal dosing of the drug using a small number of patients in various controlled clinical trials. After the demonstration of safety and initial efficacy, Phase III studies begin in large numbers of patients in controlled trials. Phase III studies are conducted to gather additional evidence for specific indications and usually are considered to be the pivotal safety and efficacy studies that support a new drug application (NDA).

The results of these three phases of studies, along with preclinical results, are compiled into an NDA or International Registration Dossier (IRD) and submitted to the FDA and other regulatory agencies worldwide with requests for approval to market the drug. While regulatory agencies are reviewing the data contained in the NDA/IRD, most companies initiate Phase IIIB studies to provide additional information regarding use of the drug. These studies usually involve large number of patients, with safety and efficacy as major endpoints. They also address practical questions regarding the drug's use in more realistic situations.

Although this traditional method of evaluating drugs via safety and efficacy studies is well-established, from an outcomes measurement perspective, it is incomplete. Because of the controlled nature of clinical trials, the safety and efficacy data obtained are likely to only approximate the effectiveness of the drug under real world, or less controlled, conditions. When conducting and interpreting clinical trials, it must be kept in mind that efficacy information indicates whether a drug can work under controlled conditions; it is the effectiveness of a product that is a measure of how the drug works in the real world, under average conditions created by, for example, noncompliance, use of concomitant therapy, or lack of access to care. Results obtained early in controlled trials may be compared and contrasted to results from Phase IV studies, which may have fewer controls, to determine the consistency of outcomes results. Pharmacoeconomic researchers and evaluators must keep in mind that data collected within any controlled study may not be representative of the drug effects experienced by all patients who take the drug. Study design and the pharmacoeconomic methods used will help to determine the degree to which data gathered will approximate what might be observed in the healthcare setting.

The shifts that are now occurring in the basic foundation of the medical care system necessitate incorporating pharmacoeconomic research within the context of clinical trial research. However, there are advantages and disadvantages with conducting this research. This chapter will identify issues and discuss considerations surrounding the incorporation of pharmacoeconomics into clinical trials. Baseline factors, design issues, instrument selection and administration, data management, analysis and interpretation, and reporting of results will be discussed.

Determining the Baseline

It is difficult to know whether or not a treatment has been successful if the natural course (condition without treatment) of the disease is unknown. The absence of baseline information markedly reduces the value of any information generated by the incorporation of pharmacoeconomics into an isolated clinical study since there is no benchmark with which to compare the results. Thus, it is crucial that a baseline be established before beginning the clinical research. Incorporating epidemiologic research and methods into the drug development and pharmacoeconomic research plans early on will aid in the interpretation of later study results. Epidemiologic research methods can be used to identify the natural course of the disease and current treatments as well as to provide information that will be useful in determining the burden of the disease to patients, healthcare systems, and society.

Before developing the research plan, a thorough review of the literature should be conducted. The literature search can be generated via MEDLINE using typical clinical search terms. Literature sources such as *Social Science Abstracts, International Pharmaceutical Abstracts,* government documents, and other databases also should be considered. However, not all information desired will be found in the literature; knowledge gaps can be identified from the literature review, providing a platform for the researcher to expand.

Identifying what is known about the condition and its current treatments helps focus the research effort. Questions of interest typically include "Who does the condition most affect? In what ways? Who bears the burden of the illness?" For example, asthma may affect a child clinically, and in terms of lost school days, but in an economic sense it may also affect a working parent or the parent's employer. Likewise, Alzheimer's disease has tremendous economic and humanistic consequences on the caregivers. Additionally, some diseases have no effective treatment and the healthcare system can provide only minimal care for the patient. However, these conditions may incur costs outside of the healthcare system. Depending on the perspective taken, those costs may be as important as the costs incurred within the system. For example, the cost of AIDS is great in terms of the morbidity costs incurred outside of the healthcare system.

Early on, it is important to assess the humanistic factors affected by the disease to capture the total burden of the illness and establish baseline information. Likewise, patient satisfaction with specific aspects of current treatments or interventions should be considered and measured. These baseline humanistic (satisfaction and quality of life [QOL]) assessments may indicate the degree to which there is "room for improvement" from the patient's perspective. If baseline scores indicate minimal dissatisfaction or impairment, it is unlikely that an intervention will result in significant improvement in satisfaction or health-related (HR) QOL, assuming valid, reliable, precise instruments are used. Osterhaus et al.[5] compared patients with migraine with age- and gender-adjusted samples and demonstrated that even between migraine headaches, the condition had a significant impact on patient HRQOL. Lindley et al.[6] measured the QOL of patients before and after highly emetogenic chemotherapy and demonstrated the impact of nausea and vomiting on patient perceptions. Baseline HRQOL assessment may involve cross-sectional data collection or longitudinal collection. Cross-sectional data collection provides a fingerprint of HRQOL at one point, with patients reporting their health status during the past week or month. Following a group of patients over time to collect longitudinal data can provide information about changes in health status during the measurement period.

It also is valuable to establish baseline levels of resource use. The basis for economic evaluation is an appropriate and complete assessment of the resources being used as opposed to dollars being spent. This is particularly true when collecting data from multiple locations and within environments where costs are subject to change. Resources used also represent, in part, the processes of care involved in patient diagnoses and treatment. Until recently, there have been only minimal attempts to link such processes of care to patient outcomes. If resources are limited, it is important for decision- and policy-makers to ensure that providers are using resources efficiently and effectively. If it is not known what or how much is being used to achieve an endpoint, it is impossible to know whether or not efficiencies are being attained. As resource use comes under greater scrutiny, it becomes more important to know what resources are involved in treating a condition to make proper use of the existing resources and ensure that new treatments are properly framed.

Although prospective studies may be required to capture the baseline data, there are other sources to consider. Some of these sources include patient diaries, government surveys, and medical charts. These sources can be used to conduct longitudinal studies to capture resource use over time. Various databases exist that can provide some information regarding resources used to treat conditions. These databases exist because many healthcare providers, including health maintenance organizations, have been paid based on the resources they use, so there is an incentive to provide such data. However, administrative databases do have shortcomings since they were not designed to provide complete outcomes information; they were designed to pay claims. If the condition is clearly and easily defined by a disease or treatment computer code, claims databases may provide information regarding the processes of care. However, medical claims data should never be assumed to be accurate. Appropriate validation techniques should be used to demonstrate the accuracy of the claims.

The importance of establishing appropriate and rigorous baselines for pharmacoeconomic assessment cannot be overstated. The management of outcomes is dependent on the ability to measure them, and measurement must have a frame of reference.

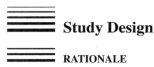 **Study Design**

RATIONALE

After benchmarks have been established, the next critical step is to incorporate pharmacoeconomic parameters into clinical trials. The goal of this step is to provide data that will determine the value of the product or intervention from various perspectives. Pharmacoeconomic research attempts to answer the "so what" question to the observed clinical change; that is, it documents the economic and humanistic consequences of pharmacotherapy. Ideally, pharmacoeconomic and clinical study plans should be developed in tandem. The degree of pharmacoeconomic involvement will most likely be a function of the phase of research in which the study is being conducted, the clinical study design, the condition of interest, and the information gathered at baseline regarding the condition and its impact. Key questions to address include, What is the primary purpose of the study? Are economic and QOL measures of primary or secondary importance? Why does this study need to be conducted? The process defined to address these questions should be clear and transparent so that any potential issues surrounding study design or bias are easily addressed.

OBJECTIVES

The pharmacoeconomic research question(s) should be defined in consideration of the clinical research question(s) raised. The questions should be clearly stated so that the study can be designed to answer the questions. Pharmacoeconomic research may be incorporated into a clinical trial as a secondary objective or as a primary objective. For example, if the study is a pivotal, Phase III study in which the primary goal is to measure safety and efficacy for an NDA/IRD submission, pharmacoeconomics may be considered as an "add on," and it is unlikely that the study will be (or should be) modified to make it more "appropriate" for a pharmacoeconomics study.[7] On the other hand, a Phase IIIB or Phase IV study, with the primary intent of measuring HRQOL or resource use in a general population with the condition under study, should be designed with the objective of answering a pharmacoeconomic question.[8] Having a study designed primarily to collect pharmacoeconomic parameters does not mean that safety and efficacy are ignored; clinical data must be collected in order to associate resource use and HRQOL changes with the clinical response.

DESIGN ISSUES

The pharmacoeconomic endpoints should be clearly identified a priori in the protocol. The protocol should be closely adhered to and standard precautions should be taken to minimize any potential biases or systematic error that may lead to erroneous conclusions. If the major purpose for conducting the study is to assess pharmacoeconomic changes with treatment, then the completion of baseline evaluations also should be part of the inclusion criteria in the protocol.

When designing pharmacoeconomic studies, it is critical to adhere to sound scientific principles. Randomized controlled trials are generally considered to provide the strongest level of evidence of efficacy. Hence, clinical trials, especially those intended to be part of an NDA or an sNDA are typically randomized, double-blind, and placebo-controlled. However, other study designs (observational, pretest/posttest, modeling) may be better suited to evaluating a pharmacoeconomic question, where blinding may mask the actual use of resources or the impact of a means of drug administration on HRQOL. Observational studies are sometimes used by health services researchers if the goal is to evaluate resource use in a realistic setting for various populations using one intervention or another. The results must be interpreted cautiously and should not be reviewed in isolation.

If resource use assessments are incorporated into the study, the perspective, (e.g., patient, society, employer) must be identified as well. Several perspectives may be of interest, given the current healthcare system. As the system undergoes further shifts, some perspectives will no doubt be of greater interest than others. Clearly, society and patient perspectives are of interest, because as a society, certain types of healthcare resources, such as vaccinations, are highly valued in part because of their external benefits. Third party payer perspectives are of interest because of the decision-making power that they have in the current healthcare system.

It is difficult to collect resource use and other economic data that are representative of realistic situations in a clinical study designed primarily to assess safety and efficacy. This is particularly true for chronic conditions such as hypertension or studies designed to prevent disease that use intermediate outcomes as endpoints (cholesterol reducing studies designed to reduce coronary artery disease, or studies to prevent sequelae of osteoporosis). On the other hand, some clinical trials of acute conditions may very closely mimic reality (treatment of sepsis, for example). The researcher must be aware of the extent of the limits imposed by the clinical trial design and document them in subsequent publications or presentations.

Likewise, the extent to which humanistic data collected in controlled clinical trials are indicative of expectations in the true population of patients is a function of the type of patients enrolled in the trial and whether the study design reflects a realistic use of the drug. For example, an antihypertensive clinical trial may include only individuals with mild-to-moderate hypertension and exclude those with other preexisting conditions. Conversely, a study of migraine with strict enrollment criteria may enroll only those with the most severe symptoms. The patients participating in a clinical trial may serve as a proxy or may provide an indication of what to expect in future use outside of trial conditions. If mildly affected patients show some improvement, one might expect to see larger improvements in more severe patients. If the intervention is linked with the improvement, results will indicate what aspects (economic or humanistic) have changed; this can be predictive of the expected results of future studies. The results from pharmacoeconomic evaluations in early clinical trials will allow for more focused research in later studies.

SAMPLE SIZE

In planning the design of a study, it is essential to determine the appropriate sample size. Sample size may be a function of efficacy parameters, specific HRQOL parameters, or economic parameters. If pharmacoeconomics is the primary objective of the study, the sample size should be estimated based on changes expected in those parameters. Currently, there is little information about sample size based on pharmacoeconomic parameters. Norms for the SF-36 Health Survey scales in the general US population have been published by age and gender.[9] However, until more information becomes available, pilot studies with pharmacoeconomic parameters, or previous trials, also may provide useful data. As an alternative, clinical parameters may be used to generate sample sizes; however, such an approach does not guarantee an appropriate estimate. For example, the number of subjects needed to show a clinical difference in asthma treatment might be 40 based on forced expiratory volume in one second; however, a cost-effectiveness study might require 140 subjects if the power calculation is based on the expected difference in number of emergency room visits. Post hoc power calculation will provide support for future studies. Additionally, in cases where pharmacoeconomic measures were not used to estimate sample size, sensitivity analysis should be used to place the results obtained from a study in proper perspective.

INSTRUMENT SELECTION

Selection and design of the data collection instrument is another important aspect of this research plan. Recognizing the symptomatology of the condition, and how the population is affected, will enable the researcher to select or create an instrument to measure how an intervention might lessen the economic and humanistic burden of the specific condition in question. The decision of instrument selection is critical. If HRQOL measures are to be included, the condition in question will be the determinant of whether or not a disease-specific instrument is required. If no appropriate instrument exists, an existing instrument may have to be modified or a new instrument designed. If it is not clear whether a disease-specific HRQOL instrument is needed, it is better to err on the conservative side and use one. A feasible approach is to use a standardized, validated core instrument to collect HRQOL measures, with customized additions to address the specific considerations warranted by the condition under study.

The issues of validity, reliability, and instrument sensitivity should be considered before an instrument is selected for use in baseline measurement and in a clinical trial. It is certainly possible to use a new instrument in a clinical trial without previous knowledge of its validity or reliability; however, the risk the researcher takes is that, after the fact, the instrument may be shown to lack those desired properties. Before using an instrument in a controlled trial, if possible, one should consider conducting a pilot test to verify that it is valid, reliable, and sensitive. If time does not permit it, one needs to consider the risks involved in ending up with data that are not usable.[10] Resource utilization questionnaires, too, also should be carefully developed and tested prior to use within a clinical trial. Data to be collected directly from patients by use of these instruments require special considerations. Some points to consider before the instruments is selected are literacy and translation of clinical terms into language that the patients will understand. The number of items one intends to include will be a function of the disease of interest.

Proper administration of the data collection instruments also is important. The protocol should specify how data will be collected, who will collect them, the specific time(s) during the study data will be collected, and who will provide the information. Investigators need to be informed of their responsibilities in providing and/or collecting data. Anticipating these questions and addressing them before data collection starts is important to the success of the data collection and, therefore, the study results.

Selection of investigators is another important consideration that affects the success of the study. The number of sites involved in a study may vary. Increasing the number of sites increases the potential complications from a management perspective. However, multiple sites are often needed so that sufficient numbers of patients can be enrolled within a reasonable time frame.

If the patient is the main source of pharmacoeconomic information, the burden placed on the patient needs to be considered. Most patients will not object to providing information. However, if the patients are going to be asked to provide information, they must be notified via informed consent. Patients should be told how much is expected of them, what they are to do, who will answer their questions, and other facts about the study and its effect on them. These issues must be clearly stated in the patient consent form.

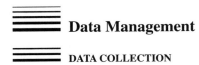

Data Management

DATA COLLECTION

In most traditional clinical trials, data are collected in the practitioner's office, hospital, or clinic. Since the physician is usually the investigator and may be making decisions about clinical efficacy, this method is appropriate. Pharmacoeconomic data are frequently, but not always, collected from the patient. Knowledge of the disease helps indicate who can provide the most reliable information about its burden. The patient and the physician are often respondents of choice. However, if the trial involves children or the elderly with cognitive dysfunction, or patients with other mental impairment, the patient may not be the most ideal source of information. Rather, caregivers or parents may be more appropriate respondents.

There are also trade-offs between asking for information at the healthcare provider's site (e.g., office, pharmacy) versus collecting it at home. Collecting data at the provider's office means that pharmacoeconomic data are collected at the same time that clinical data are collected. If questionnaires are completed at home, the ability to link the response with a clinical response may be a bit more difficult. On the other hand, patients or caregivers may feel rushed at the provider's site, especially if they are asked to provide additional information during the visit. The likelihood of obtaining complete responses is higher if the data collection forms are completed before the patient leaves the site, and the completeness can be checked by the investigator or another staff member. Also, if questions arise, someone is close by to answer them.

Another potential concern of asking questions at the provider's site is that the patient or caregiver may respond in the manner that they think will please the provider as opposed to how they really feel. The issue of social response bias should not be ignored, but it should be kept in perspective. It is, in part, a function of what questions are being posed. If patient satisfaction with the provider is the issue, a social response is of concern. But, if the questions focus on the patient's ability to work or attend school, response bias may not be as significant. Response bias is not limited to a physician's office, it also could occur in a home where a spouse may coach a patient as to the "right" responses. Social response bias may be reduced by changing the data collection medium. A personal interview in a waiting room is not likely to generate any information that the patient considers confidential. Patient self-report via a paper-and-pencil format or computer may provide a better sense of security. There is no generally agreed upon means to collect such data, as each method has its pros and cons, but whatever method is used, it is important to be consistent across all patients, and throughout the study. For example, the SF-36 Health Survey, a commonly used, validated instrument, consistently generates higher scores when data are collected over the telephone as opposed to a paper-and-pencil completion.[11] If change over time is of interest, consistent use of one approach is most appropriate.

═══════ **FREQUENCY OF DATA COLLECTION**

How often should pharmacoeconomic data be collected? If change is to be measured, a baseline and final assessment are required, at a minimum. Additional data collection points will be a function of the trial design and the condition being evaluated. When making the frequency decision, one should consider the pattern of intervention, and whether measures can be concentrated on where the maximum response to treatment is expected. Distinguishing between early and late effects of an intervention may be useful. The frequency with which data are to be collected should be stated in the protocol. Conservative estimates are recommended as data can always be aggregated, but cannot be disaggregated any finer than the original data collection points. Patient burden should also be considered when making these decisions. For an acute treatment, a baseline and final assessment may be appropriate; for a long-term trial, more frequent measures may be necessary to reduce the time period for which patients are asked to recall drug effects.

DATA ENTRY

Proper procedures must be in place to assure that data being analyzed are of acceptable quality. As with most studies, expected problems in the analysis of such data will surround missing data, multiple responses to single-item questions, illegible items, and stray marks. As the data proceeds through data entry, quality assurance, and quality control, procedures such as how missing data are to be handled should be identified and then adhered to scrupulously. A code book should be developed addressing each variable to be entered, and decisions made beforehand of how to deal with likely problems. When new problems arise with data entry (and they will), decide the response, be consistent, and note it in the code book. In the case of HRQOL analysis where several items may comprise a scale, it will be important to state at what point missing items will negate the use of an observation. In the case of economic data, missing items may reduce the usable sample size. Lack of critical demographic information may mean that work status cannot be identified. Missing data can be minimized by using appropriate questionnaires that are easy to complete with minimal burden on the patient or caregiver.

Analysis and Interpretation

An analysis plan also should be developed and either stated in the protocol or maintained as a separate document. The data analysis methods included in the statistical section of the protocol will be dictated by the types of data collected. Variables should be identified that are hypothesized to change over time. As is the case for the clinical component of many studies, a single variable may not suffice as "the answer" for a pharmacoeconomic study. Therefore, primary and secondary measures should be identified. The more measures identified to be of primary importance, the larger the sample size needed and the greater the likelihood of having one measure reach statistical significance due to chance. In the case of resource use, variables of interest may be length of hospital stay or intensity of resource use. Economic variables need to be evaluated as was determined before the study started. In the case of HRQOL measures, an index, a profile, or a battery of measures may be primary variables. If HRQOL is evaluated via a standard instrument, the instrument should be scored according to the developer's instructions. Multiple analysis of data not specified or planned for in the original study protocol is inappropriate, unless it is a pilot study intended to generate hypotheses as opposed to testing hypotheses.

The patients to be included in the analysis need to be identified. In some cases, the "intent to treat" sample is the appropriate choice—this includes all patients enrolled in the study—whether or not they actually followed the protocol. The intent to treat analysis is considered to most closely reflect actual use of a drug. Not everyone is compliant, and not every patient provides data for all collection points. Another option is to analyze only those patients who completed the study "per protocol." This subgroup may be of interest if HRQOL of an intervention is being evaluated (e.g., there is interest in evaluating only patients who took the drug properly). Analysis of both intent to treat and per protocol groups and a comment on the similarities and differences also is an option, but it is more time consuming.

There are a variety of methods by which pharmacoeconomic data may be analyzed. Clearly, which analytic method to use will be a function of what level of data are collected (e.g., nominal, ordinal, interval), its distributional properties, and the number of time points at which data are collected (cross-sectional or longitudinal). Direct comparisons, trends, percent successes, survival analyses, repeated measures, and multivariate analyses all have been used. Whichever method is chosen, it should be stated and justified in the protocol. In general, it is best to keep the analysis as simple as possible. Results should be reported in unweighted averages, in standard form. If HRQOL is measured using a profile, each dimension should be reported separately. Treatment groups should be separated and analyzed by treatment.

Potential confounders of data also need to be considered. Before one can attribute an effect to a specific intervention, it is important to minimize the likelihood of that effect being due to other variables. Randomization into groups, control groups, adequate sample sizes, and appropriate control of baseline parameters helps to minimize confounding, although one can never be entirely sure. Uncertainty can be addressed in two ways. Statistical methods can be used to address uncertainty that may be due to sampling techniques. Sensitivity analysis can be used to address uncertainty due to lack of knowledge. Sensitivity analyses ask "What if?" and test the robustness of the data. When assumptions are made about certain parameters, sensitivity analysis quantifies how comfortable one can be with those assumptions.

For example, there is no general agreement on the precise discount rate that should be used to discount future health benefits or future health costs. Since the precise rate is unknown, it is reasonable to test study results with a low, high, and middle value. If study results vary widely, one can have less confidence in any single set of results. Sensitivity analysis can demonstrate the dependence of a conclusion on a certain assumption, or that an assumption does not affect results significantly. It also can be used to establish a minimum or maximum value that a variable must possess for study results to be positive.

If the study is multinational, cross-cultural differences must be considered. Before clinical data such as blood pressure and laboratory values can be pooled for analysis, the data must be evaluated for homogeneity. In the same vein, neither HRQOL nor economic data should be pooled without cultural and homogeneity issues being taken into consideration. There may be substantial differences in HRQOL responses across cultures.[8] Thus, instruments need to be translated to assure linguistic and conceptual equivalence. From an economic perspective, different countries may have different pricing policies and the decision as to what monetary value to use is not always clear. It may be more simple to express economic evaluations in terms of resources used rather than in monetary increments. Despite attempts to control for various parameters, differences may still exist, and in those cases, data should not be aggregated.

Reporting the Results

When reporting pharmacoeconomic data that were collected in clinical trials it is useful to keep the presentation simple. If the initial questions asked were clearly stated, such an approach is realistic. One should avoid discussions of individual patients; rather, summary measures should be used to discuss the differences between treatments over time. One should be aware of potential censoring of HRQOL or economic results by death and/or early drop outs. For example, if patients in a duodenal ulcer prevention trial who have more than two relapses are dropped from the study because the treatment is considered a failure, these patients may be using up significantly more resources than patients who are doing well and still in the study. If the patients in whom treatment fails are lost to follow-up, it will be very difficult to trace the real impact of treatment due to limited knowledge of what happens to people in whom the treatment does not work. Likewise, the value of treatment may be underestimated if the patients in the placebo group are dropping out. The components of variance should be discussed and sensitivity analyses should be conducted so the reader can have an idea of the robustness of the data.

Summary

The decision to incorporate pharmacoeconomic parameters into a clinical trial depends on the healthcare environment and what information is being requested to make rational decisions about healthcare choices. Some regulatory agencies require and others are considering requiring economic information as a component of the drug approval and/or reimbursement process. Just as resource availability may limit a pharmaceutical company's ability to develop all of the potential drugs it has in its pipeline, resources also may limit the extent to which pharmacoeconomics will be incorporated into specific drug development programs. Realistically, some pharmaceutical products and healthcare interventions will be in greater need of pharmacoeconomic support than others. For example, drugs that are expected to be used for chronic conditions, to palliate symptoms, or slow the spread of an illness, but not cure it, are more likely to generate queries regarding their pharmacoeconomic benefit than a drug that cures an acute condition. Marketplace competition and demands also play roles in the decision. If a company plans to enter a market in which a number of similar drugs already exist it may be sufficient to compete only on the basis of price, as long as equal efficacy and safety can be demonstrated. HRQOL studies may be of interest only if there is a reason to suggest a difference in the adverse effects or functional status as a result of the intervention.

Pharmacoeconomics is a valuable tool used for making rational choices about pharmaceutical care interventions. Data can be collected in controlled trials before a drug has been approved and such data can be very useful as long as certain caveats are acknowledged. Whatever pharmacoeconomic assessment is chosen, it is imperative that all aspects of the study be transparent and able to stand the tests of reproducibility and appropriate criticism.

References

1. Letsch SW, Lazenby HC, Levit KR, Cowan CA. National health care expenditures 1991. Health Care Financ Rev 1992;14(2):1-30.

2. Wennberg JE. Improving the medical decision making process. Health Affairs 1988; 7:99-106.

3. Wechsler J. Re-evaluating clinical trials: devices, outcomes, and efficacy. Appl Clin Trials 1993;2:14-8.

4. Spilker B. Designing the overall project. In: Guide to planning and managing multiple clinical studies. New York: Raven Press, 1987: 36-62.

5. Osterhaus JT, Townsend RJ, Gandek B, Ware JE Jr. Measuring the functional status and well-being of patients with migraine headache. Headache 1994;34:337-43.

6. Lindley CM, Hirsch JD, O'Neill CV, Transau MC, Gilbert CS, Osterhaus JT. Quality of life consequences of chemotherapy-induced emesis. Qual Life Res 1992;1:331-40.

7. Cady RK, Dexter J, Sargent JD, Markley H, Osterhaus JT, Webster CJ. Efficacy of subcutaneous sumatriptan in repeated episodes of migraine. Neurology 1993;43:1363-8.

8. Hurny C, Bernhard J, Gelberg RD, Coates A, Castiglione M, Isley M, et al. Quality of life measures for patients receiving adjuvant therapy for breast cancer: an international trial. Eur J Cancer 1992;28:118-24.

9. Ware JE Jr, Snow KK, Kosinski M, Gandek B. SF-36 health survey manual and interpretation guide. Boston: The Health Institute New England Medical Center, 1993.

10. Young TL, Kirchdoerfer LJ, Osterhaus JT. A development and validation process for a disease specific quality of life instrument. Drug Info Assoc J (in press).

11. McHorney CA, Kosinski M, Ware JE. Comparisons of the costs and quality of norms for the SF-36 health survey collected by mail versus telephone interview. Med Care 1994;32:551-67.

11

Pharmacoeconomic Research in Medical Centers

Nelda E. Johnson
Jan D. Hirsch
David B. Nash
John J. Schrogie

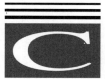onducting pharmacoeconomic analyses in a medical center setting can be beneficial for several reasons. Not only can these analyses contribute to the ever-growing body of published research, but the results can be used by decision-makers within the medical center to guide drug policy decisions for the formulary system[1] and can be incorporated into the institution's budgeting process.[2] By generating and using pharmacoeconomic data, medical center decision-makers can be better informed about the overall impact of drug use and become less reliant on data based solely on pharmacy drug expenditures.

As purchasers of health care increasingly demand to know the value of healthcare services, providers will experience increasing pressure to provide efficient, effective care while maintaining high-quality medical services. Data from pharmacoeconomic analyses that demonstrate the value (economic and humanistic) of interventions may prove essential as third party payers increasingly negotiate fixed payment rates with healthcare providers. No longer can medical centers allow new technologies to diffuse rapidly into clinical practice without regard for evaluations of their cost-effectiveness and impact on patient quality of life.

This chapter describes some of the specific processes involved in designing and conducting pharmacoeconomic analyses in medical centers and illustrates some projects that have been successfully completed in this setting. Additional discussion provides insight into the challenges that may be encountered when conducting pharmacoeconomic analyses in medical centers and highlights the future for this type of research.

Project Selection

Because of possible limitations that may exist for dedicating resources and personnel to pharmacoeconomic research projects in medical centers, it may be necessary to prioritize and select from a variety of potential topics. Highest priority should be given to products with very high acquisition costs or with high volume of use. Newer products that offer a greater clinical benefit but cost significantly more than the comparative therapy should be evaluated to see if the positive clinical outcomes offset the higher cost of the product. Drugs with higher benefit but lower costs than comparative therapies probably do not require additional study. Final selection of a project should be based on discussions with clinicians likely to use the product and pharmacists involved with developing drug use policies. The medical center's clinical programs also should be taken into consideration when selecting a project.

Research Team Members

Because investigators conducting pharmacoeconomic analyses need access to a variety of confidential data from different sources, it is essential to involve an interdisciplinary group whose members have a broad range of expertise. Such a group should consist of clinicians, pharmacists, pharmacoeconomic researchers, data analysts, information systems personnel, and representatives from hospital administrative staff. Each team member should bring sufficient expertise to the project to ensure appropriate design of methodology, drug therapy comparisons, interpretation of clinical conditions and outcomes, financial data management, and statistical analyses. Additional input may be required from specialty coders in the medical records department or from pharmacy data managers, depending on the study design used.

Models for establishing teams of clinicians, pharmacists, and pharmacoeconomic researchers to conduct economic analyses in the hospital setting have been described previously.[3] For instance, at Johns Hopkins' Office of Practice Evaluation a variety of studies have been conducted, including an analysis of the cost-effectiveness of clinical decision making and evaluations of new hospital-based technologies.[4]

By conducting well-designed, sophisticated investigations, it is expected that the results of such projects will be of sufficient quality to be acceptable for publication in peer-reviewed journals. Such high-quality research not only provides recognition for the investigators but provides the institution with a valuable resource to help decision-makers understand and assess the overall impact of pharmaceutical products. As noted by Lipsy,[5] it is hoped that joint ventures between pharmacoeconomists and clinicians will provide results that are applicable to the hospital setting.

Designing a Study

Many different types of analyses fall under the umbrella of pharmacoeconomic research including cost minimization, cost-benefit, cost-utility, and cost-effectiveness analyses. No single analysis type would be considered the most "correct" for determining the value of an intervention used in a medical center because the analysis type for each study is dependent on the clinical question posed. Pharmacoeconomic analyses may range from complex research projects to less involved forms of analyses that are often sponsored within an institution. When time or budgetary constraints within a medical center dictate that a less involved form of analysis be used, the researcher must be cognizant of the specific caveats and limitations that will apply to interpretation of the data generated.

Because pharmacoeconomic techniques and methodologies are still evolving, it is imperative that investigators are knowledgeable of current methodologies and select the most appropriate technique for each analysis. This is especially true for quality-of-life analyses where new instruments are being developed and tested for reliability and validity. As with any other research project, pharmacoeconomic analyses should be carefully planned evaluations designed to test a specific research hypothesis. Guidelines for conducting good economic evaluations should be followed to help ensure that the results obtained are valid and free from unintentional bias.[6,7] In conducting pharmacoeconomic analyses, specific attention should be given to the points outlined in Table 1.[6]

There may be numerous decision-makers in a medical center who come from varied backgrounds, so there may be several unique perspectives from which the pharmacoeconomic data will be evaluated and incorporated into the decision-making process. Both economic and humanistic evaluations may be needed to fully express a variety of relevant perspectives and assess the value of an intervention. The perspective included in the research design may differ greatly depending on whether the study will be conducted for inpatients or outpatients. Research conducted with an inpatient population will focus on the consequences of an intervention that are immediate

Table 1. Conducting Pharmacoeconomic Analyses[a]

• Clearly define the research question
• Specify the viewpoint or perspective of the analysis
• Determine the alternative therapy for comparison
• Evaluate the clinical effectiveness of the therapy
• Identify all relevant costs and consequences to be measured
• Select the appropriate methodology for the study
• Measure and analyze all costs and consequences
• Interpret and communicate study results

[a]Adapted from ref. 6.

and primarily visible to health professionals, hospital administrators, or healthcare purchasers. Inpatient studies offer the investigator an opportunity to create a well-controlled study in which all consequences related to an intervention can be measured. These types of studies frequently focus on acute illness with short-term clinical and economic outcomes and are viewed from the perspective of the hospital administrator.

In contrast, research conducted on an outpatient population will focus on longer term consequences that are generally removed from the immediate domain of the healthcare system, but are more relevant to the individual patient. The ability to account for variance within this population becomes less precise since an observer cannot report and verify all patient behavior. Instead, there is increased reliance on patient self-report for measurements that focus on outcomes such as health-related quality of life or functional ability (return to work or increased mobility). These studies are usually viewed from the patient or societal perspective.

Prospective Data Collection

The design selected for the study will depend not only on the research question and the perspective used, but on the time and resources allocated to the project. In general, randomized prospective pharmacoeconomic analyses are likely to take longer to complete although they offer the greatest opportunity to control variables in the study. Investigators may find opportunities to collect pharmacoeconomic data in conjunction with randomized clinical trials being conducted in the medical center. This offers the investigator an opportunity to conduct the pharmacoeconomic evaluation early in the development of a drug and provides the medical center and the pharmaceutical company with economic data for the new drug.[8] However, because drug use in a clinical trial setting usually differs from how the drug is used in routine clinical practice, the relevance of the alternative therapies being compared and the costs that are part of the study protocol requirements must be considered.[9] In addition, the investigator may need to use modeling techniques to extrapolate the results to settings outside the clinical trial.

Retrospective Data Collection

Depending on the sophistication of the medical information system available, investigators may find that these databases offer one of the most efficient ways to collect clinical and economic data. Information systems that are designed to support clinical financial decision-making models can serve as a comprehensive data source by providing the investigator with both clinical as well as financial data.

Some of these information systems use a repository system to extract data from various existing departmental databases such as pharmacy, laboratory, medical records, and billing systems.[10] These data are then automatically merged into one integrated database, creating a data-rich source of information for pharmacoeconomic analyses. Ideally, the key data elements in such a system would include information of sufficiently high quality and detail that minimal chart review would be required for validation. Some of the key data elements likely to be retrievable from such a system are listed in Table 2.

Clearly, it is an advantage for an institution to have a database resource that combines both clinical and financial data in an interactive mode. Two primary alternatives for centers without this resource are to (1) merge data from existing but separate databases or (2) combine clinical data from chart reviews with financial data obtained from a patient-based accounting system.

The limitations of using data from hospital information systems may include the loss of data due to aggregation of the information[11] or lack of clinical detail because of limits in the medical record abstracting process. In addition, the hospital information system may store only data that relates to certain departments or only to inpatient admissions. For instance, drugs or other resources used in areas such as emergency or operating rooms may be missing from the database. Because of these limitations, it is imperative that the investigators have a thorough understanding of the origin and limitations of the data in the system before designing the study. It should be kept in mind that hospital cost accounting systems are designed for financial decision making, and additional work may be required to accurately characterize the clinical parameters and economic outcomes of interest. The use of time and motion studies in conjunction with standard cost accounting techniques may be helpful in determining the specific cost components of an intervention not captured in sufficient detail in the database.

Table 2. Important Data Elements

- Length of hospital stay
- Intensity and cost of resources used in various hospital departments
- Patient charges
- Drug therapies and doses administered
- Demographic information
- Payer status
- Admission/discharge dates and status
- Admitting and discharge diagnoses
- Medical service
- Severity of illness measures

The search strategies used for economic analyses will vary depending on the study design, but an initial search may involve preliminary investigations to identify the total patient population of interest or the number of patients who received the therapies being compared. The clinical homogeneity of the patient population identified should be assessed to determine whether refinements to the population need to be made or to identify comparable patient populations for the study. In cases where computer codes for the clinical condition of interest are inadequate, algorithms or proxy measures may have to be developed to adequately select patients for inclusion. Additional steps such as validation of the computer-generated data may need to be made through audits of the primary medical records. See Jones[11] for a more complete discussion of the methodology for searching hospital databases using pharmacoepidemiology study designs.

Example Projects

Highlights of two example studies are described below as a means of discussing some of the practical applications, issues, and potential compromises faced when conducting pharmacoeconomic studies in a medical center. The framework used to compare and contrast each study is based on the methods for evaluating economic analyses proposed by Drummond et al.[12]

EXAMPLE 1

This first example focuses on an analysis of the overall economic impact that a novel antiemetic therapy (ondansetron) had on the use of hospital resources for inpatients admitted for maintenance chemotherapy treatment.[13] This product was selected for evaluation because it was considered to offer clinical advantages over traditional therapies, but the acquisition cost was considerably higher than the traditional therapies it replaced. At the time the study was conducted, there were no published data about the overall pharmacoeconomic impact of this drug in a medical center setting.

Perspective of the Study. This study used the hospital's perspective and was conducted from the viewpoint of a hospital administrator. Therefore, direct and indirect overhead costs from all departments and the overall total costs to the institution were considered.[13]

Evidence of Clinical Effectiveness. Several randomized clinical trials had confirmed the efficacy of ondansetron for the specified indication. However, clinical trials measure efficacy (Does the drug work?) while the question of effectiveness (Does the drug work in a given patient/prescriber population?) had not yet been documented in a systematic way in this institution. Therefore, the study design also included a prospective evaluation of the clinical effectiveness of ondansetron in the medical center.[13]

Study Methodology. The study used primary data collected by nurses taking care of patients undergoing chemotherapy to determine the frequency of nausea and vomiting and a time and motion study to determine the costs associated with episodes of nausea and vomiting. These data were combined with historical (retrospective) data obtained from an integrated database for the clinical and financial parameters associated with hospitalizations of patients admitted for maintenance chemotherapy.[13]

Using the hospital's information system, patients were identified who had been coded as having an admission for Diagnosis-Related Group 410 (chemotherapy) during the six months prior to and the six months after the introduction of ondansetron. Although comparisons across time without control groups may be considered less than ideal from a research design standpoint, this is the natural course of diffusion for new technologies and appropriately reflects the hospital administrator's perspective. Thus, describing the course of events in terms of changes in total hospital costs and changes in length of stay over the two time periods was appropriate. However, this approach required the researchers to consider possible effects associated with changes in severity of illness over time and changes in prescriber treatment patterns that could have affected the primary outcome measure: length of stay.[13]

Interpretation and Communication of Study Results. Results showed that hospital costs and length of stay decreased after the introduction of ondansetron. But, as ondansetron became more widely used, the P&T committee implemented guidelines to encourage the appropriate use of the product.

The use of summary data for this study represented a compromise between the validity of the data collection and the real-time constraints present at the medical center. Although these types of trade-offs are essential to implement studies within a patient care environment, the potential impact of the limitations should be clearly examined when results are interpreted and reported. The advantage of using this study methodology is that it presented hospital administrators with data about the actual financial impact of a drug therapy and did not rely on theoretical probabilities of the clinical and financial outcomes.

EXAMPLE 2

The second example illustrates how a pharmacoeconomic analysis was used by a medical center to estimate the impact an expensive new product would have on total hospital costs once the product became commercially available. In this example, a decision tree model was used to predict the clinical and financial impact of nebacumab, a monoclonal antibody under investigation in the US for the treatment of gram-negative septic shock. This biotechnology product was selected for evaluation not only because of its high acquisition cost, but because clinical trials showed that it demonstrated efficacy only in a subgroup of patients with sepsis who had documented gram-negative bacteremia. It seemed likely that in routine clinical practice, clinicians would employ less stringent criteria for use of the product and many patients might receive the product with little opportunity for clinical benefit but at great additional expense to the institution. To control the use of nebacumab, clinical guidelines with specific criteria for using the drug were developed by an expert panel convened by Thomas Jefferson University Hospital in conjunction with the University Hospital Consortium, an alliance of 60 academic medical centers.[14] The pharmacoeconomic analysis was designed to evaluate the potential benefits of adopting the guidelines for the use of nebacumab.[15]

Perspective of the Study. The analysis used the hospital's perspective and was conducted from the viewpoint of the hospital administrator. Therefore, direct and indirect overhead costs from all departments and overall total costs to the institution were considered.[15]

Evidence of Clinical Effectiveness. Because nebacumab was not approved by the Food and Drug Administration at the time the analysis was conducted, there was no information about its effectiveness in routine clinical practice. Therefore, the analysis used efficacy data from a published randomized controlled clinical study designed to evaluate safety and efficacy.[16]

Study Methodology. A decision tree was constructed to compare the total hospital costs and number of lives saved for each of three alternatives: treat all, treat none, or treat by guidelines. Data for the analysis were obtained from several different sources. Survival rates were obtained from published clinical trial data; hospital costs and number of patients with gram-negative sepsis were obtained from the medical center's medical information system. The basic model required a set of assumptions, including (1) the proportion of patients who would meet the guideline criteria for treatment with nebacumab (assumption based on retrospective data on characteristics of patients with sepsis), (2) the proportion of patients with sepsis who would actually have gram-negative bacteremia (obtained retrospectively from the hospital database), and (3) the impact of nebacumab therapy on length of hospital stay and thus total hospital costs.[17]

Interpretation and Communication of Study Results. This analysis showed that the marginal cost for each additional survivor in the treat all branch was more than twice that in the treat by guidelines branch. Both of these branches resulted in the maximal number of sepsis survivors, but the treat by guidelines option would cost the hospital significantly less than the treat all option because it results in a lower marginal cost per life saved. Although the treat none branch was the least costly option to the institution, it resulted in fewer lives saved, an outcome the institution did not consider acceptable.[15] By calculating the potential benefits of using the guidelines, the medical center could evaluate whether the potential benefit of using the guidelines offset the costs associated with implementing and monitoring their use. This analysis gave the medical center a more rational basis for making a decision on whether it was beneficial to implement clinical practice guidelines for an expensive new technology.

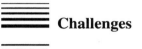 ## Challenges

FINDING SUPPORT FOR PROJECTS

One of the primary challenges that may face investigators in medical centers is finding the time and resources necessary to conduct full-scale pharmacoeconomic analyses. Because of this, some medical centers may find it desirable to create a separate, full-time office dedicated to conducting these types of analyses. In this way, high-priority, but time-consuming, projects identified by hospital committees or administrators can be channeled to the medical center's fully staffed office. They in turn can conduct the analysis in a timely fashion and provide results relevant to the institution. This facilitates the use of consistent methodology as well as efficiency in training of staff.

Some academic medical centers have successfully supported projects for evaluating the cost-effective use of hospital resources by initiating internally funded grant programs. For example, Strong Memorial Hospital in Rochester, NY, initiated a number of internally funded cost-effectiveness studies in 1987; they resulted in annual marginal cost savings of nearly $600,000 in the first year of the program alone.[18] Several academic medical centers, including the Brigham and Women's Hospital in Boston, the University of Texas at Galveston, and the Cleveland Clinics have previously funded full-time positions for specialists in pharmacoeconomics.

Pharmaceutical and medical device companies are increasingly willing to sponsor economic analyses because of the recognized need to assess the economic as well as clinical outcomes of a product. This increased interest in industry-sponsored collaborative research has been described in the literature.[19] Hillman et al.[20] outlined ethical standards and guidelines to help investigators minimize the potential for bias in the conduct and reporting of economic analyses. In a survey conducted by the Center for

Outcomes Information in San Francisco, 26 of 42 drug manufacturers reported that they were involved in outcomes research and predicted that they would be paying more attention to outcomes and cost-effectiveness research in the future.[21]

The federal government also has funded pharmacoeconomics research. The impetus for this funding may date back to the Omnibus Budget Reconciliation Act of 1986, which mandated analysis of the cost-effectiveness of medical treatments. The government has since commissioned the Agency for Health Care Policy and Research to study the clinical and economic outcomes of pharmaceutical therapies so that guidelines can be established for the appropriate, cost-effective treatment of patients.

SELECTING OUTCOME MEASURES

The selection of appropriate outcome-based measurements is essential for pharmacoeconomic studies and need to accurately reflect the perspective taken for the study. For instance, using length of hospital stay as an outcome measure is appropriate for studies using the perspective of the hospital or third party payer, especially since length of hospital stay is the single most important determinant of hospital costs.[22] But, because length of stay can be altered by a patient's clinical condition, severity of illness, or physician practice patterns, careful consideration must be given to these measures throughout the design, analysis, and interpretation of the study results.

Outcome measures such as health-related quality of life are important components of pharmacoeconomic analyses. These studies require extensive follow-up by trained study personnel for patients outside the hospital setting with chronic illnesses. The selection of appropriate, valid, and reliable quality-of-life questionnaires that are sensitive to changes associated with the medical intervention of interest is key to conducting a successful analysis.

COMMUNICATING STUDY RESULTS

Once the data have been collected and analyzed, investigators need to effectively communicate the study results both internally within the institution and externally. The methods used to disseminate the study results will vary depending on the organization's structure and culture, but certain key personnel within a healthcare organization should receive the results of the economic analyses. For example, the chair of the pharmacy and therapeutics committee, the director of the pharmacy, and others involved in setting policies for formulary drug use should have immediate access to the results of pharmacoeconomic analyses. In addition, study results should be interpreted and communicated to medical staff leaders and administrative staff throughout the healthcare organization.

Organizations that have committees designed to receive and act on pharmacoeconomic analyses may find that the acceptance and use of such information will be greatly simplified. However, for organizations without this avenue, economic analyses may represent new concepts that require additional education about the methodology used and ways to incorporate the results into the decision-making process. Interest in the results of economic analyses can be fostered through newsletter briefings, presentations at research meetings, and discussions at departmental meetings. The publication of study results in peer-reviewed journals and presentation at national symposiums also can foster greater interest and respect for the economic analyses.

EXTERNAL VALIDITY OF RESULTS

Caution should be exercised in the direct extrapolation of the economic results from one setting to another because of differences in the costs and alternative regimens used in different settings.[9] By reporting the actual resource quantities measured in the study, the results may be more useful to others who wish to apply them in settings where price levels may be different. The value of quality-of-life evaluations to outside organizations may be enhanced by providing thorough descriptions of the study population, including factors that may influence quality-of-life scores such as demographics (e.g., age, sex, comorbidities). The external validity of the study may be further enhanced by including sufficiently large enough numbers of patients in the analyses or by conducting multicenter studies.

Future Directions

BIOTECHNOLOGY DRUGS

Hospital pharmacy managers as well as healthcare administrators, insurers, and government payers are sufficiently concerned about the high costs of new biotechnology drugs to commit resources to evaluate their potential cost and benefits. For instance, within four months of a journal publication describing the use of human antiendotoxin monoclonal antibodies for gram-negative sepsis, 80% of hospitals surveyed by the University HealthSystem Consortium in Chicago, IL had a mechanism in place to study their fiscal impact even though no product had yet received Food and Drug Administration approval.[14] Several researchers in academic health centers used modeling techniques to conduct cost-effectiveness analyses for the new agent in the treatment of gram-negative sepsis.[17,23,24] These studies and other pharmacoeconomic analyses for recombinant granulocyte colony-stimulating factor[25] and epoetin[26] have stimulated additional interest in using pharmacoeconomic data to assist in formulary[2,5] and pharmaceutical benefit coverage decisions. It is anticipated that the assessment of pharmacoeconomic data will become an integral part of managing pharmacy drug budgets as biotechnology products continue to consume ever-increasing portions of pharmacy budgets.

In some institutions, special subcommittees of the pharmacy and therapeutics committee have been created to assess expensive new technologies such as biotechnology drugs.[27] These committees can help focus formulary deliberations on ways in which healthcare providers can use expensive drugs in a cost-effective manner by identifying the types of patients most likely to benefit and the clinical conditions under which a product's value may be greater than or equal to its acquisition price. These committees can obtain and use pharmacoeconomic data to produce technology assessment documents that review the literature and delineate policies or guidelines for the use of these products.

NETWORKING AMONG HOSPITALS

Technology assessments that incorporate data from economic analyses conducted in the medical center setting may prove crucial for organizations attempting to control costs while maintaining high-quality care. According to a 1992 survey reported in *Hospitals,* only one-fifth of the responding hospitals had formal technology assessment programs.[28] In the future, institutions that lack the resources to conduct their own assessments of technology may find it beneficial to network with other similar institutions.[29] For example, the University HealthSystem Consortium has a program specifically designed to aid its member hospitals in their efforts to evaluate and compare the cost and value of technologies. Thus, the medical centers can pool their resources and draw on expertise from within the network of academic medical centers. This network also offers researchers opportunities to conduct multicenter pharmacoeconomic studies, thereby increasing the potential external validity of the medical center–based studies.

LINKING OUTPUTS TO PURCHASERS

Over the past few years, pharmacoeconomic data have gained added importance in decisions on to how to best use and reimburse for products and services in the clinical setting. Those who pay the healthcare bills are interested in such research because it may help eliminate unnecessary or ineffective treatment or identify areas where early treatment is valuable. As spending on health care continues to rise and as purchasers of health care demand increased value, it is expected that pharmacoeconomic analyses for pharmaceuticals will become an increasingly important part of the hospital decision-making process. Drug use policies and clinical guidelines designed to foster cost-effective, high-quality care may eventually be linked to third party reimbursement, as indicated by several initiatives undertaken by the federal government.[30]

The Health Care Financing Administration already requires hospitals to provide discharge data that are used to calculate hospital mortality rates and hospital charges for certain medical interventions. Some managed care organizations have the ability to analyze claims data and provide monetary incentives to physicians and hospitals who provide cost-effective care according to clinical guidelines. As payers demand more information about the costs and benefits of healthcare services, medical centers will need to become more sophisticated in retrieving and analyzing their own data to compete effectively on the basis of cost and quality of services provided. Those who work in the clinical setting have begun to understand that we have entered a new era of assessment and accountability with regard to the quality and cost of care delivered.[31]

Summary

As pharmacoeconomic analyses become more sophisticated and data for drugs become more widely available, the use and value of this information will undoubtedly increase. It is also likely that medical centers will need to become more involved in conducting their own clinical economic analyses for important planning and purchasing decisions. The advent of sophisticated hospital information systems may facilitate the collection, analysis, and use of pharmacoeconomic data for important planning and purchasing decisions as medical centers strive to provide high-quality, cost-effective care. Pharmacoeconomic analyses should be seen as a powerful tool that can be used to help at least partially rationalize the selection and use of pharmaceutical agents in the medical center setting.

References

1. Nash DB, Catalano ML, Wordell CJ. The formulary decision making process in a U.S. academic medical center. PharmacoEconomics 1993;3:22-35.

2. Johnson NE. Pharmacoeconomics and biotech drugs. Pharm Ther 1992;17:1402-12.

3. Nash DB. Creating centralized clinical evaluation units. In: Lord JT, ed. The physician leader's guide. Rockville, MD: Bader and Associates, October, 1992:85-8.

4. Steinberg EP, Graziano S. Integrating technology assessment and medical practice evaluation into hospital operations. Qual Rev Bull 1990;6:218-22.

5. Lipsy RJ. Institutional formularies: the relevance of pharmacoeconomic analysis to formulary decisions. PharmacoEconomics 1992;1:265-81.

6. Drummond M. Australian guidelines for cost-effectiveness studies of pharmaceuticals. PharmacoEconomics 1992;1(suppl 1):61-9.

7. Jolicoeur LM, Jones-Grizzle AJ, Boyer JG. Guidelines for performing a pharmacoeconomic analysis. Am J Hosp Pharm 1992;49:1741-7.

8. Copley-Merriman C, Egbunonu-Davis L, Kotsanos JG, Conforti P, Franson T, Gordon G. Clinical economics: a method for prospective health data collection. PharmacoEconomics 1992;1:370-6.

9. Drummond MF, Davies L. Economic analyses alongside clinical trials: revisiting the methodological issues. Int J Technol Assess Health Care 1991;7:561-73.

10. Cavanaugh F. Information architecture: the repository alternative. Comput Healthcare 1992 (Nov):16-8.

11. Jones JK. Inpatient data bases. In: Strom BL, ed. Pharmacoepidemiology. New York: Churchill Livingston, 1989:213-27.

12. Drummond MF, Stoddart GL, Torrence GW. Methods for the economic evaluation of health care programmes. New York: Oxford University Press, 1987.

13. Johnson NE, Nash DB, Carpenter CE, Sistek CJ. Ondansetron: costs and resource utilisation in a U.S. teaching hospital setting. PharmacoEconomics 1993;3:471-81.

14. Nash DB, Johnson NE, Gottlieb JE, Vlasses PH. Monoclonal antibodies for septic shock: in or out of the barn door? Qual Rev Bull 1991;17:310-3.

15. Carpenter CE, Nash DB, Johnson NE. Evaluating the cost containment potential of clinical guidelines. Qual Rev Bull 1993;19:119-23.

16. Ziegler EG, et al. Treatment for gram-negative bacteremia and septic shock with HA-1A human monoclonal antibody against endotoxin. N Engl J Med 1991;324:429-36.

17. Schulman KA, Glick HA, Rubin H, Eisenberg JM. Cost-effectiveness of HA-1A monoclonal antibody for gram-negative sepsis: economic assessment of a new therapeutic agent. JAMA 1991;266:3466-71.

18. Franklin PD, Panzer R, Brideau LP, Griner PF. Innovations in clinical practice through hospital-funded grants. Acad Med 1990;65:355-60.

19. Cuatrecasas P. Industry-university alliances in biomedical research. J Clin Pharmacol 1992;32:100-6.

20. Hillman AL, Eisenberg JM, Pauly MV, Bloom BS, Glick H, Kinosian B, et al. Avoiding bias in the conduct and reporting of cost-effectiveness research sponsored by pharmaceutical companies. N Engl J Med 1991;324:1362-5.

21. Drug manufacturers study cost effectiveness, quality of life. In: Report on medical guidelines and outcomes research. Alexandria, VA: Capitol Publications, 1991;2:1-6.

22. Kukull WA, Koepsell TD, Conrad DA, Immanuel V, Prodzinski J, Franz C. Rapid estimation of hospitalization charges from a brief medical record review. Med Care 1986; 24:961-6.

23. Chalfin DB, Holbein MEB, Fein AM, Carlon GC. Cost-effectiveness of monoclonal antibodies to gram-negative endotoxin in the treatment of gram-negative sepsis in ICU patients. JAMA 1993;269:249-54.

24. Barriere SL. The economic impact of HA-1A (Centoxin) against endotoxin. PharmacoEconomics 1992;2:408-13.

25. Faulds D, Lewis NJ, Milne RJ. Recombinant granulocyte colony-stimulating factor: pharmacoeconomic considerations in chemotherapy-induced neutropenia. PharmacoEconomics 1992;1:231-49.

26. Leese B, Hutton J, Maynard A. A comparison of the costs and benefits of recombinant human erythropoietin (epoetin) in the treatment of chronic renal failure in 5 European countries. PharmacoEconomics 1992;1:346-56.

27. Selzer JL, Wordell CJ, Nash DB, Johnson NE, Gottlieb JE. P & T committee response to evolving technologies: preparing for the launch of high-tech, high-cost products. Hosp Formulary 1992;27:379-92.

28. Lumsdon K. Beyond tech assessment: balancing needs, strategy. Hospitals 1992; August 5:20-6.

29. Wagner M. Hospitals will have their own assessment efforts. Modern Healthcare 1991;December 2:38.

30. Shulman SR. The reimbursement factor in pharmaceutical regulation: rebates, cost-effectiveness, and practice guidelines. PharmacoEconomics 1992;1(suppl 1):21-7.

31. Relman AS. Assessment and accountability. The third revolution in medical care. N Engl J Med 1988;319:1220-2.

12

Pharmacoeconomics and Community Practice

C. E. Reeder
Jean Paul Gagnon

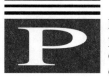harmacoeconomics is an emerging and dynamic discipline. As with most emerging disciplines, the pharmacoeconomic literature has been conceptual in nature, defining terminology and developing guidelines necessary for conducting quality research. Few articles detail how pharmacists can use the principles of pharmacoeconomics within their practice settings, especially pharmacists practicing in a community environment. It is possible that some community pharmacists will design or conduct cost-minimization, cost-benefit, cost-effectiveness, cost-utility, or cost-consequence analyses. However, trends in health care indicate that community pharmacists are more likely to be participating in these studies and using the data generated through pharmacoeconomic analyses to evaluate manufacturers, products, and services.

The profession of pharmacy has begun to espouse the concept of pharmaceutical care. With the adoption of this concept comes increased responsibilities for measuring the value of products and services. "Value" is the trade-off of costs versus clinical and humanistic (quality-of-life) outcomes.[1] Through the provision of pharmaceutical care, pharmacists must be concerned not only with providing patients the highest quality of care (i.e., assuring the best outcomes for patients), but also with providing this quality to a cost-conscious patient. The combination of quality and cost is the underlying principle of pharmacoeconomics and suggests that community pharmacists do have an important role to play in these analyses.

Recent trends in health care, such as the movement toward a system of managed competition and an increased emphasis on cost containment, indicate that quality and cost containment are concerns not only at the individual level but also at the state and national levels. Assuring that quality care is provided at the least cost is not a role relegated only to third party administrators or government agencies; other healthcare practitioners, including the community pharmacist, also are involved. If community pharmacists are to assume this important role, they must understand the principles of pharmacoeconomics and be able to apply them in their practices. Finally, community pharmacists must be prepared to document the value of their professional services in terms of costs versus clinical and humanistic outcomes.

Sometimes the pressures of daily routines restrict our ability to recognize changes taking place in society. Few of us take the time to think of our profession as it might be in the not too distant future. As Levitt[2] pointed out in his classic article "Marketing Myopia," many businesses fail because they define themselves too narrowly and do not adapt as technology advances. Levitt's example of the railroad industry provides an interesting comparison for the state of community pharmacy practice.

> The railroads did not stop growing because the need for passenger and freight transportation declined. The railroads are in trouble today not because the need was filled by others, but because it was not filled by the railroads themselves. They let others take customers away from them because they assumed themselves to be in the railroad business rather than in the transportation business. The reason they defined their industry wrongly was because they were railroad-oriented instead of transportation-oriented; they were product-oriented instead of customer-oriented.[2]

The lesson for community pharmacy is clear: to continue to grow and be a viable part of the future healthcare system, pharmacy must recognize and act on customer wants and needs and not be satisfied with the status quo. Pharmacists must realize they are not in the pharmacy business but rather in the "patient management" business. Community pharmacy must not limit itself by focusing on the short-term; it must look into the future to determine if changes in the way pharmacists practice will make pharmacoeconomics and outcomes management an important part of what community pharmacists will do.

The fact that nearly all major pharmaceutical associations have embraced pharmaceutical care as a practice philosophy certainly portends a future of change for the profession. Smith,[3] in his teaching of leadership, uses the concept of the "Merlin factor." This approach refers to the legendary wizard who lived backward in time (Merlin was born in the future and aged as he proceeded into the past). He influenced the behaviors of kings by drawing on his foreknowledge of their destinies. In other words, Merlin had the amazing ability to assess the potential of the present moment from the perspective of a clearly envisioned point in the future. Because he knew what was going to happen in the future, he could instill direction and knowledge into those whose actions could achieve the future that he had envisioned.

Although the application of pharmacoeconomics and outcomes management within community pharmacy practice may not seem feasible at present, the future holds endless possibilities. What is needed is the Merlin approach, a look into the future to envision the practice of community pharmacy and where pharmacists will use pharmacoeconomic data. Once we see the future, we can think and plan backward from that vision to generate effective action in the present. Moreover, by practicing the Merlin approach the profession can dedicate itself to a future that is strategically alluring, but very improbable if evaluated solely from a historical perspective.

The Future of Community Pharmacy Practice

One way to determine what community pharmacy will look like 10 years from now is to examine current trends in our society. Popcorn,[4] the founder of Brain Reserve, continually examines general consumer trends and their unique relationships to the future marketplace. She has identified current trends that forecast future lifestyle, wants, and needs. Melby,[5] author of several published articles on the future of pharmacy, studied Popcorn's predictions and their implications for pharmacy. Listed below are some of Popcorn's societal trends that relate to pharmacy and Melby's assessment of their potential impact on pharmacy practice.

Cocooning. Consumers seek to protect themselves from a harsh, unpredictable world by searching for a safe, familiar environment. Consumers want to stay home. Melby[5] sees cocooning manifested as a demand by patients for treatment at home whenever possible. As a result there will be a surge of high-technology devices that can be used by the critically ill. In addition, there will be a movement toward having prescriptions delivered to patients at home and having pharmacists make house calls to discuss medication use and management.

Fantasy Adventure. The modern age whets our desire for the road not taken. Experimentation and safe risk taking are on the rise. Melby[5] predicts that pharmacists will become more adventurous in their approaches to patient education. Pharmacists of the future may use holograms to demonstrate how to use medications and home care products. Virtual reality techniques may be used to allow patients to feel how a product will work.

The Vigilante Consumer. Consumers will manipulate the marketplace through pressure, protest, and politics. Pharmacists will have to protect the safety and welfare of the patient or they will be admonished or abandoned by consumers. Pharmacists will become even more responsible for selecting the manufacturers of pharmaceutical products. Consumers will rely on pharmacists to evaluate quality and cost of pharmaceuticals and to pick the manufacturers of high-quality, cost-effective products.

Staying Alive. Patients are beginning to accept responsibility for their own health and fitness. Melby[5] notes that self-care will be the norm in 10 years and patients will be measuring their own blood pressure and self-treating minor seasonal disorders. Pharmacists will need to assist patients with their self-care needs.

Cashing Out. Patients want a better quality of life with more meaningful work activities, back-to-basic values, and more leisure time. Pharmacies will use robotics to become more automated, thus reducing the time patients have to spend in pharmacies. Correlated with a decline in the time used for the dispensing function will be an increase in time spent on patient counseling. Pharmacists will be challenged to demonstrate to employers and payers that patient counseling is valuable to the patient's well-being.

Save Our Society. The 1990s will be the decency decade as this country experiences a reawakening of social conscience. Consumers and payers will hold pharmacists accountable for the outcomes related to drug therapy. Pharmacists will use the power of their computerized databases to monitor patient outcomes and will take an active role in drug utilization review and drug protocol management.

Clanning. Consumers are forming tighter alliances with others who have similar desires. Patients will be looking for personal pharmacies that offer valued, cost-effective products and services.

MANAGED COMPETITION

Other important environmental changes are focused on the healthcare delivery system. Because of the growth of managed care, interest in healthcare reform, and ever-rising costs, the scope, role, and structure of payers, providers, and suppliers are changing. A scan of the healthcare environment reveals that networks or alliances of hospitals and providers, fueled by the concept of managed competition, are proliferating at a rapid rate. Hospitals and other healthcare providers are banding together to achieve economies of scale. In the very near future instead of 10 to 15 hospitals and a number of primary care practices in a city there will be two or three systems or integrated networks comprised of hospitals and providers. To push this concept along, the Federal Trade Commission has published guidelines that allow networks to form without violating antitrust laws.[6] Formation of networks is part of an overall trend toward integration of the healthcare system. This process of integration and consolidation is being accelerated by coalitions of employees who are leveraging the healthcare distribution system.

After hospitals are united into systems, they begin to look for ways to reduce costs and improve or maintain quality. One of the first steps administrators take after forming a system is to identify areas where costs can be reduced. Favorite targets are redundancies: for example, three different formularies and pharmacy systems. Obviously, costs can be saved by having one formulary among the hospitals with one pharmacy and therapeutics committee. One of the goals of such systems will be to develop a formulary that provides cost-effective pharmaceuticals.

At the same time hospitals and other providers are networking, suppliers are vertically integrating to prepare themselves to provide products and services to the new systems. Good examples are the Medco–Merck alliance, Lilly and PCS, and SmithKline Beecham and DPS. These alliances will probably be composed of a number of pharmaceutical companies, wholesalers, and networks of pharmacies which will ultimately offer a formulary to the integrated health system. It is quite conceivable that in the future four or five vertically integrated networks of manufacturers, wholesalers, and retailers will be selling formularies and pharmacy services instead of products. Under this scenario pharmacists will need the skills to build a cost-effective formulary, select a vertically integrated group, evaluate the quality/cost of a formulary, and change prescriber behavior using drug utilization evaluation and drug protocols. All of these skills require extensive training in pharmacoeconomics and outcomes management.

In summary, using the Merlin approach to envision the future of community pharmacy practice reveals that future pharmacists will be held accountable for managing drug use through compliance programs, drug utilization review and drug protocol management, monitoring and assessing pharmaceutical outcomes, determining the value of the pharmaceuticals dispensed and the pharmaceutical care services rendered, and selecting suppliers. New roles and niches for monitoring cost-effectiveness and outcomes will arise as payers begin to compensate pharmacists on the basis of their services, what they have done to improve the quality of health care, and how well they evaluate, monitor, and manage the demand for the products and services they deliver.

Future Uses of Pharmacoeconomic Principles by Community Practitioners

As Weinstein and Fineberry[7] have stated, it is not the results of a pharmacoeconomic analysis that will impact a decision, it is the process of structuring information in a systematic framework that brings to light the key uncertainties and the most important value trade-offs. Given the review of important trends in society and where community pharmacy might be in the future, the remainder of this chapter will focus on how pharmacists will apply pharmacoeconomic principles and data in their practices to allow them to meet the wants and needs of their patients.

HEALTH STATUS MONITORING

Health status measurement will have an important role in optimal patient treatment in the future. As the most accessible health professional, community pharmacists are in an ideal position to collect health status data from their patients. A number of general- and disease-specific instruments discussed in an earlier chapter will be perfected and readily available for use by pharmacists. The Sickness Impact Profile[8] and Quality of Well-Being Scale[9] are examples of the type of instruments that provide an easy and valid measure of a patient's functional and social well-being. The Medical Outcomes Study SF-36, a general measure of a patient's health-related quality of life, provides a profile of the patient's quality of life along eight dimensions.[10] Changes in a patient's health status and quality-of-life profile are important indicators of how well the patient is responding to medications and will be used to manage and improve patient therapy. Such information will be used routinely in patient counseling and physician communications. Coupled with traditional physiologic measures, such as blood pressure, and serum glucose or lipid concentrations, these measures of health status will provide a clearer picture of the patient's overall health and progress.

Consider, for example, the patient who receives an antihypertensive medication. The medication is successful in lowering the patient's blood pressure but has the undesirable effect of persistent sedation. As a result of sedation, the patient becomes noncompliant and blood pressure increases. The use of a quality-of-life index could have assisted the pharmacist in identifying the decline in the patient's well-being and social functioning. The patient could have been counseled and the physician contacted, if necessary, to consider alternative treatments or dosage adjustments. To survive and prosper in the future, pharmacists must become responsible for proactively monitoring patient medication use and outcomes. Identification of under- and overuse of medications and their consequences for therapeutic, economic, and quality-of-life outcomes will be an integral part of the future pharmacist's role.

Technologic advances will allow the pharmacist to automate data collection and management tasks associated with health and quality-of-life assessments, thus allowing the pharmacist to conduct prospective drug utilization review. Pharmacy computer systems will be enhanced to read optical scan forms, store patient data, and print patient health and quality-of-life profiles. This information can be linked to a physician database to keep the patient's physician informed of treatment outcomes and problems with therapy. In addition, pharmacists will be responsible for collecting economic data on the indirect costs and consequences for pharmaceutical therapies and services. Documentation of costs related to lost productivity and caregiver opportunity costs represent significant aspects of patient outcomes from pharmaceuticals and pharmaceutical services. An important role for the pharmacist will be total medication management. Success in this capacity will depend on the pharmacist's ability to collect and maintain comprehensive databases on patient outcomes and to use this information to improve decisions about appropriate therapy.

Great opportunities will exist in the future for pharmacists to use health status and quality-of-life indices to improve patient care, enhance the image of their pharmacies, and increase interprofessional communication. With increasing interest in patient health outcomes, it will be important for pharmacists to demonstrate the value of their services to the healthcare system.

EVALUATING PHARMACY SERVICES

Another area where community pharmacists will apply the principles and tools of pharmacoeconomics is in justifying the value of their professional services. This will be done by documenting the effects of pharmaceutical care on patient health outcomes. With healthcare spending exceeding 14% of the gross domestic product, individuals, governments, and third party payers will want a cost-effectiveness impact statement for all new services. In allocating scarce resources, everyone will be cognizant of where the most benefit can be gained for each dollar spent. For pharmacy, the major question will be "What difference do pharmacists, pharmaceuticals, and pharmaceutical services make in patient health outcomes?" Several societal trends identified earlier point to the consumer's desire for valued services. To justify future existence, community pharmacists must be prepared to answer this question on an on-going basis. Pharmacists will create and maintain patient databases that relate their functions to positive, cost-effective patient outcomes.

Efforts are underway to evaluate the impact of pharmaceutical care on patient health and well-being. This is just the first step in the broader quest to establish the added value of pharmacists. Third party and government payers will refuse to reimburse for any functions that do not offer benefits in excess of costs. As they move their practices toward the next century, community pharmacists will begin to think in terms of costs and consequences. Although making these justifications may appear onerous if not impossible tasks, pharmacists can team with researchers at local schools of pharmacy to conduct pharmacoeconomic analyses of pharmaceutical services. Such cooperation and mutual interests should facilitate the development of the requisite database.

POSTMARKETING SURVEILLANCE

Another potentially productive and rewarding area of pharmacoeconomics that community pharmacists might consider is participation in Phase IV postmarketing surveillance studies. These studies are typically sponsored by pharmaceutical companies as part of the drug approval and marketing process. Experience has shown that while clinical testing of drugs under controlled conditions is important, the real value of a new drug or device is its effectiveness in general patient populations. Numerous examples exist of drugs completing the elaborate and time-consuming premarket drug approval process only to be recalled shortly after marketing because of untoward effects not detected during clinical trials.

Community pharmacists will be involved in and reimbursed for participation in postmarketing studies. To do so typically will require collaboration with a sponsoring pharmaceutical firm and working with researchers in a school of pharmacy that might coordinate study conduct, data collection, and analysis. Postmarketing studies follow the consequences of using a therapy in general practice. Community pharmacists are in an ideal position to identify patients who are receiving a medication and to collect pertinent information regarding patient status and therapeutic outcomes. Because postmarketing studies are conducted under specified research protocols, the major functions of the pharmacist in these types of studies are to identify patients, discuss the use of the medicine, and document consequences of therapy. Community pharmacists have an advantage in this regard in that they can not only identify a patient receiving a drug for the first time, but also can perform follow-up surveys to determine compliance, side effects, adverse reactions, and ultimately therapeutic and quality-of-life outcomes. Networks of research-oriented community pharmacies are likely to evolve to accommodate the need for large-scale postmarketing studies of pharmaceutical products and services.

Participation in postmarketing studies meshes nicely with monitoring patient health outcomes in that the structure necessary to perform either activity is similar. Pharmacy computer systems can be modified or adapted to identify potential subjects and alert pharmacists to collect the appropriate information. Moreover, pharmacists can use the system to follow scheduled refill dates and collect data on medication use at some point after the medication is prescribed. Postmarketing studies can become a routine part of a pharmacy's medication and health status monitoring program.

Determining the Value of Pharmaceuticals

Most major pharmaceutical firms are establishing medical outcome or pharmacoeconomic research units within the company. Health insurance companies, benefits managers, and government agencies are demanding evidence that their premium dollars are well spent. Other countries, including Germany, Canada, and Australia, have already begun to require pharmacoeconomic analyses for reimbursement of new products. The US is certain to follow in questioning the value of all components of the health-care delivery system. As a consequence, more emphasis will be placed on conducting studies on cost-effectiveness and therapeutic outcomes to justify the acceptance of and payment for new pharmaceutical therapies.

To survive in the marketplace, a pharmaceutical manufacturer must demonstrate the superiority of its products over existing therapies. The development and introduction of drugs with little or incremental therapeutic benefit will become increasingly difficult to justify, whereas products that offer therapeutic advantages or improvement in patient outcomes will find success. It will be important for community pharmacists to scientifically evaluate new treatment modalities and to make recommendations on their value and cost to patients, prescribers, and payers. Moreover, pharmacists must prepare themselves to assume additional responsibility for pharmaceutical therapy selection. This role goes beyond the traditional concept of drug product selection where the pharmacist simply chooses a reliable generically and therapeutically equivalent drug product. In this expanded role, pharmacists will need to be able to tailor pharmaceutical therapy to specific patient clinical, economic, and quality-of-life needs.

Formularies

In the not-too-distant future pharmacists will not only be responsible for evaluating specific pharmaceutical entities but also formularies of drugs offered by integrated systems. It is conceivable that instead of offering products, networks of suppliers and retailers will be selling formularies or drug management systems. Teams of pharmacists will be responsible for evaluating the cost-effectiveness of formulary offerings from these groups. These formularies will have to be cost-effective and produce positive quality-of-life effects on patients.

Sophisticated cost-effective analysis models and computer software will be available for use in evaluating these formularies. Pharmacists will have to be educated in computer as well as traditional pharmacoeconomic skills. Serving on these evaluation teams will require considerable analytic and decision-making skills because the effects of the choice of a formulary will dramatically impact the operation of the health partnership and its network of hospitals. These same skills will be required as pharmacists participate in the development and implementation of treatment guidelines, protocols, and disease state management programs.

Pharmaceutical Care Services

Community pharmacists can use the knowledge of pharmacoeconomics and patient outcomes to their advantage, but to do so will require creativity and a proactive posture. Community pharmacists are accustomed to receiving contracts from third parties that at best offer to pay part of the pharmacy's usual prescription charge. Why have these contracts been so arbitrary and unprofitable? Possibly because third party administrators see little added value in the services and care pharmacists provide. Not recognizing quality differences among therapies and services, much less the consequences of inappropriate therapy, the primary cost-containment strategy of third party payers has been to reimburse for the lowest cost product. Most of the evidence offered in support of higher professional fees and charges has been anecdotal or self-anointed without any justification for the value of the pharmaceutical services provided.

Rather than having a third party administrator dictate a formulary or fee schedule, community pharmacists will work together with other healthcare providers or third party administrators to develop a pharmaceutical care package that can be marketed to benefit managers, employers, managed care plans, and insurers in their local area. This coalition will develop, in conjunction with local physicians, its own formulary based on the most cost-effective therapies. Group buying will then be practiced to secure the lowest product cost for members. The pharmacy group will market itself on the outcomes it can offer the patients it serves.

Such an endeavor will require pharmacists to evaluate products based on clinical, economic, and humanistic outcomes and decide which bundle of services will optimize therapeutic outcomes. As part of a buying group or managed competition network, pharmacists will be in the position of evaluating pharmaceutical manufacturers not only on the quality of their products but also on the value of the services they supply to pharmacists and patients.

Pharmacists must position themselves to manage not only their business but also their patients' health outcomes. The impact of prospective and retrospective drug utilization review and drug protocol management on patient well-being, use of medical sources, and cost must be documented at the community pharmacy level. Do we have all the information needed to do this? Not at the present, but community pharmacists do have the background, ability, and resources to perform these new functions and to apply pharmacoeconomic principles to evaluate and document pharmaceutical outcomes.

Skills Needed to Compete in the 21st Century

What skills do community pharmacists need to successfully integrate these new opportunities into their current practice? Certainly, pharmacists need to be able to interpret and evaluate findings from pharmacoeconomic studies. A major portion of this book is devoted to helping the reader critically evaluate the quality and applicability of this literature. As part of their future practice, community pharmacists using published guidelines will be required to evaluate studies provided by pharmaceutical manufacturers or published in the medical literature regarding the cost-effectiveness, cost-benefit, or cost-utility of pharmaceuticals. Likewise, community pharmacists will work with researchers who are interested in conducting pharmacoeconomic evaluations and pharmaceutical outcome studies. Pharmacists also will be responsible for selecting manufacturers using a number of important variables including policies regarding returned goods, reputation, and liability protection.

Pharmaceutical outcomes manager will be an apt descriptor of the pharmacist in the 21st century. Therapeutic success will be measured not only in clinical terms but also in terms of the ability of pharmacists to balance the cost and consequences of therapy. Perhaps the most important duty that pharmacists will assume will be managing humanistic outcomes, assuring that the patient's quality of life, the most important outcome, is the focus of therapy.

Lastly, community pharmacists must market their value and contributions for patient well-being to the public, healthcare payers, and other decision-makers. This means developing a proactive marketing campaign based on sound pharmacoeconomic studies and a cooperative effort among all community pharmacists to establish their cost-effectiveness to the healthcare system. Controls on utilization and costs are essential components of a well-managed healthcare system and will not be abolished simply because community pharmacists demonstrate their value to the healthcare system. The real challenge of the future will be to convince healthcare payers and decision-makers to consider the full impact of pharmaceuticals and pharmaceutical care on patient outcomes and the total cost of care.

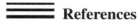 **References**

1. Kozma CM, Reeder CE, Schulz RS. Economic, clinical, and humanistic outcomes: a planning model for pharmacoeconomic research Clin Ther 1993;15:1121-32.

2. Levitt T. Marketing mopia. Harvard Bus Rev 1960;38(4):45-56.

3. Smith CE. The Merlin factor. Washington, DC: Leadership and Strategic Intent, 1991.

4. Popcorn F. In: The 21st century: hospital pharmacy in a changing health care delivery system. Orlando, FL: Lederle Laboratories, December, 1992.

5. Melby M. In: The 21st century: hospital pharmacy in a changing health care delivery system. Orlando, FL: Lederle Laboratories, December, 1992.

6. Federal Trade Commission, Justice Department announce joint policies for health care antitrust enforcement. FTC News, September 15, 1993.

7. Weinstein MC, Fineberry HV, eds. Clinical decision analysis. Philadelphia: WB Saunders, 1980.

8. Bergner M, Bobitt RA, Pollard WE, et al. The sickness impact profile: validation of a health status measure. Med Care 1976;14:57-67.

9. Kaplan RM, Bush JW, Berry CC. Health status: types of validity and the index of well-being. Health Serv Res 1976;11:478-507.

10. Ware JE, Sherbourne CD. The MOS 36-item short-form health survey (SF-36) I. Conceptual framework and item selection. Med Care 1992;30:473-83.

13

The Application of Pharmacoeconomics in Managed Healthcare Settings

Andy Stergachis
Sean D. Sullivan
Peter M. Penna

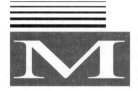anaged healthcare plans have been among the most aggressive managers of cost, utilization, and quality of pharmaceuticals in the US. They have generally been more successful than traditional fee-for-service plans in implementing a variety of drug use management programs to control drug costs, quality, and access. Managed healthcare plans use a variety of strategies to administer prescription drug benefits, including the use of drug formularies, generic and therapeutic interchange, use of preferred provider networks, financial incentives to promote appropriate drug use, member cost-sharing, drug utilization review programs, enhanced clinical and utilization information systems, pharmaceutical care services, and disease management programs.

Managed care plans attempt to achieve numerous goals, including improvements in the appropriate use of medications, the enhancement of favorable patient outcomes, and improvements of the cost-effectiveness and cost-efficiency of health care. To carry out these responsibilities, managed care plans need to make high-quality decisions regarding the appropriate use of pharmaceuticals. These decisions are strengthened through the conduct and application of credible, relevant pharmacoeconomic research.[1] Pharmacoeconomic data also offer the opportunity to better judge the value of pharmaceuticals and pharmaceutical services in achieving desired outcomes for managed care plans. This chapter describes the current and future role of pharmacoeconomics in the management of pharmaceuticals, pharmaceutical services, and drug policies in managed care organizations, with a particular emphasis on staff-model health maintenance organizations (HMOs), considered to be the most tightly controlled managed care model type.

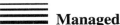 Managed Health Care

Although the term "managed care" lacks a commonly accepted definition, it is used to characterize health plans that incorporate mechanisms designed to review and control the cost, quality, and use of health services and to generally limit enrollees' choice of providers to a specified network of healthcare providers. In essence, managed care involves the delivery of a predetermined level of healthcare benefits to a defined population on a prepaid basis. Examples of managed care plans include HMOs, and the continuum of plans with less restrictive controls over choice of providers and utilization of services: preferred provider organizations (PPOs), network models, exclusive provider organizations, triple option plans, fee-for-service insurance programs with active utilization quality management programs (e.g., managed indemnity programs), and various hybrids.[2,3] At least two types of HMOs exist: the staff model and the individual practice association (IPA) model. In the staff-model HMO, physicians are employees of the HMO, are usually paid by the HMO on a salaried basis, and are a part of the formal administrative structure of the organization. Many staff-model HMOs also own clinics, hospitals, and pharmacies for the exclusive use of their enrollees. In an IPA model HMO, physicians are usually reimbursed by the HMO on the basis of a contracted, discounted fee-for-service, or capitated at-risk payment. Here, community-based physicians serve the managed care plan enrollees as well as fee-for-service patients. Compared with staff-model HMOs, IPAs typically offer greater patient access at the expense of reduced control over utilization, cost, and quality.

PPOs are characterized by the presence of incentives for patients to use a network of providers on a "preferred basis." PPO network providers commit to accepting fixed reimbursement and to observing an appropriate, effective, and cost-efficient practice style. Network model plans are a network of several independent, multispecialty medical groups. Like IPAs and PPOs, network plans serve managed care plans and fee-for-service patients. It is common for IPA, PPO, and network physicians to be involved with several managed care plans simultaneously.

Managed healthcare organizations have become a dominant force in the US healthcare system. As of 1992, an estimated 70% of physicians in the US were affiliated with managed care programs, and often with multiple programs.[4] In less than a dozen years, the percentage of the population covered by managed care plans has grown considerably. In 1980, managed care plans represented only 5% of the private health insurance market. By 1991, however, approximately 80% of the insured population was directly or indirectly influenced by managed care. Over 49 million people, or approximately 19% of the US population, were enrolled in the nation's 540 HMO plans alone in 1993, with the greatest concentration of HMO enrollees in the Pacific region of the US.[5] Approximately 90% of HMO members belong to non–staff-model HMO plans.[6] Over the past 10 years, PPOs have become the most prevalent approach to managed health care. An estimated 122 million people in the US are eligible to enroll in PPOs.[6] We are likely to see enrollment in managed care organizations grow even further by the year 2000 as a consequence of the effect of market forces and healthcare reform packages being considered at the state and national levels. The stimulation of the growth of managed healthcare organizations has been noted repeatedly as a mechanism for controlling healthcare costs in the private and public sectors.

Managed healthcare organizations are characterized by their use of strategies for controlling healthcare costs. They also have been leaders in attempts to assess and assure the quality of care, including patient outcomes. Overall strategies include the use of prepaid financing arrangements for a full range of services, a focus on primary care and prevention, and the use of information technologies and other managerial approaches to optimize the utilization of services. Prepaid financing arrangements place an organization and its providers at financial risk because a capitation amount is actuarially computed to cover the expected cost of care for the average enrollee over a defined period of time, typically one year. Such a risk-based method of payment provides incentives to control provider overutilization. Additionally, managed care organizations have monitoring mechanisms for provider underutilization as well. The General Accounting Office recently summarized that most managed care plans include the following cost control features: use of provider networks, with explicit criteria for selection of providers; alternative payment methods and rates that often shift some financial risk to providers; and utilization controls over hospital services and specialist physician services.[7]

Managed Care Pharmacy Benefits Programs

An estimated 40% of sales of pharmaceuticals in the US are made on behalf of managed healthcare plans (Table 1). In 1991, approximately 75% of HMO plans offered prescription drug coverage and 14% provided coverage for over-the-counter medications.[5] Although HMOs spend an average of only 11% of their total expenditures on pharmaceuticals, this segment is one of the fastest growing expenses for HMOs. In 1991, HMOs paid an average of $103 per member per year for drugs, up 17% from 1990 and 47% from 1989. In contrast, the 1991 overall average annual expenditure for prescription drugs in the US was approximately $200 per person.

Table 1. Outpatient Pharmaceutical Benefits by Payer Type[a]

TYPE	INDIVIDUALS[b]	DRUG COVERAGE[b]	PHARMACEUTICAL BENEFITS MANAGEMENT (%)
Indemnity	66.0	60.3	15
PPO/POS provider	47.5	28.7	20
HMO	41.5	37.4	65
Medicare/Medigap	34.0	19.8	15
Medicaid	28.0	28.0[c]	100
Uninsured	37.0		
Total	254.0	174.2	40

[a]HMO = health maintenance organization; POS = point of service; PPO = preferred provider organization. Data obtained from Shearson Lehmman Brothers and Health Industries Research Center, newsletter, New York, February 10, 1993. Some overlap exists in these figures. For example, 2 million Medicare enrollees are covered by HMOs.
[b]Data given per million persons.
[c]Only 12.8 million Medicaid patients are believed to be covered by a pharmaceutical benefits program. However, all are included because all Medicaid programs receive price discounts through the Omnibus Budget Reconciliation Act of 1990.

The number of prescriptions filled per HMO enrollee was 5.8 per year in 1991, up slightly from 5.7 in 1990.[5]

To better understand the factors responsible for the increase in expenses for pharmaceuticals, Group Health Cooperative of Puget Sound (GHC), a staff-model HMO, separates the increases into two components: inflation and utilization or volume of prescribed drugs, including new drugs added to the formulary. For example, in 1992 GHC's $38.3 million budget for outpatient and inpatient drugs amounted to approximately $104 per enrollee per year (Table 2). New drugs added to the formulary typically account for 1–2% of the increases from year to year. In 1993, however, new drug additions amounted to a 6% increase from the previous year. Current

Table 2. Factors Resulting in Increase in Drug Expenditures for 1992: Group Health Cooperative of Puget Sound

1992 Drug expenditures ($)	
total	38,595,414
per member per month	8.74
Factors responsible for increase from 1991 to 1992[a] (%)	
utilization	13.55
inflation	0.91

[a]Relative percent contribution to change in drug expenditure, adjusted for enrollment growth.

projections are that 1994 drug costs will be 8% higher than those for 1993 on a cost-per-enrollee basis, with most of the increase due to increased drug utilization, particularly the use of newer and more expensive drugs. The contribution of prescription price inflation to drug expense can be determined by analyzing contractually determined price increases, rebate programs, and the availability of generic alternatives to drugs losing patent protection. An analysis of the contribution of drug utilization to increases in drug expenses takes into account major drugs likely to be released by the Food and Drug Administration (FDA) or added to the drug formulary. The availability of sophisticated information systems enables the assessment and projection of changes in drug use patterns. By breaking down drug expenditure increases into its component parts, a managed healthcare organization should be better able to focus its efforts at managing its drug budget.

Strategies Used to Manage Drug Benefits: Implications for Pharmacoeconomics

Managed care plans use a variety of strategies to manage the cost, quality, and access to pharmaceuticals provided to their enrollees. The basic elements of a pharmacy benefit package include a pharmacy and therapeutics (P&T) committee, a drug formulary, generic and therapeutic interchange, the use of special controls on high-cost drugs, treatment guidelines, and a variety of pharmaceutical care interventions, including drug utilization review, disease management programs, and academic detailing. Other characteristics of pharmaceutical benefits include member cost-sharing, some degree of financial risk-sharing with prescribers, and, in many cases, contracting with community-based pharmacies to provide pharmaceuticals and pharmaceutical care services to members. Managed care plans also effectively use contracting with pharmaceutical manufacturers to achieve price discounts, including the solicitation of bids from manufacturers of therapeutically equivalent drugs.

To better select and evaluate the specific strategies for managing pharmaceutical benefits, managed care plans frequently access and analyze primary and secondary data about the care received by their enrollees. Relatively new methods, such as decision analysis, have emerged as contributors to improved medical decision-making in managed health care. As more fully described in the remainder of this chapter, managed care plans are beginning to use the methodologies of pharmacoeconomics and pharmacoepidemiology to improve decision-making. Illustration of the application of pharmacoeconomics to managed care are categorized into three general areas: formulary policy, prescriber and pharmacist practices, and drug benefit design.

FORMULARY POLICY

At the center of most managed care plans' pharmacy benefits programs is the P&T committee, the committee charged with maintaining the drug formulary system. A look at the mission of GHC's P&T committee suggests how these committees evaluate information and make decisions regarding pharmaceuticals. At GHC, the mission of the P&T committee is to establish and maintain safe, effective, appropriate, and cost-effective drug therapy in a manner that facilitates optimal patient outcomes (Figure 1). Effective P&T committees do this by: (a) monitoring the on-going research and development activities of the pharmaceutical industry; (b) determining which drugs should be added, deleted, or restricted in the formulary, based on uniformly applied criteria; (c) defining criteria and/or restrictions for use of drugs within the managed care plan; (d) taking necessary organizational and educational steps to implement committee action; and (e) evaluating and measuring drug utilization and outcomes, and taking appropriate actions when opportunities for improvement are identified.

Formulary systems play a major role in facilitating appropriate drug usage, cost, and quality. They are designed in part to provide savings in pharmaceutical product expenses by facilitating the purchase of drug products at lower prices, reducing drug inventories, and increasing the use of

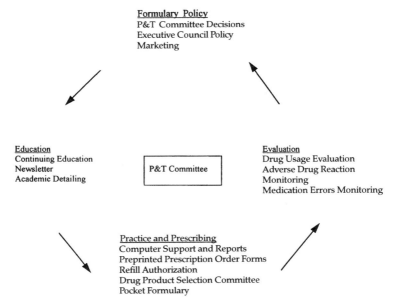

Figure 1. Group Health Cooperative of Puget Sound's medication use management program. P&T = pharmacy and therapeutics.

clinically similar but less expensive drugs. Approximately half of all HMOs used formularies in 1991, with 88% of staff-model HMOs using formularies compared with only 36% of IPAs.[5] Successful formularies restrict access to or discourage the use of those drugs for which there are lower-cost substitutes available, thereby encouraging the use of more efficient medications. Although there is considerable debate about whether formularies result in overall cost savings, there is evidence that savings are realized for particular drug categories.[8-11]

When compiling and revising formularies, the most frequently used criteria for selecting among alternative drugs are clinical efficacy, risk of adverse effects, and daily cost of drug. Too often, cost analyses focus on a search for the least costly alternative, without an explicit analysis of overall cost-effectiveness. In fact, cost-minimization analysis is the most frequently applied pharmacoeconomic method in formulary decision-making. For example, if a drug is determined to be therapeutically similar to existing drugs on the formulary, then daily cost of drug therapy is weighed heavily by the P&T committee. Additional factors, including quality of life, patient preference, and outcomes, are only now beginning to be discussed as part of the formulary decision-making process. Data from pharmacoeconomic studies are increasingly entering into formulary decision-making. P&T committees are beginning to examine cost information on a broader basis, taking patient outcomes into account. The goal of formulary management should not necessarily be to decrease the drug budget alone, but rather to improve the efficiency of care delivery and optimize patients' health status relative to resource constraints. Increasingly, emphasis is being placed on P&T committee consideration of the nonmedical economic impact of pharmaceuticals (e.g., indirect costs).[12] Unfortunately, such pharmacoeconomic data are rarely available to decision-makers in a timely manner, and when these data are available they are often misunderstood by decision-makers.

Not surprisingly, pharmaceutical companies are expanding their activities to generate data that attempt to estimate the value of their products in relation to competitors' products. In a 1993 survey, pharmaceutical manufacturers reported that they had conducted more than twice as many outcomes research studies in 1993 as in 1992.[13] These studies include economic appraisals as well as quality-of-life studies. The majority of respondents to the survey expect the number of pharmacoeconomic studies to increase. Most managed care pharmacy directors would agree that valid outcomes and cost-effectiveness data can lead to more effective formulary decisions, regardless of the source of funding. However, concerns are growing about variation in the quality of such studies leading to the development of standards for pharmacoeconomic evaluations.[14,15] Moreover, the FDA recently became more involved in the cost-effectiveness field by accelerating the development of principles for substantiation and disclosure necessary to support promotional claims.[16]

Managed care plans themselves have performed pharmacoeconomic studies in support of formulary decision-making. They can frequently access either primary or secondary health, utilization, and cost data to support pharmacoeconomic analyses. There are examples of data that have been used for cost-of-illness, cost-minimization, and cost-effectiveness studies in managed care settings. Clouse and Osterhaus[17] conducted a cost-of-illness study using United HealthCare Corporation databases. The investigators compared healthcare use and associated costs in patients with and without migraine headache to determine the cost incurred by the health plan for the care of each of these groups. Glauber and Brown[18] conducted another example of a cost-of-illness study. Using data from the Northwest Region of Kaiser Permanente, a group practice HMO, they evaluated the use and cost of drugs among patients with diabetes and found that they use a greater variety of drugs in larger quantities and at greater cost than patients without diabetes. Pharmacy expenditures accounted for 17% of the total cost of caring for that population of patients with diabetes. In yet another example, Stergachis et al.[19] used data from GHC, a staff-model HMO, to assess the medical outcomes and costs associated with the pharmacological treatment of patients with peripheral arterial disease. Among the outcomes assessed were the incidence of invasive diagnostic and therapeutic procedures, hospitalizations, and the cost of care related to peripheral arterial disease.

Another analysis strategy for making or evaluating formulary policy is the use of decision analysis. Decision analysis offers a framework for evaluating a wide variety of decisions: to select a drug for addition to a formulary; to conduct a cost-effectiveness analysis; to determine a treatment strategy; to improve clinical decision-making; and to make better policy decisions.[20] As an example, Hillman and Bloom[21] used decision analysis to help predict the economic impact of a new drug, misoprostol, in actual clinical use. A decision tree was developed, a combination of the medical and clinical literature and a panel of experts was used to assign clinical probabilities, and the rate of gastric ulcers associated with nonsteroidal anti-inflammatory drug use was used as a measure of outcomes. Other examples of pharmacy-related decision analysis can be found in the literature.[22,23]

There have been other economic appraisals of various components of formulary management,[24] including the effects of therapeutic interchange. Therapeutic interchange, within the context of a formulary, allows the pharmacist to substitute drug products that are deemed therapeutically equivalent, although not chemically equivalent. Managed care programs are increasingly allowing the interchange of one drug with another of the same pharmacologic or therapeutic class when deemed appropriate. This decision is usually made by the P&T committee. For example, cephalexin and cephradine have been determined by GHC's P&T committee as therapeutically equivalent, allowing GHC to stock only one of these drugs based on the best contract terms GHC can negotiate. There have been a few formal assessments of the cost savings associated with therapeutic interchange. McDonough et al.[25] reported the total direct cost and savings associated with a voluntary program that switched enalapril to lisinopril in patients with benign essential hypertension who were enrolled in Harvard Community Health Plan, a staff-model HMO. Direct costs included drug acquisition, office visits, laboratory monitoring, management of adverse effects, pharmacy administrative costs, and the time value of money. Using computerized pharmacy records and a review of patient medical records for a random sample of enalapril- and lisinopril-treated patients, the authors demonstrated a net savings in less than 12 months following the initiation of the voluntary therapeutic interchange program.

PRESCRIBER AND PHARMACIST PRACTICES

Ensuring appropriate drug use (i.e., prescribing, dispensing, ingestion) can maximize the benefit that enrollees receive from their medications and medical care services. One of the reasons that clinical pharmacy practice has been successful in many managed care settings is the availability of a formal structure and communication network among healthcare professionals.[26] Managed healthcare plans use a variety of approaches for improving drug prescribing and achieving improved patient outcomes, including the use of practice guidelines, pharmaceutical care services, drug utilization review programs, and academic detailing. There has been a continuing and growing effort to use economic models to evaluate the effects of programs and policies designed to influence the practice of prescribers and pharmacists. Pharmacists also are one of the most effective resources for influencing physician and patient compliance with formulary policy. The effectiveness of pharmacists in a variety of clinical roles has been demonstrated in HMO settings.[26,27]

Managed healthcare plans commonly use prescribing guidelines to promote the quality of drug therapy, while minimizing unnecessary expenditures. Often developed by the P&T committee as a component of formulary review, prescribing guidelines also are referred to as clinical guidelines, algorithms, clinical roadmaps, stepped care protocols, and drug usage criteria.[28] Preprinted prescription order forms, if structured in a preferred order-of-prescribing, also can be considered as tools to promote fomulary compliance. As noted by Schrogie and Nash,[29] the presence of a recommended guideline may have remarkable effects on pharmacotherapy. For example, by mentioning selected drugs as candidates for use, other competing and therapeutically equivalent drugs may be excluded. Stuart et al.[30] described an educational program that featured a clinical algorithm to encourage the rational use of lipid-lowering drugs at GHC. A preliminary analysis suggested that the program was associated with a $1 million cost-avoidance in this drug category. To be most effective, the development and evaluation of practice guidelines should be augmented with a pharmacoeconomic and outcomes analysis to provide more specific direction.

Numerous studies have explored the effectiveness of clinical pharmacy services on the appropriateness of drug prescribing in managed care settings.[31-34] Although many questions persist about whether such programs actually affect patient outcomes, demonstration studies conducted in managed care settings suggest that pharmacists can reduce drug costs[32-34] and, in some instances, reduce total direct medical costs.[35] An area often overlooked by pharmacists in managed healthcare plans is the potential for improving patient compliance with prescribed medication regimens.[36] The recent patient outcomes and pharmaceutical therapy initiative by the federal Agency for Health Care Policy and Research provided funding for a spectrum of research studies that will lead to more scientific knowledge about the most effective and appropriate role of pharmaceutical therapy.[37] One study funded by the agency, which is being conducted at GHC and the surrounding community, is a randomized controlled trial to determine if the delivery of pharmaceutical care can improve the outcomes of children and adolescents with asthma. Included in the study is a cost-effectiveness analysis.

One of the most common approaches to influencing practice patterns in managed care settings is the use of drug utilization review programs, including drug usage evaluation (DUE) and drug use management activities.[38] Although there are formal definitions for each of these terms, the spectrum of activities includes the ongoing review of individual and population-based drug therapy provisions to identify and correct suboptimal drug use. In a study of the development and evaluation of a drug usage evaluation program for community-acquired pneumonia in an HMO-owned hospital, Stocker et al. used a pre- and posttest concurrent control group design to assess the impact of the program on appropriateness of prescribing, cost of antibiotics, time febrile, and length of hospital stay. (Unpublished data. Stocker DE, Stergachis A, Chamberlain MC. Drug usage evaluation and the management and outcomes of community-acquired pneumonia. GHC, Seattle, WA.) This is an example of a study that included process and outcome measures as part of the evaluation.

DRUG BENEFIT DESIGN

Managed healthcare plans have considerable flexibility in determining the specific features of their drug benefits programs. The pharmacy benefit design of an intensively managed plan usually includes a drug formulary, a preferred pharmacy network (and/or in-house pharmacies), provider financial risk-sharing, member cost-sharing, coverage for FDA- or compendium-approved indications only, and prescription volume limitations.[5] As part of the drug formulary provision, plans may implement prior authorization to manage high-cost pharmaceuticals (e.g., drugs for catastrophic diseases, various products of biotechnology); exclude or restrict entire categories of drugs (e.g., over-the-counter products, contraceptives, fertility drugs, smoking cessation products, cosmetic drugs); and implement provisions for member cost-sharing. Cost-sharing can be in the form of copayments, coinsurance, deductibles, and/or some combination of the three approaches.

Soumerai and Ross-Degnan[39,40] have called attention to the need to evaluate the intended and unintended impacts of drug policies. Based on their experience with Medicaid and other state drug benefit programs, they argue for more rigorous evaluation research of several popular cost-sharing and other intervention programs. Using a historical cohort design, Harris et al.[41] analyzed how the use and cost of pharmaceuticals varied by level of drug copayment in a staff-model HMO. Based on an analysis of 19,982 enrollees aged less than 65 years, they determined that the implementation of progressively greater levels of copayments continued to have a marked effect on drug utilization, prescription unit costs, and per capita drug costs. There is a need for greater research into the effects of cost-sharing provisions on total drug costs, patient satisfaction, and patient outcomes.

Methodologic Challenges

There are a variety of methodologic challenges facing those who wish to perform pharmacoeconomic studies to meet the needs of managed care plans.[42] One of the most important considerations is the adoption of the viewpoint of the managed care plan in the design and the analysis of pharmacoeconomic studies. This perspective would influence numerous design features, including the selection of the specific comparator drug(s), the selection of meaningful clinical outcomes, the use of cost versus charge data, and the relative importance (or unimportance) of indirect consequences, such as worker productivity. As managed care plans continue to use large automated databases, there is a need to be attentive to the development of variables such as indications for use, severity of illness, comorbidities, and other potential confounding factors.[43,44] When affordable and appropriate, randomized prospective trials of the cost-effectiveness of pharmacologic interventions contribute valuable information for managed care plans.[45] In addition, controlled postmarketing observational studies provide valuable information on the effectiveness of medications under customary use conditions.[46]

Summary

Even though the term pharmacoeconomics is relatively new, managed care plans have historically scrutinized the economic value of their pharmacy benefit programs (pharmaceuticals, pharmaceutical services, and drug policies). There is little doubt that managed care plans are increasingly demanding and using pharmacoeconomic data to manage drug benefit programs. In interviews with managed care organizations, The Boston Consulting Group reported that all those with formularies stated that cost-effectiveness is one of the criteria they use in coverage decisions, a criterion that many said was not used only five years ago.[17] However, managed care pharmacy directors and employer benefit managers continue to make coverage decisions largely from a drug price perspective.

Pharmaceutical companies are responding to the demand for pharmacoeconomic data by expanding their activities in pharmacoeconomics, including quality-of-life studies,[13] and managed care plans are increasingly performing outcomes research studies, including pharmacoeconomic evaluations. However, pharmaceutical companies cannot provide complete information on the clinical and economic outcomes of drug therapy based on premarketing studies alone. Collaborative efforts between managed care, academia, government agencies, and the pharmaceutical industry can facilitate the design and conduct of valid, objective, and timely pharmacoeconomic evaluations.

References

1. Clouse JC. Pharmacoeconomics: a managed care perspective. Top Hosp Pharm Manage 1994;13:54-9.
2. 1992 National directory of HMO's. Washington, DC: Group Health Association of America, 1992.
3. Greenlick MR, Freeborn DK, Pope CR. Health care research in an HMO. Baltimore: Johns Hopkins University Press, 1989.
4. Opportunities for the community pharmacist in managed care. Washington, DC: American Pharmaceutical Association, 1994.
5. Pharmacy benefit report: HMO facts & figures. Summit, NJ: Ciba-Geigy, 1993.
6. Managed care digest: HMO edition. Kansas City, MO: Marion Merrell Dow, 1992.
7. Managed health care: effect on employers' costs difficult to measure. Washington, DC: General Accounting Office, GAO/HRD-94-3, October 1993.
8. Hazlet TK, Hu TW. Association between formulary strategies and hospital drug expenditures, Am J Hosp Pharm 1992;49:2207-10.
9. Sloan FA, Gordon GS, Cocks DL. Hospital drug formularies and use of hospital services. Med Care 1993;31:851-67.
10. Gabrowski HG, Schweitzer SO, Shiota SR. The effect of Medicaid formularies on the availability of new drugs. PharmacoEconomics 1992;1(suppl 1):32-40.
11. Schumacher GE. Multiattribute evaluation in formulary decision making as applied to calcium-channel blockers. Am J Hosp Pharm 1991;48:301-8.
12. Hatoum HT, Freeman RA. The use of pharmacoeconomic data in formulary selection. Top Hosp Pharm Manage 1994;13:11-22.
13. The Zitter Group and Technology Assessment Group. 1993 Pharmaceutical outcomes activities. San Francisco: The Zitter Group, 1993.

14. Hillman AL, Eisenberg JM, Pauly MV, Bloom BS, Citick H, Kinosian B, et al. Avoiding bias in the conduct and reporting of cost-effectiveness research sponsored by pharmaceutical companies. N Engl J Med 1991;324:1362-5.

15. Task Force on Principles for Economic Analysis of Health Care Technology. Economic analysis of health care technology: a report on principles. Ann Intern Med 1995;122:61-70.

16. Division of Drug Marketing, Advertising and Communications, Food and Drug Administration. Principles for the review of pharmacoeconomic promotion. Presented at the Center for Pharmaceutical Outcomes Research Meeting, Chapel Hill, NC, 1995.

17. Clouse JC, Osterhaus JT. Healthcare resource use and costs associated with migraine in a managed healthcare setting. Ann Pharmacother 1994;28:659-64.

18. Glauber HS, Brown JB. Use of health maintenance organization data bases to study pharmacy resource usage in diabetes mellitus. Diabetes Care 1992;15:870-6.

19. Stergachis A, Sheingold S, Luce BR, Psaty BM, Revicki DA. Medical care and cost outcomes after pentoxifylline treatment for peripheral arterial disease. Arch Intern Med 1992; 152:1220-4.

20. Barr JT, Schumacher GE. Applying decision analysis to pharmacy management and practice decisions. Top Hosp Pharm Manage 1994;13:60-71.

21. Hillman AL, Bloom BS. Economic effects of prophylactic use of misoprostol to prevent gastric ulcer in patients taking nonsteroidal anti-inflammatory drugs. Arch Intern Med 1989;149:2061-5.

22. Hillmer BE, Smith TJ. Efficacy and cost effectiveness of adjuvant chemotherapy in women with node-negative breast cancer: a decision-analysis model. N Engl J Med 1991; 324:160-8.

23. Lessler DS, Sullivan SD, Stergachis A. Cost-effectiveness of unenhanced MR imaging vs contrast-enhanced CR of the abdomen or pelvis. Am J Radiol 1994;163:5-7.

24. Lipsy RJ. Institutional formularies: the relevance of pharmacoeconomic analysis to formulary decisions. PharmacoEconomics 1992;1:265-81.

25. McDonough KP, Weaver RH, Viall GD. Enalapril to lisinopril: economic impact of a voluntary angiotensin-converting enzyme-inhibitor substitution program in a staff-model health maintenance organization. Ann Pharmacother 1992;26:399-404.

26. Stergachis A, Campbell WH, Penna PM. Clinical pharmacy and managed healthcare systems. Top Hosp Pharm Manage 1988;8:78-88.

27. The AACP Clinical Practice Affairs Committee. Clinical pharmacy in the noninstitutional setting: a white paper from the American College of Clinical Pharmacy. Pharmacotherapy 1992;12:359-64.

28. Field MJ, Lohr KN, eds. Clinical practice guidelines. Washington, DC: National Academy Press, Institute of Medicine, 1990.

29. Schrogie JJ, Nash DB. Relationship between practice guidelines, formulary management, and pharmacoeconomic studies. Top Hosp Pharm Manage 1994;13:38-46.

30. Stuart ME, Handley MR, Chamberlain MC, Wallach R, Penna P, Stergachis A. A successful HMO education program to encourage rational use of lipid lowering drugs. HMO Practice 1991;5:198-204.

31. Stergachis A, Fors M, Wagner EH, Sims D, Penna P. Effects of clinical pharmacists on drug prescribing in a primary care clinic. Am J Hosp Pharm 1987;44:525-9.

32. Forstrom MJ, Ried LD, Stergachis AS, Corliss DA. Effect of a clinical pharmacist program on the cost of hypertension treatment in an HMO family practice clinic. DICP Ann Pharmacother 1990;24:304-9.

33. Willett MS, Bertch KE, Rich DS, Ereshefsky L. Prospectus on the economic value of clinical pharmacy services: a position statement of the American College of Clinical Pharmacy. Pharmacotherapy 1989;9:45-56.

34. Report of the task force on the cost-effectiveness of pharmaceutical products and pharmacy services. Alexandria, VA: American Association of Colleges of Pharmacy, 1989.

35. Borgsdorf LR, Miano JS, Knapp KK. Pharmacist-managed medication review in a managed care system. Am J Hosp Pharm 1994;51:772-7.

36. Feldman JA, DeTullio PL. Medication noncompliance: an issue to consider in the drug selection process. Hosp Formulary 1994;29:204-11.

37. Patient outcomes and pharmaceutical therapy. AHCPR Pub. No. 94-0015. Rockville, MD: Agency for Health Care Policy and Research, 1993.

38. Lipton HL, Bird JA. Drug utilization review in ambulatory care settings: state of the science and directions for outcomes research. Med Care 1993;31:1069-82.

39. Soumerai SB, Ross-Degnan D. Experience of state drug benefit programs. Health Affairs 1990;9:36-54.

40. Soumerai SB, Ross-Degnan D, Avorn J, McLaughlin T J, Choodnovskiy I. Effects of Medicaid drug-payment limits on admission to hospitals and nursing homes. N Engl J Med 1991;325:1072-7.

41. Harris BL, Stergachis A, Ried LD. The effect of drug co-payments on utilization and cost of pharmaceuticals in a health care maintenance organization. Med Care 1990;28:907-17.

42. Luce BR, Brown RE. The use of technology assessment by hospitals, health maintenance organizations, and third-party payers in the United States. Int J Technol Assess Health Care 1995;11:79-92.

43. Von Korff M, Wagner EH, Saunders K. A chronic disease score from automated pharmacy data. J Clin Epidemiol 1992;45:197-203.

44. Saunders K, Stergachis A, Von Korff M. Group Health Cooperative of Puget Sound. In: Strom BL, ed. Pharmacoepidemiology. New York: John Wiley & Sons, 1994.

45. Oster G, Borok GM, Menzin J, Hay JF, Epstein RS, Quinn V, et al. A randomized trial to assess effectiveness and cost in clinical practice: rationale and design of the Cholesterol Reduction Intervention Study (CRIS). Control Clin Trials 1995;16:3-16.

46. Ray WA, Griffin MR, Avorn J. Evaluating drugs after their approval for clinical use. N Engl J Med 1993;329:2029-32.

47. The changing environment for U.S. pharmaceuticals. Boston: The Boston Consulting Group, 1993.

14

Pharmacoeconomics and Clinical Practice: A Physician's View

Kevin A. Schulman

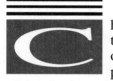hanges in health policy around the world are focusing on the goal of ensuring that the provision of medical care occurs in a fiscally rational manner. The development of pharmacoeconomics as an assessment tool is one means of developing coherent data surrounding the outcomes of pharmaceutical therapy.[1-8] Although many authors have developed metrics we can use to assess the economic impact of pharmaceutical therapies, all too few have described how these data can be understood and interpreted to improve the efficiency of clinical practice.

This chapter will discuss this implementation issue in a clinical context, both on a national and a regional health services level. In addition, this chapter will review pharmacoeconomic issues as they relate to the interpretation of published economic analyses, discuss two case examples of interpretation of pharmacoeconomic data, and finally discuss the state of the art in implementation of pharmacoeconomics in clinical practice, highlighting the possible next directions in the evolution of this clinical management tool.

 ## Economic Issues in Clinical Practice

Pharmacoeconomic analyses supply practitioners with several different types of important clinical data. Properly designed studies include an assessment of current medical practice, an assessment of the clinical efficacy of a new pharmaceutical product, and an economic analysis evaluating the impact of the product on clinical practice.

Economic analyses can report results in four different economic categories for the treatment under investigation compared with a control treatment (either placebo or an established therapy). Two of these categories are for new therapies with improved clinical outcomes, and two are for new therapies with worse clinical outcomes. These categories are: (1) the new therapy is cost saving with improved clinical outcomes, (2) the new therapy is cost additive with improved clinical outcomes, (3) the new therapy is cost saving with worse clinical outcomes, and (4) the new therapy is cost additive with worse clinical outcomes. A therapy that falls into the first category is said to be dominant in that it is always the treatment of choice. A new therapy that falls into the fourth category is dominated by the control therapy, and is never the treatment of choice. Selection of therapies in categories 2 and 3 will depend on the relationship of the costs of the therapies and outcomes achieved with the therapy. For category 2, and potentially for category 3, cost-effectiveness ratios can be calculated to allow economic assessment of these agents relative to other funded therapies.

Although pharmacoeconomic data are always interesting, and sometimes compelling, they need to be interpreted in terms of the specific clinical context being addressed before they can be used to influence the clinical decision-making process. Interpretation of these data involves several specific issues: (1) translation of treatment efficacy results to treatment efficiency results, (2) comparison of the clinical trial population to the population under consideration for treatment with the therapy, (3) translation of the costs reported to costs relevant to the perspective of the decision-maker, and (4) translation of the clinical outcome measures to outcomes relevant to the length of treatment being proposed by the practitioner. Each of these issues will be addressed separately.

EFFICIENCY

Phase III clinical trials are designed to measure the efficacy of new therapeutic products. Efficacy is the effect of an agent in the "idealized" setting of a randomized, controlled clinical trial. Efficiency of a therapy is the effect of a therapy as observed in actual clinical practice, outside a clinical protocol. Efficacy may differ greatly from efficiency.

Factors that may lead to pharmacoeconomic efficacy being greater than pharmacoeconomic efficiency include: (1) specific criteria for patient selection, (2) protocol-induced benefits for patients receiving the new medication, (3) optimization of medication dosage and monitoring of patients receiving treatment, (4) physician experience with the new medication, and (5) patient motivation and compliance with the new treatment. Factors that may lead to efficiency being greater than efficacy include: (1) a large placebo benefit to therapy (the efficacy benefit would be the benefit of therapy on an incremental basis, and would not include this placebo effect; the efficiency benefit would be the total benefit observed in patients, and would include this effect), (2) identification of a superior population for the therapy compared with the population selected for the Phase III trial, (3) increased comfort with the use of the agent resulting in reduced intensity of the new treatment in clinical practice compared with that for patients receiving the new treatment in the Phase III trial protocol, and (4) decreased efficiency of control treatment in clinical practice compared with that in the clinical trial (e.g., if physicians underdose a particular "control" medication in clinical practice, but its use is optimized in a clinical trial, the difference in effectiveness between a new treatment and the control treatment will be greater in clinical practice than that observed in the clinical trial).

Beyond these issues, one must assess whether inefficiencies in clinical practice may impact the use of the agent once it is available. To the extent that misuse of controlled therapies in clinical practice is responsible for the economic advantage of a new agent, these benefits may be achievable through less costly programs such as educational interventions. At the same time, to the extent that the demand for medical care services is not related to the clinical condition of the patient, the potential economic advantage afforded by the new therapy may not be achieved. For example, physicians can loosen their criteria for therapeutic procedures in an attempt to maintain service volume when patients experience a decrease in severity of illness with a new medication. In this case, one would not see the expected reduction in procedure volume after the therapy is introduced.

In most cases, efficacy is expected to be greater than efficiency of new therapeutic modalities. However, each therapy must be assessed individually to determine if this maxim holds.

GENERALIZABILITY

Clinical trial populations can be very specific, as discussed above. Understanding the generalizability of a pharmacoeconomic study involves two processes: understanding the generalizability from the clinical population being treated to the population for which treatment is being considered, and understanding the economic system being assessed in the study. The generalizability of the results from the clinical population under study is relatively straightforward to most clinicians. The generalizability of the economic system under consideration is a much newer activity for clinicians and policy-makers (generalizability does not include perspective, which will be discussed separately).

In the US alone, a tremendous change has occurred in the provision of healthcare services over the last decade because of changes in health insurance and government payment policies for physicians and hospitals. A pharmacoeconomic study conducted before the implementation of the Medicare Prospective Payment System may have reported significant reduction in length of stay for patients receiving a particular treatment. This finding may no longer be relevant, however, given the reduction in length of stay observed since the Prospective Payment System was implmented. Similarly, a study that reported on the reduction of inpatient costs for a disease that is now treated on an outpatient basis would have limited generalizability.

The healthcare system also can affect the intensity of services. Length-of-stay is much greater in Germany than in the US at the present time. Thus, one must review the quantity of resources used to care for both treatment and control patients to see if the intensity of resource consumption in the pharmacoeconomic study matches that expected in the system of concern to the decision-makers.

PERSPECTIVE

Perspective is the point of view from which costs and benefits are assessed for a study. The most commonly reported perspectives are patient, provider, payer, and society. Most published studies have a specific perspective. Thus, the reported costs and benefits from an economic analysis need to be translated into costs and benefits relevant to the perspective of the decision-maker for the clinical question being addressed. For example, pharmaceutical and laboratory costs can be adjusted to reflect a provider perspective (e.g., health maintenance organization [HMO] or Veterans Affairs Hospital) rather than a societal perspective. Similarly, treatment benefits can be translated from a societal perspective to a patient perspective (e.g., rather than reporting the number of physician visits for gastrointestinal adverse effects, the study can report number of days of stomach upset for patients).

OUTCOMES

Outcomes assessment is the most difficult task associated with the analysis of pharmacoeconomic data. Clinical trials are usually of short duration compared with the expected period of treatment, especially when assessing treatments for chronic disease. Although forecasting with certainty the future efficacy of therapy is impossible, one can readily identify reasonable bounds for the lifetime impact of therapy either from clinical trial data[9] or through the use of a computer model.[10]

For therapies expected to provide an improvement over current treatments, pharmacoeconomic analysis can focus on both the short- and long-term costs and benefits of therapy. Most agents do not have identical treatment efficacy, so a lifetime perspective should be maintained wherever possible for economic analysis.

Interpretation Cases

Two recent analyses reported in the medical literature will be reviewed in this section. These reports are analyzed using the four interpretation issues highlighted in the previous section.

CASE 1: COST-EFFECTIVENESS OF PHARMACEUTICAL MANAGEMENT OF HIGH BLOOD CHOLESTEROL

The treatment of high blood cholesterol was first established as a national health priority by the National Cholesterol Education Program (NCEP) in 1987.[11] This program recommended that all American adults be screened for high blood cholesterol, and that patients with elevated levels of low-density lipoprotein cholesterol (LDL-C) be treated. Treatment recommendations included two stages of diet therapy, with pharmaceutical management reserved for patients in whom diet therapy failed. The NCEP stipulates first- and second-line therapeutic agents for patients who require pharmacologic therapy. Nevertheless, these recommendations do not include any economic assessment of the different therapies, or of the cost-effectiveness of the treatment recommendations.

Schulman et al.[12] reported a cost-effectiveness analysis of the pharmacologic treatment of high blood cholesterol for patients in whom diet therapy failed. This analysis was conducted from a societal perspective and included only the direct medical costs of pharmacologic therapy. Benefits were reported as changes in total blood cholesterol, LDL-C, and high-density lipoprotein cholesterol (HDL-C) concentrations, as well as changes in an LDL-C/HDL-C index representing total reduction in cardiovascular risk resulting from treatment (including changes in both HDL-C and LDL-C concentrations). Direct medical costs included pharmaceutical costs, physician and laboratory monitoring costs, comedication (required to reduce adverse effects of specific agents), and adverse effect costs. Resource consumption for the use of these agents was based on expert opinion and literature review.

Some of the findings of this analysis are reported in Figure 1. This figure represents the costs of five years of therapy for the treatment of high blood cholesterol and the benefits of therapy in terms of LDL-C reduction. The closer the agents are positioned toward the upper left-hand portion of the curve, the more efficient they are in terms of the cost per percent reduction in LDL-C.[12]

The most efficient agents in this figure represent an efficiency frontier. Relative to agents on the frontier, nonfrontier agents (i.e., those above the efficiency frontier) for a given treatment effect have higher costs than frontier agents. Alternatively, relative to agents on the frontier, nonfrontier agents, for a given cost, have less clinical benefit than frontier agents. Agents that lie below the frontier offer less clinical benefit than agents on the frontier with the same cost or the same clinical benefit as agents on the frontier but for greater cost. The efficiency frontier allows physicians to select from a range of therapeutic agents, acknowledging that different clinical indications and adverse effect profiles exist for different therapeutic agents, and that physicians may consider these factors in making a treatment decision.

One obvious result of analysis of this figure is that while the efficiency of the agent plays an important role in clinical decision-making, other criteria are required to determine the optimal therapy for patients. This curve lends itself to three different treatment decision criteria: effect, budget, and cost-effectiveness. For patients who require a 20% reduction in LDL-C, lovastatin 20 mg achieves this clinical endpoint at the lowest cost. If it is desired to use the most effective agent that costs no more than $3,500 over five years, then colestipol 20 mg is the agent of choice. If it is desired to use the most cost-effective agent for the reduction of LDL-C concentrations, then niacin ($139 per percent reduction in LDL-C) and lovastatin 20 mg ($177 per percent reduction in LDL-C) are the agents of choice.[12]

Data Interpretation. In assessing the information provided in this study, we should review the four major analytic issues outlined in this chapter.

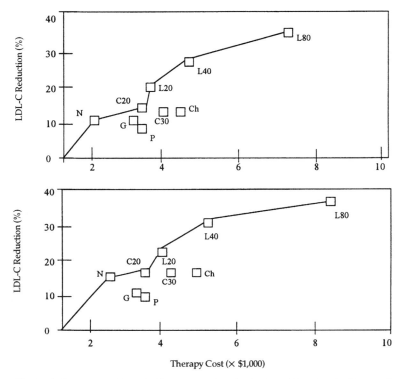

Figure 1. Cost (on x-axis) and effect (on y-axis) of reduction of low-density lipoprotein cholesterol (LDL-C) concentrations for the clinical trial model (top) and the primary care model
(bottom). The points that are higher and to the left in each figure describe an efficiency frontier,
defined as those points that produce a given effect at the least cost. These points dominate those
that are lower and rightward. An agent is dominated if it can be replaced by at least one other
agent that produces either the same or greater effect for less cost, or more effect for the same
cost. Costs are in terms of the present value of five years of therapy; effects are in nominal terms.
N = niacin; G = gemfibrozil; P = probucol; C20 = colestipol 20 g; C30 = colestipol 30 g;
Ch = cholestyramine; L20 = lovastatin 20 mg; L40 = lovastatin 40 mg; and L80 = lovastatin
80 mg. Reprinted with permission.[12]

EFFICIENCY. The first assessment was to determine whether this
analysis reported efficacy measures or efficiency measures. In this article,
the authors presented an analysis of both efficacy and efficiency. Efficacy
was represented by a clinical trial model, which is based on an intent-to-
treat analysis of the clinical and economic data. In this analysis, patients
who were noncompliant did not receive the cost or benefit of therapy other
than the therapy initiation cost. Patients who were nonresponders continued to receive the cost of therapy while they may have had little clinical
benefit from treatment.[12]

The authors also presented a primary care model, where the agent in patients who were noncompliant or nonresponders was changed to a second or third agent until 98% of patients were taking a medication they tolerated (Figure 1). This primary care model assessed the efficiency of the use of these agents in practice and resembles clinical practice more closely than the clinical trial model. Patients were to be followed by their physician until they were taking a medication that they tolerated and their blood cholesterol concentration was reduced. Noncompliant patients were to be given second and third agents to achieve their treatment goal.[12]

Compared with the clinical trial model, the primary care model may report higher costs for agents that may be difficult for patients to tolerate. In this study, these included niacin, colestipol, and cholestyramine, with the cost of niacin increasing 60% in the primary care model compared with the clinical trial model. The clinical benefit also increased, however, because more patients were receiving a therapy to which they responded in the primary care model compared with the clinical trial model. In this analysis, the authors reported that the agents on the efficiency frontier remained unchanged in either analysis.[12]

GENERALIZABILITY. This analysis was based on the results of a survey of 115 studies reported in the medical literature on the treatment of patients with high blood cholesterol. Efficacy results were reported to be for patients with type II hyperlipidemia, with total cholesterol concentrations of 6.47 mmol/L or greater. Although gender was not an inclusion or exclusion criterion for the literature review, women were greatly underrepresented in the clinical studies. Further, women had a lower relative risk of heart disease than did men of the same age.[12] Thus, these results may not be generalizable to women or to patients with disease other than type II hyperlipidemia.

PERSPECTIVE. The costs reported in the article were derived from several different sources. Resource consumption was based both on the practice patterns of a panel of medical experts in a specific geographic region and on their impressions of the intensity of resources required to treat patients before some of the treatments were widely available. Pharmaceutical costs were based on wholesale prices, and laboratory costs were based on laboratory costs in Maryland.[12] Thus, both intensity of treatment and costs of resources need to be reviewed before implementing treatment recommendations based on this analysis.

OUTCOMES. The authors based their analysis on five years of treatment costs and effects.[12] While this may be a reasonable time frame for analysis, patients probably will receive lifetime treatment with these agents. Glick et al.[13] elsewhere reported lifetime treatment analyses that support the results of this five-year treatment model.

CASE 2: COST-EFFECTIVENESS OF NEBACUMAB FOR GRAM-NEGATIVE SEPSIS—ECONOMIC ANALYSIS OF A NEW THERAPEUTIC AGENT

Despite the availability of appropriate antibiotic therapy for the treatment of patients with sepsis, this clinical syndrome still has a substantial mortality rate that may be due to the ability of a bacterial infection to overstimulate the host immune response, a process that continues despite the presence of antibiotic therapy. A new class of therapeutic agents was developed to treat this disease by tempering the host immune response. Nebacumab was the first of this class of agents that neared approval for use in the US; it was marketed in several countries in Europe. (The agent was withdrawn from the market in Europe and from clinical trials in the US in 1993.) In the original clinical trial,[14] nebacumab demonstrated efficacy in patients with gram-negative bacterial infections. However, this infection was only found in 36% of patients with sepsis in the trial. Even though this agent may never be marketed in the US, the case of nebacumab provides an excellent example of a pharmacoeconomic analysis of this class of therapeutic agents.

An economic analysis of this agent was performed to understand its potential use in clinical practice[15] and to assess whether this agent would meet funding guidelines for new therapeutic agents.[16-18] Since nebacumab was not available in the US, the base price was set at the cost of the agent in one of the European countries where it was marketed (in The Netherlands the price was $3,750 per dose[15]).

The economic analysis of this agent was based on the observed mortality of patients who received the drug versus those who received placebo, the proportion of treated patients with gram-negative infections, the cost of the agent, the cost of treating its adverse effects, and the induced costs resulting from the use of the agent.[15] Since nebacumab is only effective in the treatment of patients with gram-negative bacterial infections, the clinical effect of the agent would be a product of the expected reduction in mortality in patients with gram-negative bacterial infections and the prevalence of patients with gram-negative infections in the treated population. The data used to construct this analysis are presented in Table 1.

The effectiveness of this intervention is dependent on the long-term outcome of the patients treated with this agent. The average age of patients in this trial was 58 years, meaning the patients who benefit from this therapy would be expected to have an additional 20 years of survival based on their actuarial life expectancy. The majority of patients in this trial, however, had substantial comorbidities including cancer, liver or kidney disease, diabetes, and alcoholism. In this analysis, it was estimated that patients would survive an average of 5 years beyond hospital discharge. This estimate was examined extensively using sensitivity analysis.[15]

Table 1. Economic Analysis of Nebacumab Therapy in the Treatment of Gram-Negative Sepsis[15]

PARAMETER		95% CI
Observed mortality in patients with gram-negative infection receiving placebo (%)	0.52	0.41 to 0.62
Observed mortality in treated patients with gram-negative infection (%)	0.37	0.28 to 0.47
Proportion of patients with gram-negative infection (%)	0.36	0.32 to 0.41
Reduction in mortality in patients with gram-negative infection (%)	0.29	
Cost of therapy ($)	3,750	
Cost of adverse effects ($)	0	
Induced costs per patient ($)	1,900[a]	

CI = confidence interval.

[a]Induced costs of therapy include increased use of hospital resources for patients who would have died without nebacumab therapy, increased use of hospital resources for patients who died despite therapy, and decreased use of resources for patients who would have survived without therapy.

An analysis that examined the economic impact of a diagnostic test for gram-negative infection also was constructed. In this analysis, only patients who tested positive for gram-negative infection were treated with nebacumab therapy (the test strategy compared with the treat strategy where all patients are treated, as in this trial). The net effect of the test strategy was to reduce the number of patients with gram-positive infection treated with nebacumab therapy, while providing patients with gram-negative infection and positive tests the benefit of therapy. This strategy reduced costs while maintaining efficacy (although efficacy is dependent on the sensitivity of the test). The results of this analysis and the sensitivity analysis are presented in Table 2 and Figure 2. The results of the test analysis also are presented in Table 2 and in Figure 3.[15]

Data Interpretation. Again, in assessing the information provided in this article, we reviewed the four major analysis issues outlined in this chapter.

EFFICIENCY. This article reported treatment efficacy in the primary analysis. The authors recognized, however, that in clinical practice the patient population being treated with nebacumab may be very different from the clinical trial study population. Efficiency issues in this analysis included an assessment of the proportion of patients with gram-negative bacteremia in the treatment population and the life expectancy of treated patients.[15] The first of these two issues will be discussed in this section. The second will be discussed in the generalizability section.

The authors presented an analysis of the efficiency of nebacumab therapy. As shown in Table 3, the cost-effectiveness ratio for this therapy can vary by almost threefold under the treat strategy if patient selection varied greatly from that seen in the clinical trial.[15] Since the clinical indications

Table 2. Sensitivity Analysis[a]

INPUT	TEST STRATEGY ($)	TREAT STRATEGY ($)
Cost of base case	14,900	24,100
Cost of nebacumab therapy ($)		
2,500	12,800	18,800
5,000	17,000	29,500
Cost of acute-care hospital stay		
reduced by 50%	10,800	20,100
increased by 50%	19,000	28,200
Additional survivors only[b]	11,200	20,500
Test cost ($)		
50	14,700	24,100
200	15,300	24,100
2,160	24,100	24,100
Years of life gained		
1	67,900	110,200
20	5,200	8,400
Cost of worst-case scenario[c]	851,700	1,227,600

[a]Reprinted with permission.[15]
[b]Patients who would have died without nebacumab therapy but are expected to survive with it.
[c]Uses the most pessimistic assumptions from the analysis.

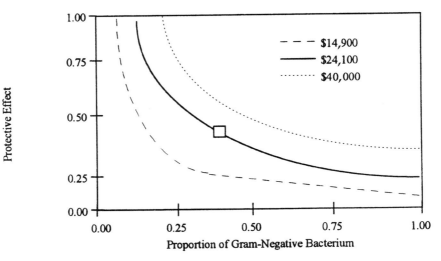

━━━ **Figure 2.** Sensitivity analysis for the treat strategy, reporting cost-effectiveness ratios resulting
━━━ when estimates of the proportion of gram-negative bacteremia in the treated population and the
protective effect of nebacumab therapy among patients with gram-negative bacteremia are varied. The curves represent combinations of these variables that have the same ratios of cost per
year of life saved. The square on the middle curve represents the proportion of patients with
gram-negative bacteremia and the protective effect used in the principal analysis. Other points
represented by this curve all have cost-effectiveness ratios that are identical to the one for the
principal analysis. Reprinted with permission.[15]

for treatment with this therapy are relatively nonspecific, the efficiency of
nebacumab therapy in clinical practice may differ from the treatment efficacy observed in the clinical trial. In this case, patient selection may increase the cost per treated patient. However, since the clinical benefit is
limited to patients with gram-negative sepsis, this additional cost was not
expected to confer any additional clinical benefit.

Similarly, different hospitals may have different rates of gram-negative
infection as a cause of sepsis. From the perspective of an economic analysis, a decrease in the rate of gram-negative infection among patients with
sepsis from 36% to a lesser percentage is equivalent to a change in prevalence of gram-negative infection from any other cause.

GENERALIZABILITY. The major issue in discussing the generalizability of these findings was that of patient selection and the life expectancy of treated patients. Ideally, this agent would be used in otherwise
healthy patients, such as those who developed infection as a complication
of surgery. These patients would be expected to return to full health and to
live out their full life expectancy. In fact, the cost-effectiveness of therapy
in otherwise healthy patients would be far greater than that reported in the
primary analysis presented in Table 2.

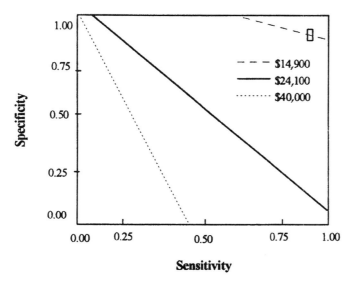

Figure 3. Sensitivity analysis of the test strategy, assessing cost-effectiveness ratios with varying combinations of test sensitivity and test specificity. The lines represent combinations of these variables that have the same ratios of cost per year of life saved. The square on the line at top right represents the sensitivity and specificity used in the principal analysis. Other points represented by this line all have cost-effectiveness ratios that are identical to the one for the principal analysis. Reprinted with permission.[15]

As discussed previously, however, most patients in the nebacumab clinical trial had substantial underlying illnesses.[15] We do not know much about the expected mortality of these patients. While reported life expectancy for patients such as these may be as long as five years, the patients receiving nebacumab therapy may be substantially more ill than

Table 3. Cost and Cost-Effectiveness of Therapy in Clinical Practice[a]

	Total Annual Costs (in Millions of $)			Cost per Year of Life Gained ($)	
PREVALENCE[b]	TEST STRATEGY	TREAT STRATEGY	SAVINGS	TEST STRATEGY	TREAT STRATEGY
0.10	1,622	6,160	4,538	18,300	65,900
0.20	1,415	3,460	2,045	15,900	37,000
0.30	1,346	2,560	1,214	15,200	27,400
0.36	1,323	2,260	937	14,900	24,100

[a]Reprinted with permission.[15]
[b]Proportion of patients with gram-negative bacteremia in the treated population, assuming relaxation of the criteria used to determine candidates for nebacumab therapy.

patients previously studied (since the patients with gram-negative infection surviving as a result of this treatment would have died without nebacumab therapy). If nebacumab therapy lengthens the dying process for these patients by only a short amount of time, then this therapy will have a much reduced clinical benefit compared with that seen in the primary analysis presented in Table 2. This would result in a substantial decrease in the efficiency of therapy and, potentially, an increase in suffering of patients and their families.

While this discussion suggests that we may wish to limit the use of nebacumab therapy to only those patients without underlying illnesses, the reality is that most patients with sepsis probably have some comorbidity contributing to their illness, and that patients with sepsis will clinically resemble those patients enrolled in the nebacumab trial. Further, as this discussion suggests, implementation of this therapy would require substantial discussion and education to ensure its best possible use. The generalizability of the results of this analysis is contingent on the success of this process and on the degree to which the therapy is used in a fashion similar to that seen in the clinical trial.

PERSPECTIVE. As in the study of cholesterol treatment, the costs reported in the nebacumab article[15] were derived from several different sources. Pharmaceutical costs were based on the price of the agent in The Netherlands, and hospital costs were based on patients treated for sepsis at the Hospital of the University of Pennsylvania in Philadelphia. Induced costs of therapy, in terms of changes in length of stay for patients treated with nebacumab, were based on a series of assumptions discussed in the article. Thus, the assumptions regarding resource costs and treatment intensity need to be reviewed before implementing treatment recommendations based on this analysis.

OUTCOMES. In this analysis, the authors assessed the impact of therapy over a patient's lifetime.[15] Quality of life was not incorporated into this analysis. Much of the discussion in the generalizability section also holds true for a discussion of an economic analysis of nebacumab therapy adjusted for quality of life.

Implementation

Both of these case examples provide means of interpreting published economic data for use in making clinical treatment decisions. Discussions based on these data are now commonly heard at formulary committee meetings on both a national (such as that being proposed in Canada and Australia[19,20]) or a local population basis (such as an HMO). Four different types of implementation strategies will be discussed in this section: treatment efficiency thresholds, formulary committee discussions, treatment decision rules, and timing of the economic evaluation.

THRESHOLDS

Treatment efficiency thresholds have been suggested for the inclusion of new therapeutic products on a national formulary.[19] In the proposed Canadian guidelines, inclusion of new pharmaceutical agents on the national formulary would be based on five grades of recommendation using pharmacoeconomic criteria (currency values are in Canadian dollars):

Compelling Evidence for Adoption and Appropriate Utilization. The new therapy has equal or improved clinical efficacy and reduced cost.

Strong Evidence for Adoption and Appropriate Utilization. The new therapy has increased clinical benefit and costs less than $20,000 per quality-adjusted life-year (QALY) gained or the new therapy has decreased clinical benefit but its use would save more than $100,000 per QALY gained.

Moderate Evidence for Adoption and Appropriate Utilization. The new therapy has increased clinical benefit and costs between $20,000 and $100,000 per QALY gained or the new therapy has decreased clinical benefit but its use would save between $20,000 and $100,000 per QALY gained.

Weak Evidence for Adoption and Appropriate Utilization. The new therapy has increased clinical benefit and costs more than $100,000 per QALY gained or the new therapy has decreased clinical benefit but its use would save less than $20,000 per QALY gained.

Compelling Evidence for Rejection. The therapy has equal or decreased clinical benefit at increased cost.

These guidelines offer a clear and consistent means of evaluating the new therapeutic products. Yet, they are not perfect. The confidence intervals surrounding cost-effectiveness estimates for new therapeutic products are generally large, and may cross these thresholds. Small differences in utilization of resources associated with the use of new agents may alter the economic analysis of the therapy as physicians become more proficient with the use of the product. Finally, the results of the economic analysis are dependent on our ability to generalize from the patient population studied in the clinical trial to the population that will eventually receive the agent.

FORMULARY COMMITTEE DISCUSSIONS

Formulary management committees now exist in most settings where physicians practice in large groups. When not used as absolute treatment criteria, pharmacoeconomic data are an important part of an informed discussion about the adoption of a new therapeutic agent by the group. Pharmacoeconomic data allow discussion of comparative efficacy and cost of specific therapeutic products, as well as explicit discussion of the clinical and ethical issues surrounding implementation of new therapeutic agents by physicians and pharmacists. More than a discussion of the cost of the product itself, pharmacoeconomic evaluation is concerned with assessment of all resources used in the care of patients including hospital treatment, outpatient medical visits, and monitoring of patients. Also, these assessments include a detailed discussion of the outcomes of therapies. From the patient perspective, these same analyses can be used to evaluate the adverse effects and the cost of the therapy to the patient.

Before adopting recommendations based on these discussions, published and other pharmacoeconomic data need to be evaluated in light of the interpretation issues reviewed previously and adapted to the specific practice setting under consideration. When comprehensive reanalysis of the data is not possible, interpretation and analysis can occur in a descriptive fashion by members of the formulary committee.

TREATMENT DECISION RULES

National pharmaceutical treatment guidelines, such as those used for the NCEP, need to incorporate pharmacoeconomic data into their treatment recommendations. Pharmacoeconomic analysis can help ensure that we achieve the greatest possible efficiency in the treatment of patients through these national public health programs.

Pharmacoeconomic analysis also can include an assessment of patient selection criteria for inclusion in a treatment program. For example, the NCEP proposed different sets of treatment recommendations based on the risk status of a patient (e.g., thresholds levels of LDL-C at which treatment should be initiated). However, these recommendations are not consistent regarding the cost-effectiveness of treating individual groups of patients.

As shown in Figure 4,[13] treating men aged 45–49 years with cholesterol-lowering agents who have no risk factors for heart disease and a total cholesterol concentration of 6.72 mmol/L results in a decrease in cardiac events at a cost-effectiveness ratio of $74,200 per year of life saved. Consistent guidelines from an economic perspective would recommend treatment of all patients who can be treated at or below this cost-effectiveness threshold. From Figure 4, that would include men who smoke and have a cholesterol concentration of 5.69 mmol/L, men with hypertension who have a cholesterol concentration of 5.69 mmol/L, and men with hypertension who also smoke and have a cholesterol concentration of less than 5.17 mmol/L.[21] Yet, patients with total cholesterol concentrations of less than 6.20 mmol/L may not meet the NCEP treatment guidelines for initiation of cholesterol-lowering therapy.

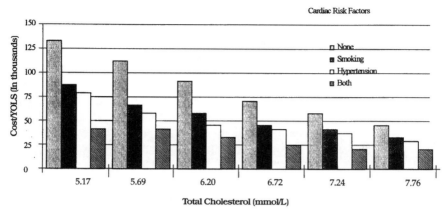

Figure 4. This figure presents the cost-effectiveness ratios for treatment of high blood cholesterol for men aged 45–49 years in whom diet therapy has failed. Pharmacologic therapy in this example is niacin. Results are presented for patients with no cardiac risk factors (other than male gender), smoking as a single risk factor, hypertension as a single risk factor, and both smoking and hypertension.[13] YOLS = year of life saved.

TIMING OF ECONOMIC EVALUATION

Pharmacoeconomic studies are currently being conducted as substudies in Phase III efficacy trials to allow decision-makers access to economic data at the time of product introduction. However, as discussed previously, clinical trials may not mirror clinical practice. Projection from efficacy to efficiency can occur as part of the evaluation of the Phase III trial economic data and as part of the treatment guideline development process on a formulary level. Phase III pharmacoeconomic evaluations are the only opportunity to collect economic information prior to the introduction of a new therapeutic agent so that decision-makers can include pharmacoeconomic assessments in their initial decision about whether to adopt the new therapy. Phase III trials also are often the only opportunity to assess economic and quality-of-life impact of the therapy in a controlled research setting. Still important to remember, though, is that pharmacoeconomic evaluation is intended as a management tool for decision-makers. Thus, pharmacoeconomic analysis will need to be revisited after the therapy is introduced into clinical practice, usually through postmarketing pharmacoeconomic studies. This is especially the case when the Phase III trial was designed to restrict the use of the agent to high-benefit populations in a manner that may not be implementable in clinical practice. For example, the nebacumab clinical trial excluded patients "with a rapidly fatal course."[14] Without a clinical trial as a mechanism for selecting patients for this therapy, clinicians may be uncomfortable in making this distinction in practice.

In one of the largest concurrent pharmacoeconomic evaluations ever conducted in a postmarketing setting, the Health Care Financing Administration (HCFA) of the Department of Health and Human Services is assessing the cost and effect of epoetin in the treatment of patients with endstage renal disease. The Medicare program, administered by HCFA, is the insurer for more than 90% of patients with endstage renal disease. For reimbursement, HCFA requires providers to record patients' epoetin doses and their blood hemoglobin concentrations at each visit where epoetin is administered. In an assessment of the program after 10 months of data collection, HCFA found that among patients who had received epoetin for 6 months or longer, fewer than 45% had ever reached a hematocrit concentration over 30%.[22] These data suggested that the efficiency of epoetin therapy is less than the reported clinical trial efficacy. The potential reasons for this difference include the following: (1) physicians were underdosing poetin in practice during this period due to the Medicare payment policy for the medication, (2) physicians were not titrating the dose appropriately when patients did not respond significantly to initial doses of therapy, or (3) the clinical trial patient population was not generalizable to the Medicare dialysis population. The assessment of this program is continuing.

This type of concurrent economic evaluation is becoming more common in European countries as well as in the US. Further, these assessments can include studies of appropriateness of patient selection in clinical practice compared with selection for the clinical trial or clinical practice guidelines.

The Future

With the increasing worldwide focus on assessing relative value of new technologies and therapies, pharmacoeconomic analysis is taking on a new importance in the pharmaceutical development process. Pharmacoeconomic data are now being developed during Phase III investigations of most new therapeutic products that are thought to have substantial market potential. Further, the quality of the pharmacoeconomic data available to decision-makers is rapidly improving, as data collection becomes more comprehensive and assessments are routinely conducted on a prospective basis. Most pharmaceutical manufacturers now hold their pharmacoeconomic assessments to the same research standards that they have developed for the treatment of clinical data, and most users of these data are now educated to the need for this level of rigor for these assessments.[23-25]

In the US, we are beginning to see the integration of pharmacoeconomics into clinical trials sponsored by the National Institutes of Health[26] and into the guideline development process sponsored by the Agency for Health Care Policy and Research.[27] One major shortcoming of the NCEP study[11] is that it did not include pharmacoeconomic data in its treatment recommendations.[21]

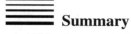 **Summary**

This chapter reviewed the interpretation of pharmacoeconomic analysis from a clinical perspective and discussed the implementation of pharmacoeconomic analysis in clinical practice. Interpretation of clinical economics studies is based on four specific issues: (1) translation of treatment efficacy results to treatment efficiency results, (2) comparison of the clinical trial population to the population under consideration for treatment with the therapy, (3) translation of the costs reported to costs relevant to the perspective of the decision-maker, and (4) translation of the clinical outcome measures to outcomes relevant to the length of treatment being proposed by the practitioner. Implementation issues include treatment efficiency thresholds, formulary committee discussions, treatment decision rules, and timing of the economic evaluation.

I would like to thank Bruce Kinosian MD for recalculating the data for Figure 4, Henry Glick MA for his ideas and suggestions, and Zesus Roulidis MD for his editorial comments.

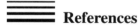 **References**

1. Detsky AS, Naglie IG. A clinician's guide to cost-effectiveness analysis. Ann Intern Med 1990;113:147-54.

2. Drummond MF. Principles of economic appraisal in health care. New York: Oxford University Press, 1980.

3. Drummond MF, Stoddart GL, Torrance GW. Methods for the economic evaluation of health care programmes. New York: Oxford Medical Publications, 1987.

4. Drummond MF, Davies L. Economic analysis alongside clinical trials: revisiting the methodological issues. Int J Technol Assess Health Care 1991;7:561-73.

5. Eddy DM. Cost-effectiveness analysis: is it up to the task? JAMA 1992;267:3342-8.

6. Eisenberg JM. Clinical economics: a guide to the economic analysis of clinical practices. JAMA 1989;262:2879-86.

7. Warner KE, Luce BR. Cost-benefit and cost-effectiveness analysis in health care: principles, practice and potential. Ann Arbor, MI: Health Administration Press, 1982.

8. Weinstein MC. Principles of cost-effective resource allocation in health care organizations. Int J Technol Assess Health Care 1990;6:93-103.

9. Schulman KA, Lynn LA, Glick HA, Eisenberg JM. Cost effectiveness of low-dose zidovudine therapy for asymptomatic patients with human immunodeficiency virus (HIV) infection. Ann Intern Med 1991;114:798-802.

10. Glick H, Heyse JF, Thompson D, Epstein RS, Smith ME, Oster G. A model for evaluating the cost-effectiveness of cholesterol-lowering treatment. Int J Technol Assess Health Care 1992;8:719-34.

11. Adult Treatment Panel. Report of the National Cholesterol Education Program Expert Panel on detection, evaluation, and treatment of high blood cholesterol in adults. Arch Intern Med 1988;148:36-69.

12. Schulman KA, Kinosian B, Jacobson TA, Glick H, William MK, Koffer H, et al. Reducing high blood cholesterol level with drugs: cost-effectiveness of pharmacologic management. JAMA 1990;264:3025-33.

13. Glick H, Kinosian BP, Juhn P, Schulman KA, Jacobson TA, Eisenberg JM. Cost-effectiveness of drug treatment for high blood cholesterol (abstract). Med Decis Making 1991;11:326.

14. Ziegler EJ, Fisher CJ Jr, Sprung CL, Straube RC, Sadoff JC, Foulke GE, et al. Treatment of gram-negative bacteremia and septic shock with HA-1A human monoclonal antibody against endotoxin: a randomized, placebo-controlled trial. N Engl J Med 1991;324: 429-36.

15. Schulman KA, Glick HA, Rubin H, Eisenberg JM. Cost-effectiveness of HA-1A monoclonal antibody for gram-negative sepsis: economic analysis of a new therapeutic agent. JAMA 1991;266:3466-71.

16. Health Care Financing Administration, Department of Health and Human Services. Medicare program: criteria and procedures for making medical service coverage decisions that relate to medical technology. 54 Fed Reg 4302-18, January 30, 1989.

17. Leaf A. Cost effectiveness as a criterion for medicare coverage. N Engl J Med 1989; 321:898-900.

18. Pear R. Medicare to weight cost as a factor in reimbursement. New York Times 1991; April 22:A-1, A-26.

19. Laupacis A, Feeny D, Detsky AS, Tugwell PX. How attractive does a new technology have to be to warrant adoption and utilization? Tentative guidelines for using clinical and economic evaluations. Can Med Assoc J 1992;146:473-81.

20. Evans D, Freund D, Dittus R, Robertson J, Henry D. The use of economic analysis as a basis for inclusion of pharmaceutical products on the Pharmaceutical Benefits Scheme. Canberra: Department of Health, Housing and Community Services, Commonwealth of Australia, 1990.

21. Kinosian BP, Glick HA, Juhn P, Jacobson T, Schulman KA, Eisenberg JM. Inconsistent guidelines: is the National Cholesterol Education Program soft on cholesterol? (abstract) Clin Res 1991;39:579A.

22. Sisk JE, Gianfrancesco FD, Coster JM. Recombinant erythropoietin and Medicare payment. JAMA 1991;266:247-52.

23. Adams ME, McCall NT, Gray DT, Orza MJ, Chalmers TC. Economic analysis in randomized control trials. Med Care 1992;30:231-43.

24. Hillman AL, Eisenberg JM, Pauly MV, Bloom BS, Glick H, Kinosian B, et al. Avoiding bias in the conduct and reporting of cost-effectiveness research sponsored by pharmaceutical companies. N Engl J Med 1991;324:1362-5.

25. Udvarhelyi IS, Colditz GA, Ri A, Epstein AM. Cost-effectiveness and cost-benefit analysis in the medical literature: are the methods being used correctly? Ann Intern Med 1992;116:238-44.

26. The SOLVD Investigators. Effect of enalapril on survival in patients with reduced left ventricular ejection fractions and congestive heart failure. N Engl J Med 1991;325: 293-302.

27. Eisenberg JM. Cost-effective medical practice. In: Kelley WN. Textbook of internal medicine. Philadelphia: JB Lippincott, 1991:30-1.

15

Assessing Pharmacoeconomic Studies

JoLaine R. Draugalis

Several authors have written guides to assist the healthcare practitioner in understanding and assessing economic analyses as applied to healthcare programs.[1-3] More recently, the methods have been applied specifically to the evaluation of drug therapies.[4-6] To use the results of pharmacoeconomic studies in decision-making, it is important that the pharmacist be able to critically read the published works in the area. Judgments must be made regarding methodologies used, validity of conclusions, and ability to generalize findings.

Assessing the Pharmacoeconomic Literature

Reading and using the results from pharmacoeconomic studies is much like using the results of any research in that a critical assessment of methods, assumptions, limitations, and the like is required. Moreover, criteria specific to economic evaluations such as discounting, sensitivity analysis, and incremental analysis also are important. The following criteria were assembled based on guidelines and checklists previously published.[4,7-9]

This inquiry list is not provided to make readers hypercritical and unaccepting of articles; few if any reports would meet these criteria in total. However, as a guide they can be useful in determining whether it is worth the reader's time to continue and, if so, whether results and conclusions are deemed valid based on the methodologies used. Some journals stipulate section headings, length, and content requirements. This may need to be considered when critiquing a report. Many of these are important when assessing any type of research report/article. Another caveat is the misuse of terminology in the pharmacoeconomic literature. For example, cost-benefit has been inappropriately used as a synonym for a cost-analysis or cost-minimization study. Additionally, cost-saving is not always equal to cost-effective, yet many authors have equated the two.[10] Earlier chapters contain critical information on economic variables to integrate with this checklist. Finally, not all categories will apply to each and every report.

CRITERIA FOR EVALUATING PHARMACOECONOMIC STUDIES

I. Title
    A. Is it interesting?
    B. Is it informative?
II. Abstract or Summary
    A. Are the following addressed: purpose, methodology, results, conclusions?
    B. If appropriate, are hypotheses clearly stated?
    C. If the results were valid, would they be useful in your institution/practice site?
III. Introduction
    A. Are the problem statement and resultant study questions clearly and precisely stated?
    B. Where appropriate, are the hypotheses to be tested stated in a testable form?
    C. Whose perspective is considered? Society, healthcare payer, patient, healthcare provider?
IV. Literature Review
    A. Is/are the relationship of the study question(s) clearly related to previous research?
    B. Is the significance of the inquiry discussed with resultant justification of the research?
V. Methodology
    A. Alternatives
        1. What alternatives are compared? Were the options described in sufficient detail?
        2. What is the primary content? Most beneficial use of limited resources (cost-benefit analysis), least costly way to achieve an objective (cost-effectiveness analysis), demonstrating equivalency in comparative groups (cost-minimization analysis), or natural units adjusted for quality-of-life (cost-utility analysis).
        3. Are the appropriate alternatives compared? Does the analysis compare the new entity against a current standard? Are all relevant alternatives considered?

B. Economic Variables
  1. Are all relevant costs and consequences considered? If an important variable is excluded, is justification given?
  2. Which variables are included? Medical resources (basic and intermediate), nonmedical resources, productive capacity, effectiveness variables (clinical indicators, cases treated, life-years saved, other), health status variables (quality-adjusted life-years)?
  3. How are the costs and consequences measured or counted?
  4. How are the costs and consequences valued? Acquisition costs, hospital services (per diem, room and board plus ancillary, charges, cost-to-charge ratio), wages (plus benefits)?
  5. What is the source of data? Medical records, data collection form (retrospective, concurrent)?
  6. Are the options compared in terms of additional costs and additional benefits (incremental analysis)?
C. Subjects
  1. Are the sampling frame and method described?
  2. If applicable, are sources of sampling bias considered?
D. Instruments
  1. Is the instrument valid for the study setting and research questions?
  2. Does the instrument yield reliable observations for the study setting and research questions?
  3. If a nonstandardized instrument is being used, what information is given regarding its development?
E. Design
  1. Is the design appropriate when considering the literature review and research hypotheses?
  2. Is the design internally valid?
  3. Is the description complete enough to allow replication?
F. Assumptions and Limitations
  1. Are assumptions and limitations clearly stated?
G. Analysis
  1. How are data analyzed?
  2. If used, are statistical methods appropriate?
VI. Results
  A. Are the results of the analysis clearly presented?
  B. Is there sufficient evidence to answer the study questions?
  C. If used, are the reported statistics relevant to the research hypotheses?
  D. Is the pictorial representation of data complete and readily understood?

VII. Sensitivity Analysis
    A. Is a sensitivity analysis conducted for those variables that may not be measured with certainty?
    B. Do the results change when factors are varied?
VIII. Discounting
    A. Are future costs and consequences discounted?
    B. Is any rationale given for the rate chosen?
IX.   Discussion and Conclusions
    A. Are results in light of the original problem statement(s)?
    B. Are results compared with those of previous inquiries?
    C. Are conclusions substantiated?
    D. Are generalizations appropriate?
    E. Are implications and recommendations presented?
X.   Overall Considerations
    A. Is the report organized and clearly written?
    B. Is an unbiased, impartial attitude portrayed?

Review of Economic Evaluations in the Literature

In 1986, Doubilet et al.[11] pointed out the misuse of the term "cost-effective." Their editorial concluded by suggesting less frequent and more precise use of the term to improve communication. The misapplication of terminology and inappropriate use of the methods have been evaluated in the pharmacy[12] and medical literature.[13,14] Each of these three groups of authors adopted similar inclusion criteria, standards, and methods in their assessments. Two of the reviews are described in more detail below.

Lee and Sanchez[12] considered 65 studies published between January 1985 and December 1990 in the following journals: *American Journal of Hospital Pharmacy* (now *American Journal of Health-System Pharmacy*) (37%), *Drug Intelligence and Clinical Pharmacy* (now *The Annals of Pharmacotherapy*) (28%), and *Hospital Pharmacy* (20%). The remaining 10 articles appeared in *Hospital Therapy*, *Clinical Therapeutics*, or *Hospital Formulary*. The evaluators determined that the studies were quite deficient in four of the 10 criteria. Only 31% of the studies identified all relevant costs and consequences for each alternative. Fourteen studies should have used discounting but only two did. A single study performed an incremental analysis. Sensitivity analysis was reported in only 6% of the articles. Over half of the articles inappropriately equated cost-saving with cost-effective.

Udvarhelyi et al.[14] analyzed 77 articles published from 1978 to 1980 (31 articles) and 1985 to 1987 (46 articles) in general medical, general surgical, and medical subspecialty journals. The studies were rated on the basis of six principles deemed to be appropriate minimum standards. Only

18% of the studies explicitly stated the perspective. Nearly all of the articles (96%) contained some cost data; however, the degree to which investigators specified the costs or how they were analyzed varied considerably. Discounting was used in 14 of 29 studies that had differential timing. Sensitivity analysis was conducted in only 30% of the studies, even though limitations were frequently indicated in the articles. Forty-two percent of the studies reported a summary measurement of efficiency. Secondary hypotheses in this evaluation included assessing different time periods and types of journal in overall performance. There was no difference in adherence to principles when the two time periods were compared. Articles in general medical journals were more apt to adhere to analytic principles than were articles in either the medical subspecialty or general surgical periodicals.

A third review[13] surveyed 47 publications appearing in medical journals between January 1982 and October 1987. There is some overlap between this and the Udvarhelyi et al.[14] analysis and therefore a detailed explanation of their findings is not reported here. The conclusions of all three reviews[12-14] were similar in that existing literature was found not to comply with basic methodologic guidelines. The findings of these reviews lend further support to the conclusion that each pharmacy practitioner must be able to critique the published literature and reject invalid conclusions.

Example Critique

In this section, a review of a journal article will be presented. The critique was written following the outline of questions presented in the "Criteria for Evaluating Pharmacoeconomic Studies" section. The article demonstrates that a decision-maker could arrive at a different formulary or prescribing decision based on using outcome measures in addition to drug acquisition cost information. The citation is:

Rice TD, Duggan AK, DeAngelis C. Cost-effectiveness of erythromycin versus mupirocin for the treatment of impetigo in children. Pediatrics 1992; 89: 210-4.

The title is quite specific and would allow the reader to determine if the article is of interest. The abstract provides the stipulated information and readers could decide if results would be useful in their setting. The problem statement, resultant study questions, and hypotheses are addressed in the introduction and/or the abstract, whereas the patient perspective is specifically stated in the discussion section. The literature review clearly relates the study question to previous research. The significance of the inquiry was portrayed via the following statement: "some physicians may hesitate to use mupirocin because of concerns about its expense."

The two treatment alternatives (mupirocin and erythromycin) were described in sufficient detail. Oral erythromycin was the current standard because of effectiveness and low cost. Mupirocin was the new topical entity.

Because the primary concern was to determine the least costly way to achieve resolution of impetiginous lesions (clinical and bacteriologic cure), a cost-effectiveness analysis was conducted. However, while not formally incorporating all estimated economic benefits and including them in a cost-effectiveness analysis as negative costs, this study combined the merits of cost-benefit and cost-effectiveness analyses by retaining a non-monetary effectiveness measure (clinical cure) and conducting additional willingness to pay (WTP) analyses and other comparisons across treatment groups. WTP is "the amounts of money people would be willing and able to pay for various possible benefits."[15] It has been suggested as a method to quantify outcomes that are difficult to value in dollars.[16] In lieu of valuing adverse effects monetarily (as costs), WTP analyses were substituted.

The costs to the patient included physician's visit fee, transportation expenses, and the medication cost. The effects were clinical and bacteriologic response, time to resolution, adverse effects, change in activities (child missed school and/or parent missed work), parental satisfaction with therapy, compliance rates, and how likely the parent would be willing to pay more for a different medicine to avoid adverse effects. The economic variables were richly described and specific descriptions were provided for valuation sources. For example, the medication costs were based on the average found in a poll of local pharmacies and the value of a missed school day was based on the Baltimore City School 1989 budget; the value of one workday was derived from 1987 US Census data.

Potential subjects were all children, 3 months to 16 years of age, who presented with impetigo to two specified sites from April through November 1989. A power analysis was conducted. Exclusion criteria were stated. Parental informed consent was obtained prior to randomization to treatment groups. Data collection mechanisms were fully described. To assess the construct validity (whether the item truly measured what it purported to measure) of their WTP measure, the researchers correlated the parents' WTP with parental assessment of the importance of each effect. Their expectations were confirmed in that, the more important an effect was judged to be by the parent, the greater the WTP to avoid or ensure the effect.

The design is appropriate when considering the literature review and research hypotheses. Because an experimental design was used (random assignment to treatment groups), nearly all threats to internal validity were controlled, with patient attrition being of primary concern. In the results section, the authors gave sufficient information to determine that attrition from groups was not preferential.

The results of the analyses were clearly presented in the text and in accompanying tables to answer the study questions. For instance, one table was titled "Comparison of Side Effects by Treatment Group" and listed the two regimens, percentage reporting adverse effects, and resultant p values. A WTP conclusion was as follows: "Of those patients who experienced at least one side effect, 56 percent of the parents in the erythromycin group compared with 11 percent in the mupirocin group were willing to pay more for a different medication that would not produce the same side effect (p = .04)." The statistical analyses were appropriate. However, the authors should have conducted a power analysis and indicated how many additional patients would be needed to detect a significant difference in the likelihood of adverse effects rather than stating that the differences "approached significance." Because the study could not be blinded, the researchers attempted to minimize bias by adhering to strict definitions for clinical outcome variables.

Sensitivity analyses were implicit regarding medication costs, as they took an average price charged by local pharmacies and dosage strength dispensed was based on weight. They subjectively assigned transportation costs of $10 per visit. No formal sensitivity analyses were conducted. Discounting was not a concern because of the time frame.

The results were considered in light of the original problem statements and when possible were compared to previous inquiries. The conclusions were substantiated and generalizations appropriate. In fact, caveats were addressed in the final section of the paper regarding generalizability and decision-making possibilities. Nevertheless, the researchers should have reminded the readers that the majority of patients were receiving medical assistance. This is an important consideration in generalizing the WTP analyses. The authors concluded that because treatment effectiveness, compliance, and overall satisfaction were not different between treatment groups, medication choice can be based on parental preference. The authors reasoned that the increased cost of mupirocin was offset by increased adverse effects and effect on parent/child activities associated with erythromycin. Overall, the report was clearly written and well organized. Finally, no funding source was mentioned leaving the readers to speculate about any financial agreements and potential sources of bias.

Additional Methodologic Considerations

Because the field of pharmacoeconomic inquiry is still developing, a number of methodologic questions and philosophic issues remain. There are also the considerations of standardization of methods and funding sources. Some of these topics have been considered in the appropriate chapters throughout the book; however, here they will be reconsidered as an overriding theme.

There is increased interest in evaluating patients' quality of life in clinical trials. Measurement issues include: (1) conceptual versus operational definitions, (2) generic versus disease-specific instruments, (3) profile versus battery versus index score aggregation, and (4) psychometric versus decision theory-based scaling.[17] Measurement criteria including reliability, validity, validation, as well as technical qualities such as instrument selection and ease of administration must be considered. Instruments must be evaluated for responsiveness; that is, sensitivity to change in certain patient populations. The choice of instruments may affect quality-of-life determination and, ultimately, a cost-effectiveness or cost-utility analysis if data are incorporated in said analyses. In fact, one study[18] showed that correlations among assessment methods were poor and the authors recommended the application of a variety of instruments when making program decisions. An analogy was drawn between using a variety of instruments in determining quality of life and conducting a cost-effectiveness analysis for each method versus conducting sensitivity analyses in other economic evaluations.

Drummond and Davies[19] provided suggestions for economic analyses that accompany clinical trials: (1) compare alternatives with practical relevance, (2) identify resource consumption unique to trial and differentiate from normal clinical practice, (3) be aware of small sample sizes and that economic hypotheses may require more subjects than clinical comparisons, (4) report the enumeration of resources consumed separately from valuation, (5) use a range of instruments and thereby assess convergent validity, (6) report net direct costs, and (7) increase generalizability by including data from other sources to go beyond simply measurement in one setting and arrive at modeling in additional settings. Future research and additional discussion must address these types of issues.

Potential for Bias and Ethical Dilemmas

In an editorial, Hillman et al.[20] made eight recommendations to decrease possible sources of bias in industry-sponsored economic evaluations: (1) written agreements should be grants to universities, rather than contracts with individuals; (2) the alternatives selected for comparison should be based on clinical relevance, rather than on potential advantageous findings; (3) the investigator should have the freedom to modify the firm's design; (4) if funding is in stages rather than one lump sum, publication rights should be guaranteed regardless of results; (5) sensitivity analyses should be used; (6) researchers should publish results irrespective of their promotional value and journal editors should consider publishing negative results; (7) journals should require disclosure of financial arrangements between authors and sponsors and the researchers should not provide consultation if conflict of interest is a concern; and (8) to ensure sound methodology and clinically relevant results, adequate funding must be secured.

Many academic and industry researchers would agree with the intent of these suggestions; however, at least one industry group took issue with several specific points. Boyer et al.[21] put forth the following: (1) they have successfully used both grants and contracts to fund academic research; (2) they have found it appropriate to fund smaller separate phases of large projects; (3) it is not always possible to alter clinical trial protocols to accommodate the economic researcher; and (4) economic evaluations are not marketing departments' exclusive domain, and economic researchers, regardless of setting, must be responsible for methodologic integrity.

Summary

Although pharmacoeconomic inquiry has no gold standard methodology such as the randomized clinical trial, there are widely accepted principles such as those put forth earlier in this chapter (e.g., the importance of considering appropriate alternatives, establishing perspective, the need for discounting, the importance of considering analyses at the margin, appropriate use of terminology, and the application of sensitivity analysis). According to Drummond et al.,[22] the motivations for standardization are threefold: to maintain methodologic standards, to facilitate the comparison among a variety of interventions, and to increase generalizability. However, rebuttal points also are provided for each of the motivations in that even with perfect standardization, we must consider technical judgments versus value judgments; that analytic viewpoints differ from setting to setting; and that complete generalizability is not possible across cultural settings. Additionally, too much rigidity may promote an unrealistic and simplistic "recipe" approach as well as suppress methodologic development and improvement.

Hillman et al.[20] promoted standardization to minimize bias in the conduct of economic evaluations supported by the pharmaceutical industry. However, if investigations are undertaken by scientists who are both competent and ethical, why should we necessarily suspect these as being more susceptible to marketing-injected bias than efficacy or effectiveness studies?[23,24] As one researcher has said of industry-sponsored funding, "they are supporting a study, not buying results."[25] US pharmaceutical firms are increasing their support of basic biomedical research, awarding more grants and contracts, and funding fellows in universities.[26] It appears that this type of funding will increase in support of pharmacoeconomic programs as well. In many cases, the only source for methodologic research such as instrument development and validation has been the pharmaceutical industry.[24] What is essential is that financial arrangements be disclosed and that researchers submit their findings to reputable peer-reviewed journals.

The underreporting of negative results is not unique to pharmacoeconomic inquiry, as journal editors historically shy away from reporting negative (i.e., not significant) results. The relative "hardness" of clinical data compared with economic endpoints has been considered as a potential source of bias.[22] An analogy to be drawn here is the use of confidence intervals with clinical data versus simply reporting a p value. Clinical endpoints may not be as hard as one would first think. The decisions of when, how often, and on what variables to conduct analyses are critical (and not absolutely standardized) in clinical research as well as in economic evaluations. Finally, why should we assume that practitioners would be swayed by a faulty cost-effective argument that is contrary to their clinical knowledge? "Pharmacoeconomic inquiry aids in decision making; however, it does not make the decisions. Most decisions cannot be made on technical factors alone, and many require value judgments."[27]

In moving the pharmacoeconomic research agenda forward, Lewis and Patwell[28] have called for communication among the interested parties: the funding sources, the research community, and the practitioners and other healthcare decision-makers. A key will be the provision of educational programs so that pharmacoeconomic research can be appropriately assessed and ultimately used in providing improved patient care. In conclusion, as Drummond[29] has pointed out, if the results of pharmacoeconomic inquiries are to be used by healthcare decision-makers, the field must be seen as science, rather than simply a marketing tool.

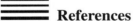 **References**

1. Drummond MF, Stoddart GL, Torrance GW. Methods for the economic evaluation of health care programmes. New York: Oxford University Press, 1987.

2. Drummond M, Stoddart G, Labelle R, Cushman R. Health economics: an introduction for clinicians. Ann Intern Med 1987;107:88-92.

3. Detsky AS, Naglie IG. A clinician's guide to cost-effectiveness analysis. Ann Intern Med 1990;113:147-54.

4. Drummond M, Smith GT, Wells N. Economic evaluation in the development of medicines. London: Office of Health Economics, 1988.

5. Freund DA, Dittus RS. Principles of pharmacoeconomic analysis of drug therapy. PharmacoEconomics 1992;1:20-32.

6. Jolicoeur LM, Jones-Grizzle AJ, Boyer JG. Guidelines for performing a pharmacoeconomic analysis. Am J Hosp Pharm 1992;49:1741-7.

7. Ward MJ, Fetler ME. Research Q & A: what guidelines should be followed in critically evaluating research reports? Nurs Res 1979;28:120-6.

8. Sackett DL. How to read clinical journals: part I. Why to read them and how to start reading them critically. Can Med Assoc J 1981;124:555-8.

9. Larson LN. Pharmacoeconomics and formulary decisions. Dyn Health Care 1989; 1:11-4.

10. Draugalis JR, Bootman JL, Larson LN, McGhan WF. Current concepts—pharmacoeconomics. Kalamazoo, MI: Upjohn, 1989:7.

11. Doubilet P, Weinstein MC, McNeil BJ. Use and misuse of the term "cost effective" in medicine. N Engl J Med 1986;314:253-6.

12. Lee JT, Sanchez LA. Interpretation of "cost-effective" and soundness of economic evaluations in the pharmacy literature. Am J Hosp Pharm 1991;48:2622-7.

13. Ganiats TG, Wong AF. Evaluation of cost-effectiveness research: a survey of recent publications. Fam Med 1991;23:457-62.

14. Udvarhelyi IS, Colditz GA, Rai A, Epstein AM. Cost-effectiveness and cost-benefit analyses in the medical literature: are the methods being used correctly? Ann Intern Med 1992;116:238-44.

15. Warner KE, Luce BR. Cost-benefit and cost-effectiveness analysis in health care. Ann Arbor, MI: Health Administration Press, 1982:89.

16. Thompson MS. Willingness to pay and accept risks to cure chronic disease. Am J Public Health 1986;76:392-6.

17. MacKeigan LD, Pathak DS. Overview of health-related quality-of-life measures. Am J Hosp Pharm 1992;49:2236-45.

18. Hornberger JC, Redelmeier DA, Petersen J. Variability among methods to assess patients' well-being and consequent effect on a cost-effectiveness analysis. J Clin Epidemiol 1992;45:505-12.

19. Drummond MF, Davies L. Economic analysis alongside clinical trials: revisiting the methodological issues. Int J Technol Assess Health Care 1991;7:561-73.

20. Hillman AL, Eisenberg JM, Pauly MV, Bloom BS, Glick H, Kinosian B, et al. Avoiding bias in the conduct and reporting of cost-effectiveness research sponsored by pharmaceutical companies. N Engl J Med 1991;324:1362-5.

21. Boyer JG, Hirsch JD, Osterhaus JT, Townsend RJ. Correspondence. N Engl J Med 1991;325:1385.

22. Drummond M, Brandt A, Luce B, Rovira J. Standardizing methodologies for economic evaluation in health care-practice, problems, and potential. Int J Technol Assess Health Care 1993;9:26-36.

23. Luce BR, Simpson K. Methods of cost effectiveness analysis: areas of consensus and debate. Washington, DC: Battelle Medical Technology Assessment and Policy Research Center, 1993.

24. Freeman RA. Minimizing bias in industry-sponsored outcomes research. Med Interface 1994;7:130-4.

25. Hamilton JO. Sure the drug works. But is it worth it? Business Week 1991;3228(August 26):62-3.

26. Clemmitt M. US drug industry's research support. Nature 1993;361:757-60.

27. Draugalis JR. Evaluating pharmacoeconomic research. In: Outcomes & cost effectiveness—new directions in managed care pharmacy. San Francisco: The Center for Outcomes Information, 1991:9-11.

28. Lewis JWL, Patwell JT. Pharmacoeconomics—consensus and controversy. Pharmaco-Resources 1994;5:3-5.

29. Drummond MF. Economic evaluation of pharmaceuticals—science or marketing? PharmacoEconomics 1992;1:8-13.

Appendix

Pharmacoeconomics: Further Practical Considerations

Lisa A. Sanchez

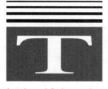he use of pharmacoeconomics by the pharmaceutical industry has been widespread. Pharmacoeconomics is used during various stages of the drug development process as well as during postmarketing phases to assist in justifying the value of specific agents within this highly competitive environment. Rigorous pharmacoeconomic research efforts also have been prevalent in academia. In this setting, the methods of pharmacoeconomics have been defined and refined. However, pharmacoeconomics can go beyond the walls of industry and academia and be applied in a traditional pharmacy setting. In fact, the most substantial benefits offered by this discipline can be realized in pharmacy practice environments including hospitals and managed care organizations. Some of these benefits are summarized in Table 1. Today's pharmacy practitioners can use pharmacoeconomics as a tool to justify the value of the goods and the services they provide.[1]

This appendix highlights the practical relevance of pharmacoeconomics. The purpose of this appendix is to summarize the practical application of pharmacoeconomic principles and methods in institutional and/or managed care pharmacy practice. Presented are how these methods can assist in various medication decisions, different strategies to put pharmacoeconomics into practice, and case studies to illustrate the application of pharmacoeconomics to real-world pharmacy practice.

Table 1. Potential Benefits of Pharmacoeconomics for the Pharmacy Practitioner

- Pharmacoeconomic analysis can be used to assess the value of pharmaceutical products and services practitioners provide
- Pharmacoeconomic data can be used when choosing between competing treatment alternatives
- Pharmacoeconomics can provide data necessary to make better drug use decisions
- Pharmacoeconomic data allow pharmacists to balance cost with quality and patient outcome

Pharmacoeconomics for Medication Decision-Making

The use of pharmacoeconomics can assist institutional and managed care pharmacists in determining the most appropriate and efficient use of drugs. These data can be a powerful tool to support various clinical and policy drug use decisions. Examples of decisions supported by pharmacoeconomics include formulary management, drug use policy (or guidelines), resource allocation, and individual patient treatment.[1] An example of each decision will be presented in a case-study format.

Complete medication decisions in today's healthcare environment should include (if appropriate) an assessment of different types of outcomes. Figure 1 contains suggested components of contemporary clinical decisions. The outcomes of medical care can be divided into three categories: clinical, economic, and humanistic.[2,3] Traditionally, medication decisions primarily assessed the clinical outcomes (e.g., efficacy, safety) of drug therapy. Over the past 5 to 15 years, some medication decisions also have included an assessment of economic outcomes (e.g., direct, indirect, intangible costs) of drug therapy. Most recently, the trend is to include an assessment of the humanistic outcomes (e.g., quality-of-life effects) of drug therapy. Thus, contemporary medication decisions should be multidimensional and the application of pharmacoeconomic principles and methods can assist in incorporating these outcomes.

Strategies to Put Pharmacoeconomics into Practice

The transition from theory to practice, or the practical applications of pharmacoeconomics, can be challenging. Many pharmacists are familiar with pharmacoeconomic principles and methods but are unclear on how to incorporate pharmacoeconomic data into everyday practice. Not all pharmacoeconomic data must come from a randomized clinical trial in order to be meaningful. Various strategies to aid pharmacists in putting pharmacoeconomics into practice include (1) critically evaluating, interpreting,

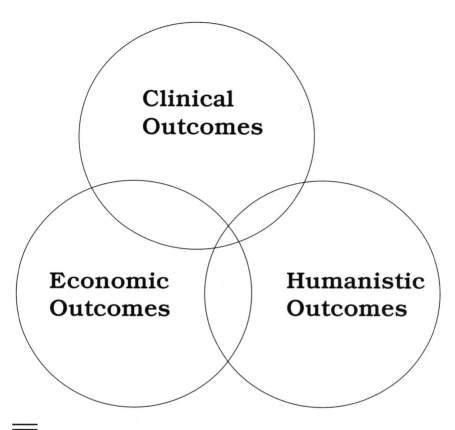

Figure 1. Components of contemporary clinical decision-making.[3]

and using the results of published studies; (2) using economic modeling techniques; and (3) conducting institution- or plan-specific pharmacoeconomic studies.[4] Table 2 lists the advantages and disadvantages of these strategies, and each is briefly discussed below.

The most obvious and seemingly user-friendly approach to put pharmacoeconomics into practice is to search medical, pharmacy, and health economics literature sources for any previous studies conducted on the treatment alternatives in question. It is advisable to try this strategy first as it can provide results quickly and inexpensively. However, there are disadvantages to this strategy, the primary one being the documented variations in the quality of pharmacoeconomic studies published to date.[5-7] All published studies should be critically evaluated using published guidelines and check lists[5,7-10] prior to using the results. Table 3 contains 11 basic criteria that can be applied to published reports to assist in evaluating the quality of a study.

**Table 2. Advantages and Disadvantages of Strategies to Put
Pharmacoeconomics into Practice**

STRATEGY	ADVANTAGE	DISADVANTAGE
Use published literature	inexpensive readily available provides data quickly subject to peer review results may be from a large population RCT	data may be from RCT (protocol-driven) difficult to generalize results may not be comparative variations in quality of analyses published
Build an economic model	relatively inexpensive provides data quickly can bridge efficacy and effectiveness can be plan- or institution-specific	results are dependent on assumptions researcher bias may be introduced controversial provides only a simulation
Conduct an institution- or plan-specific study	usually comparative data will be plan- or institution-specific designed to reflect "usual care" can be prospective or retrospective	expensive time-consuming can be difficult to randomize and control patient selection bias may be introduced potential for small sample size

RCT = randomized clinical trial.

The use of economic modeling techniques is another strategy for putting pharmacoeconomics into practice.[4,11] This strategy also can be relatively inexpensive and provide results in a timely manner. When used appropriately, these models can forecast the economic impact of a medication decision on a patient or organization. Additionally, models can be populated with institution- or plan-specific data, generating results that better reflect the "usual care" delivered at a practice setting.[12] The primary disadvantage to this approach is that the results generated are highly dependent on the assumptions made when building the model. These assumptions must be tested using sensitivity analysis prior to using the results.

Conducting an institution- or plan-specific pharmacoeconomic study is another strategy to put pharmacoeconomics into practice. There are numerous advantages associated with conducting your own pharmacoeconomics research project. The reader is referred to various published guidelines and standards for conducting and reporting pharmacoeconomic research.[12-15] Because this strategy can be challenging and costly (in both time and monetary resources), this strategy should be reserved for medication decisions that may be significant in terms of cost and quality of care.

Case Studies

Presented are four case studies in which economic evaluation methods are used to determine the value of various pharmacy products or services. In each case, the most appropriate pharmacoeconomic method (defined in previous chapters) and strategy (described above) was applied to real-world problems that may occur in daily pharmacy practice.

CASE 1: INDIVIDUAL PATIENT TREATMENT DECISION

Drug A and drug B are third-generation cephalosporins. Published studies have shown that they are therapeutically equivalent with respect to safety and efficacy. However, the agents do differ in a few respects:

	Drug A	Drug B
Drug cost	$7 dose	$16 dose
Dosing regimen	qid	bid
Pharmacist preparation time ($30/h)	9 min	2 min

As a clinical pharmacist rounding with the infectious disease team, you are asked to recommend the best treatment alternative for a particular patient on your service. Given the above information, which drug would you recommend be prescribed?

Analysis. This case consists of comparing agents within the same therapeutic category, with a documented equivalency in outcome, for a patient treatment decision. After searching pharmacy and medical literature sources, the claims of comparable efficacy and safety are confirmed. Now the primary focus for this evaluation becomes the determination of the least expensive treatment alternative.

If two agents are equal with respect to safety and efficacy, then it is probably not necessary to perform cost-effectiveness or cost-utility analysis. If it was appropriate to measure and compare benefits of patient outcome in monetary terms, then cost-benefit analysis might be appropriate. When there are documented claims of therapeutic equivalence, cost-minimization analysis is the most appropriate pharmacoeconomic tool to use.

When determining the least expensive alternative, it is not appropriate to simply compare the acquisition costs of the agents. All relevant costs associated with the therapies must be identified, measured, and compared. The alternative with the least expensive drug acquisition cost may not always represent the least costly alternative when all utilization costs to the institution are considered.

Examples of cost categories to be considered include drug acquisition costs, administration costs, and pharmacist labor costs, given that the therapies differ in these areas. When quantifying the three cost categories listed above, the cost per day of therapy is approximately $46 and $34 for drugs A and B, respectively, making drug B the obvious choice for this patient.

CASE 2: FORMULARY MANAGEMENT DECISION[15]

Drug A and drug B are histamine$_2$-antagonists used to treat peptic ulcer disease. The medical literature contains the following information:

	Drug A	Drug B
Drug cost (per episode)	$60	$120
Effectiveness (pain relief)	70%	90%
Adverse drug reactions	1%	2%

Drug B is an agent newly approved by the Food and Drug Administration (FDA) that is available at twice the acquisition cost of drug A. The pharmacy and therapeutics (P&T) committee at your managed care plan is concerned because of the higher acquisition cost of drug B. Which drug would you recommend to the committee for formulary inclusion and promotion for patients with ulcers covered by your managed care plan?

Analysis. This case also consists of comparing treatment alternatives from the same therapeutic category. However, this case differs from the first one in that the agents being compared differ in safety, efficacy, *and* cost. Also, the comparison is now for the purpose of a formulary management decision for a managed care plan. To appropriately compare agents that differ in these areas, the pharmacist must use a tool that weighs costs and clinical outcomes concurrently.

Cost-benefit, cost-effectiveness, and cost-utility analyses may be theoretically appropriate. Since the costs of the treatment alternatives are measured in monetary units, and effectiveness is measured in terms of achieving a specific clinical objective (relief of pain), then the most appropriate method to use is cost-effectiveness analysis. A literature search may reveal a published cost-effectiveness analysis comparing drugs A and B from a managed care perspective. However, this analysis should be critically evaluated using published guidelines[8-10] prior to generalizing the results to your plan. The questions listed in Table 3 should be applied to this study.

For example, the primary effectiveness measure might be quantified in terms of patient outcome of time to heal or relief of peptic ulcer pain. The research question for this problem would essentially become, "Which drug provides the most pain relief or the quickest time to heal per dollar spent?" The costs identified, measured, and compared in this analysis should include total drug utilization costs, costs associated with the difference in effectiveness (cost of retreating a treatment failure), and costs of treating adverse effects associated with the two drugs. Thus, the total cost also may include the costs for clinic or emergency room visits, hospitalization, and diagnostic procedures (e.g., barium swallow, endoscopy).

On the surface, when comparing acquisition costs of drugs A and B, it may appear that the least expensive alternative is drug A (half the acquisition cost of drug B). However, by using a thorough cost-effectiveness analysis published in the literature, the superior effectiveness profile and

Table 3. Summary of Criteria for Evaluating Published Pharmacoeconomic Studies[10]

1. Objective
What is the question being considered?
Is the question clear, defined, and
  measurable?

2. Perspective
What is the perspective of the analysis
  (e.g., patient, provider, payer, society)?
Is it appropriate given the scope of the
  problem?

3. Type of analysis
What pharmacoeconomic tool was used?
Is it appropriate given the problem?
Is it what was actually conducted?

4. Study design
What was the study design?
What were the data sources?
Is the study suitable if carried out in
  an RCT?

5. Choice of comparators (interventions)
Were all appropriate treatment alternatives
  considered and described?
Were any appropriate alternatives
  omitted?
Are the alternatives relevant to the
  perspective and clinical nature of the
  study?
Was a do-nothing approach considered?

6. Costs and outcomes
What are the costs and outcomes
  included?
Are the costs and outcomes relevant to
  the perspective chosen?
Do they include positive and negative
  outcomes?
How were costs and outcomes valued?
Were costs and outcomes measured in the
  appropriate physical units?

7. Discounting
Was the study performed over time?
Were future costs and outcomes
  discounted to their present value?
Was justification given for the rate used?

8. Results
Are the results accurate and practical for
  medical decision makers?
Were the appropriate statistical analyses
  performed?
Was an incremental analysis performed?
Are the assumptions/limitations
  discussed?

9. Sensitivity analysis
Are cost ranges for significant variables
  tested for sensitivity?
Are the appropriate and relevant
  variables varied?
Do the findings follow the anticipated
  trend?

10. Conclusions
Are the study conclusions justified?
Is it possible to extrapolate the conclu-
  sions to daily clinical practice?

11. Sponsorship
Was the study conducted by a pharmaceutical company?
Was the study sponsored by a pharmaceutical company?
Was any bias introduced because of
  study sponsorship?

RCT = randomized clinical trial.

the relatively low incidence of serious adverse effects associated with these agents might actually make drug B the more cost-effective alternative. Thus, drug B may be the best choice for inclusion to the formulary.

CASE 3: JUSTIFICATION OF A SERVICE FOR RESOURCE ALLOCATION[15]

As Director of Pharmacy for a 750-bed teaching hospital, you want to establish an ambu-latory chemotherapy infusion pharmacy. You believe that this program will improve the quality of patient care and save money for your institution. After negotiations with your hospital administrator, the funding is approved. However, approval is contingent for a one-year trial basis, after which you must document and justify the value of this program to the hospital. How do you demonstrate the value of the ambulatory chemotherapy infusion pharmacy to the administrator?

Analysis. Case 3 illustrates how a resource allocation decision could be supported with pharmacoeconomic data. In today's hospitals, requests for additional funds from one department are often at the expense of the budget of another department.[16] With increased competition for these resources, justifying the value of new or existing services is often necessary.

Showing that a chemotherapy infusion pharmacy will yield a high return on investment will increase the probability of funding by the institution. By identifying and measuring all relevant costs and benefits associated with this program, the program may be justified to administrators. If the costs and benefits of this service can be converted into dollars, then cost-benefit analysis may be the most appropriate pharmacoeconomic method to use.

If valuation of this service needs to be performed prior to the allocation of any funds, then it may be appropriate to construct an economic model using pertinent values from a meta-analysis of the literature. This could also be populated with institution-specific data to yield an estimate of the impact of this service on your hospital. If valuation of this service can be done after funding (during the one-year trial period), then it may be advisable to design a prospective evaluation to be conducted during the course of the trial year. The 10-step process developing by Jolicoeur et al.[13] should provide the pharmacist researcher with a research process.

To use cost-benefit analysis, the cost of providing this service must be identified and measured in monetary units. The cost of providing this service will include the pharmacist's salary and any additional drug and supply costs, all of which can be easily converted into dollars. Similarly, the benefits of this service need to be identified and converted into dollars. Theoretically, the benefits will include decreased total drug costs, reduced drug loss and waste, decreased nursing time, and perhaps decreased need for retreating treatment failures and treating adverse drug reactions associated with inappropriate chemotherapy and antiemetic dosing. In addition, a pharmacy located in the chemotherapy clinic may make it viable to increase the number of patients going through the clinic each day, possibly resulting in increased hospital revenues.

Since it is feasible to convert these potential benefits into monetary units, cost-benefit analysis is a practical option. With careful documentation, one might make a strong case that the benefits of an ambulatory chemotherapy infusion pharmacy outweigh the costs of providing this service, and may even generate revenue for the hospital.

CASE 4: DRUG POLICY DECISION

Drug A is a new antiemetic agent. The use and total pharmacy expenditures for this agent have been high (more than $300,000). The P&T committee at your institution wants to develop and approve a policy regarding the institutional use of the agent to attempt to decrease total expenditures for this agent while maintaining high-quality patient care. The following dosing regimens are being used in the institution:

	Regimen 1	Regimen 2
Drug dose	30 mg	20 mg
Dosing schedule	qd	qd

No published information regarding efficacy and safety is available comparing the two dosages. Which dosage would you recommend be the regimen of choice for the institutional drug usage policy?

This decision, given its potential impact on quality of care and total costs, may warrant a prospective pharmacoeconomic evaluation. Again, published guidelines for conducting a pharmacoeconomic evaluation should be used to guide the completion of this study.[12-15]

Analysis. This case involves a comparison of different dosing regimens of the same drug for an institutional drug use policy decision. Although the drug is the same, there is no evidence that the two regimens are equal in effectiveness and safety. Thus, initially applying cost-effectiveness analysis is the most appropriate method. Following study development, implementation, and data collection, the regimens' cost-effectiveness profiles are as follows:

	Regimen 1	Regimen 2
Effectiveness	75%	79%
Safety (primary headache)	11%	10%
Cost per day	$128.00	$96.00
Average cost-effectiveness ratio	$170.67	$121.52

Upon collecting and analyzing these data, it appears that the two regimens are comparable in effectiveness and safety, given a modest sample size (due to time limitations). However, they differ in their cost-effectiveness ratios and cost per patient day. Given that regimen 2 appears to be the one of choice, obtaining the desired therapeutic effect at the least cost per patient per day, this dosing regimen can now be incorporated into institutional usage guidelines and brought to the P&T committee for approval. It may be advisable, however, to calculate the annual cost savings associated with promoting the use of regimen 2 to your hospital staff (total cost per patient × total eligible patients per year).

Once the drug use policy is approved, it is imperative to appropriately implement the policy. For maximum acceptance by the medical staff it is recommended that a large educational effort aimed at primary users be pursued. By offering inservice education programs to oncologists and oncology nurses, the study rationale, pharmacoeconomic data, and drug use policy can be presented. Other educational strategies include written (pocket cards) and computerized (on-line messages) communications. It is also important to be available for any questions, comments, or concerns that might arise upon implementation of the new dosing regimen. Lastly, it is important to monitor the effect of this policy on the institution and patients. Therefore, three to nine months after implementation, follow-up data should be collected on a random sample of approximately 10% of the patients who received the drug under the new treatment guidelines. Completion of this process may increase the acceptance of the drug policy by physicians and nurses. Furthermore, promoting this policy as a means to provide the highest quality patient care, at a potential cost-savings to the institution, may increase the probability of a high acceptance rate.

Summary

Pharmacoeconomics provides the tools necessary to quantify the value of goods and services pharmacists provide. Although pharmacoeconomics has been used primarily by the pharmaceutical industry and academic institutions, it also may be used by traditional pharmacy practitioners, regardless of the setting. By using pharmacoeconomic principles and methods appropriately, the practitioner can reap the many benefits that pharmacoeconomics offers. With pharmacy budgets continuing to decrease while healthcare costs soar, pharmacists are challenged to justify the products and services they provide. Pharmacoeconomics assists pharmacists in meeting this challenge by providing the means to quantify the value of pharmacy to the rest of the healthcare system and to society.

References

1. Sanchez LA. Expanding the role of pharmacists in pharmacoeconomics: how and why? PharmacoEconomics 1994;5:367-75.

2. Coons SJ, Kaplan RM. Quality of life assessment: understanding its use as an outcomes measure. Hosp Formul 1995;30:412-6.

3. Kozma CM, Reeder CE, Schulz RM. Economic, clinical, and humanistic outcomes: a planning model for pharmacoeconomic research. Clin Ther 1993;15:1121-32.

4. Sanchez LA. Pharmacoeconomics and formulary decision making. PharmacoEconomics 1996;8(suppl 2):16-25.

5. Lee JT, Sanchez LA. Interpretation of 'cost-effective' and soundness of economic evaluations in the pharmacy literature. Am J Hosp Pharm 1991;48:2:622-7.

6. Udvarhelyi S, Colditz GA, Rai A, et al. Cost effectiveness and cost benefit analyses in the medical literature. Ann Intern Med 1992;116:238-44.

7. Bradley CA, Iskedjian M, Lanctôt K, Mittman N, Simone C, St Pierre E, et al. Quality assessment of economic evaluations in selected pharmacy, medical, and health economics journals. Ann Pharmacother 1995;29:681-9.

8. Drummond MF, Stoddart GL, Torrance GW. Methods for the economic evaluation of health care programmes. Oxford: Oxford University Press, 1987:5-38,74-111.

9. Sacristán JA, Soto J, Galende I. Evaluation of pharmacoeconomic studies: utilization of a checklist. Ann Pharmacother 1993;27:1126-33.

10. Sanchez LA. Pharmacoeconomic principles and methods: evaluating the quality of published pharmacoeconomic evaluations. Hosp Pharm 1995;30:146-52.

11. Milne RJ. Evaluation of the pharmacoeconomic literature. PharmacoEconomics 1994; 6:337-45.

12. Clemens K, Townsend R, Luscombe F, et al. Methodological and conduct principles for pharmacoeconomic research. PharmacoEconomics 1995;8:169-74.

13. Jolicoeur LM, Jones-Grizzle AJ, Boyer JG. Guidelines for performing a pharmacoeconomic analysis. Am J Hosp Pharm 1992;49:1741-7.

14. Task Force on Principles for Economic Analysis of Healthcare Technology. Economic analysis of healthcare technology: a report on principles. Ann Intern Med 1995;122:61-70.

15. Sanchez LA. Pharmacoeconomic principles and methods: conducting pharmacoeconomic evaluations in a hospital setting. Hosp Pharm 1995;30(5):412,415-16,428.

16. Sanchez LA, Lee JT. Use and misuse of pharmacoeconomic terms: a definitions primer. Top Hosp Pharm Manage 1994;13(4):11-22.

17. McGhan WF. Pharmacoeconomics and the evaluation of drugs and services. Hospital Formulary 1993;28:365-78.

Index